LEARNING TO LOVE

LEARNING TO LOVE

Intimacy and the Discourse of Development in China

Sonya E. Pritzker

University of Michigan Press
Ann Arbor

Copyright © 2024 by Sonya E. Pritzker
All rights reserved

For questions or permissions, please contact um.press.perms@umich.edu

Published in the United States of America by the
University of Michigan Press
Manufactured in the United States of America
Printed on acid-free paper
First published July 2024

A CIP catalog record for this book is available from the British Library.

Library of Congress Cataloging-in-Publication data has been applied for.

ISBN 978-0-472-07686-4 (hardcover : alk. paper)
ISBN 978-0-472-05686-6 (paper : alk. paper)
ISBN 978-0-472-22176-9 (e-book)

DOI: https://doi.org/10.3998/mpub.11743065

Contents

Acknowledgments / ix

Introduction / 1
    Learning to Love / 3
    Entangling Differently / 8
    Implicit Justice? / 15
        Justice in a Hantopia / 20
    Situating the Research / 23
    Overview of Chapters / 25

CHAPTER 1
    Suffering/Desire / 31
        The Tentativeness of Desire / 33
            Telling Suffering / 35
            Telling-in-Relation / 38
        The Feeling of Home / 39
        Space Invasion / 44
        The Timid and Weak Type / 53
        Awkward Introductions / 58
        Concluding Reflections / 66

CHAPTER 2
    Home/Horizons / 69
        Atmospheres / 71
        Textuality and the Agency of Atmospheres / 75
        Boundary Making / 83
            Opening the Space / 83
            Closing the Space / 85
        Concluding Reflections / 90

CHAPTER 3
   The Great Self / 93
      Reconfiguring the Body-Self / 94
      Big Self, Little Self / 97
      The Distributed Body / 100
      Enacting the Inner Other / 103
      Time Travel / 105
      The Madhouse / 110
         Dis-concert / 114
      Concluding Reflections / 121

CHAPTER 4
   Considering Culture / 124
      Chinese Education Methods . . . or What? / 126
      Western Methods / 133
      Progress Plus Social *Daode* / 139
      Fake Flowers / 143
      Concluding Reflections / 148

CHAPTER 5
   Wrangling with Ghosts / 152
      Conversations with Ghosts / 154
      The Agency of Images / 160
      The Indexicality of Ghosts / 166
      Cultural Time in *Jiapai* / 172
         Big Data Cloud / 176
         Frameworks of Thought / 180
      Concluding Reflections / 184

CHAPTER 6
   These Burdens We Carry / 188
      "We Have So Much Hurt" / 191
      Speaking of Shame / 197
      The Hate in My Heart / 201
      "Those Things That Are Collective" / 210
      Concluding Reflections / 216

CHAPTER 7
   Tinkering with the Patriarchy / 220
      The Permeability of Patriarchy / 222
      Men's Work / 228

"That Home in Your Inner Heart" / 233
Rethinking the Yijing / 242
Concluding Reflections / 252

CONCLUSION / 255
Perplexing Particulars in the Era of COVID / 258
"Stay with Us" / 261
Concluding Reflections / 267

Notes / 271
References / 275
Index / 297

Digital materials related to this title can be found on the Fulcrum platform via the following citable URL: https://doi.org/10.3998/mpub.11743065

Acknowledgments

All that you touch, you change. All that you change, changes you.
—OCTAVIA BUTLER

This book represents over ten years of thinking, experiencing, writing, responding, and communicating. With such temporal breadth, it is difficult to name everyone who has had an impact on this volume. I'll start, however, by expressing my deepest gratitude and respect to all of the people who participated in this research, no matter how small or large a role they played. The vulnerability and intimacy involved with this project constituted a true journey of the soul, so to speak, the result of which adds up to far more than this book.

I would also like to express my immense gratitude to the Wenner-Gren Foundation, who offered a generous Post-PhD Research Award to fund the bulk of this research. I was also lucky enough to receive funding for various parts of the project from the UCLA Center for East-West Medicine and the University of Alabama.

An extra special thanks also goes to my colleague and dear friend, Professor Di Luo. Having joined the small Asian Studies faculty at the University of Alabama in the same year, we very quickly established a unique and broad-ranging intellectual collaboration that very explicitly led to the (co)creation of this book. This book would not have been possible without the vast historical perspectives offered by Di, who never ceased to challenge, push, and expand my ideas.

The core concepts at the heart of this book, it is also important to note, have developed in countless conversations with mentors, colleagues, and coauthors conducted in writing, on Zoom, and in person over many years. This is where I find it particularly difficult to generate a complete list of specific names, especially because—following Octavia Butler—my ideas were utterly changed by each encounter. In alphabetical order, however, I would like to thank the following individuals for engaging deeply, at various stages, with the ideas presented here: Emily Baum, Jason DeCaro, Whitney Duncan, Gareth Fisher, Gili Hammer, Marta Hanson, Tony Hu, Claudia Huang, Judith Irvine, Graham Jones, Teresa Kuan, Kiki Liang, Christopher Lynn, Elinor Ochs, Sabina Perrino, Suzi Roberts, Bambi Schieffelin, Hsuan-Ying Huang, Samuel Wade, Lesley Jo Weaver, Jing Xu, Mei Zhan, and Li Zhang. Here, I want to also give a shout out to all of my University of Alabama students—both graduate and undergraduate—who have discussed and sometimes even adopted and expanded the central concepts I present here: Baili Gall, Amanda Guitar, Larry Monocello, Michael Smetana, and students in the annual seminar in linguistic anthropology (ANT401-50) between 2015 and 2023. Thank you for the challenges you've offered me, the trust, and the willingness to take it all further than I could have ever imagined.

It would be remiss not to further mention the radical and deep influence, throughout this text, of scholars, activists, and students who I have become more recently acquainted with in my recent research on the field of embodied social justice. Again, too many to name. Special thanks, however, to Kesha Fikes, Sam Grant, Staci Haines, Tessa Hicks Peterson, Rae Johnson, Sará King, and all fifty-four collaborators involved with the Living Justice Project (livingjusticeproject.com). Thank you, finally, to the two anonymous reviewers who took the time and care to comment on this book as well as the amazing team at University of Michigan Press.

Last but certainly not least, a very special thank you to my family: Jeremy Bailin, Nadya Boynton-Pritzker, Steve Pritzker, Blythe Tannahill, Mary Hawkins, and Craig Tannahill (also, of course: Meowleau-Ponty, Mitzvah, and Pumpkinhead). To Jeremy and Nadya especially, who endured the daily trials and tribulations inevitably involved with finalizing a book during COVID: thank you, from the bottom of my heart, for (most of the time) heeding the "Disturb at your own risk" sign often hanging outside my office door as I wrote.

Introduction

In the realm of the political, among the religious, in our families, and in our romantic lives, we see little indication that love informs decisions, strengthens our understanding of community, or keeps us together. This bleak picture in no way alters the nature of our longing. We still hope that love will prevail. We still believe in love's promise.
—BELL HOOKS

To learn to live ... Who would learn? From whom? To teach to live, but to whom? Will we ever know? ... To live, by definition, is not something one learns. Not from oneself, it is not learned from life, taught by life. Only from the other and by death. In any case from the other at the edge of life.
—JACQUES DERRIDA

It was early summer 2015, the fourth day of a five-day inner child retreat offered by the New Life Center for Holistic Growth, a small but growing center offering numerous courses, salons, and retreats focused on holistically healing and "psychospiritual self-development" (心灵成长 xinling chengzhang). About sixty of us were seated in a circle in the large banquet room of an upscale hotel, which had been transformed with pink sheets covering the carpeted floors and hundreds of pastel pillows scattered throughout the room. The room felt familiar by that point. Over the past four days, we had danced wildly, cried profusely, and played with abandon in the space. We had traveled in time to multiple pasts and had become one another's mothers, fathers, grandmothers, and even our grandmothers' long-deceased ancestors. We sat that afternoon, gazing toward our instructor, Teacher Johann or "Teacher Jo." A white, Australian psychologist and devoted practitioner of a deeply embodied form of spiritual practice that he had cultivated with a South Asian teacher for over a decade. Teacher Jo had by that time also been leading workshops at various sites throughout (urban) China for almost the same amount of time.

Teacher Jo looked around the room and smiled at each of us, seemingly individually.

"We are going to do an exercise," he said, finally, pointing to the pillows, going on to explain that we would be addressing the cushions as if they were our parents: first our mothers and then our fathers.

"You are going to hold the cushion at the ends, and you are going to express frustration," he said, telling us that we would be hitting the pillows, punching them as we uttered whatever came up: "Stop controlling me! Or stop criticizing me! Where were you when I needed you?," he offered as examples. "I'm never good enough for you!"

Teacher Jo then paused and looked around, grinning broadly and evoking smiles from several participants, some of whom seemed to be more nervous than mirthful. Many looked like they were holding their breath. Others looked skeptical, as if he was making a bad joke and calling it "science." After remaining quiet for what seemed like a long time, however, he spoke seriously, reminding us that it was completely normal to harbor anger and resentment, even toward our parents. If we still had trouble remembering specific incidents or reasons for being angry, he guided us to let our bodies lead. Our bodies would guide us toward whatever needed to be expressed. This would be easier, he noted, if we did not compare ourselves to others who seemed more skilled at expressing emotion.

"The important thing is what you feel inside and your sincerity," he assured us, telling us we had license to express "whatever came up" provided we didn't harm anyone else within the space.

"Pay attention to your fists during the exercise" he said, "and don't hit the person in front of you. He or she is not your mother."

More laughter. Teacher Jo then told us to spread out throughout the room with one pillow each. We shuffled around and landed about two feet apart from one another and began engaging with the cushion as if it was our mother. A few participants who had attended previous workshops closed their eyes and immediately entered a passionate dialogue with the pillow, which they then proceeded to punch. Others stared blankly at their pillows or began tapping them lightly.

"I want to feel a big wind coming towards me!," Teacher Jo shouted, lifting his hands up repeatedly as if attempting to stir up the *qi* in the room.

Several people suddenly began screaming loudly and hitting their pillows vigorously. A few began to weep. One woman started shivering, while another held her hand over her mouth as if she was going to vomit. Yet others remained silent and unmoving, some gazing around the room as if in a dream, others staring down at their cushions with an intense glare.

After about ten minutes of this, Teacher Johan rang a small bell and asked us to sit with our backs straight, eyes closed. After several minutes of silence, he spoke again. "Ask yourself, if I am not defined by my past, who am I?," he said gently. "If I am not my negative feelings, who am I? If I leave all of that behind, who am I now? Who am I? Remain in this openness. In this curiosity. Who am I? Who am I?" He paused. "Try to hear the echo. What is the echo within you when you say 'I'? Who is this I that is beyond these images that you created?"

Several more minutes of silence passed as we breathed and sat, some of us contemplating our teacher's words, others drifting off into a state somewhere between sleep and wakefulness.

LEARNING TO LOVE

The first time I found myself in a ballroom of more than fifty Chinese adults hitting pillows, crying, and yelling at their "parents," it was striking. In addition to being emotionally intense, the exercise directly challenged the moral norm—and, at least since 2013, the *legal obligation*—of filial piety (孝顺 *xiaoshun*) (Lin and Trevaskes 2019). Indeed, most people who came to New Life Center for Holistic Growth had what one instructor described as such a "deeply rooted" (根深蒂固 *genshen digu*) orientation to filial piety that the expression of anger toward one's parents constituted a form of embodied *betrayal*.[1] For most of these individuals, in other words, filial piety was far from simply a set of "rules" enacted within a preordained structure of relational hierarchies. It was, rather, an intimate, embodied *orienting device* structuring their affective, physiological, and social experience of themselves in the world (Williams 1977; Ahmed 2007). Alongside other culturally salient concepts that I discuss throughout this book, filial piety was also an intimate experience that extended across space and time and made other relationships in their lives both possible and pleasant.

What, then, were these apparently successful, middle-class, predominantly Han Chinese citizens doing pounding their fists at pillows and screaming at their mothers and fathers? Had they bought into "the stereotypical therapy story" within which one's personal past is framed as the sole cause for suffering (Wright 2011, 192)? Were they immersing themselves in the kinds of therapeutic individualizing and "familializing" (Ivy 1993) narratives that, in China and elsewhere, are often seen as a strategy for directing attention away from more collective sociopolitical concerns (J. Yang 2018a-b)? Or were they engaged in a culturally transformative, alchemical process of some kind? To even begin to answer such questions, more ethnographic context is necessary.

During the summers of 2014–16, when I conducted the formal research on which this book is based, the New Life Center for Holistic Growth was a small bookstore and space for spiritual practice and natural healing in the heart of a large city in northeast China. The overall genre of both texts and practices at the center was referred to formally as "body-mind-spirit" (身心灵 *shen-xin-ling*), an adaptation of what had previously been established as "New Age" (新时代 *xin shidai*) for more than forty years in Taiwan (Farrelly 2017, 2019a-b). Many weekday evenings, the center, which had been open for about five years, hosted free reading groups, "salons," and workshops in a range of modalities and experiential practices, including yoga, inner child work, family constellation therapy (or *jiapai* as I refer to it throughout this book), Chinese medical massage, and call-and-response Indian chanting (kirtan or 唱诵 *chansong*). Longer retreats were hosted at a large hotel at the outskirts of the city, usually costing around RMB 5–7,000 (USD 800–1,000 at the time). In 2015, the center also began to offer guided spiritual travel to destinations such as Indonesia, India, and Tibet.

At free events, the clientele at New Life was somewhat diverse in terms of age and socioeconomic status. All the participants that I encountered, however, presented as cis-gendered, heterosexual, and ethnically Han. The overall age range for all participants, who were also mostly urban dwelling, was between nineteen and seventy-nine, with most falling somewhere between twenty-five and forty-five years of age. Participants were also predominantly middle class: those who had not yet retired were usually employed as teachers, salespeople, or executives in white collar corporate positions—or they were related to someone who was. As in psychotherapeutic and holistic group practices in settings worldwide, finally, most participants at the center were women (Heelas 1996, 2008; Duncan 2017, 2018; Matza 2018; L. Zhang 2020). Most of the teachers and lead interns were, however, men and, within a given workshop, usually about 20 percent of participants were men.

Regardless of age, gender, or socioeconomic status, it is however important to center that most participants arrived at New Life experiencing the kind of *anxiety* (焦虑 *jiaolu*) that Li Zhang suggests constitutes the "pulse" beating at the heart of Chinese society in the early twenty-first century (2020, 4). Like others attracted to novel psychotherapeutic or religious practices in China, they often used terms that underscored an embodied, relational sense of disorientation in the world, including 迷茫 *mimang*, "confused," 不平 *buping*, "off balance," and 馄饨 *huntun*, "chaotic and blurred" (Zhang 2020, 119; see also Fisher 2014; Hizi 2018). They were all also deeply affected, though often in distinct ways, by the kind of spatiotemporally jarring *mood* that Farquhar and Zhang (2012) have observed as characterizing early twenty-first century China. Many scholars have thus engaged with a collective experience of the kind of "ungroundedness" resulting from a simultaneous lack of social consensus and attendant search for new discourses and new pathways to agency (Xiang and Wu 2022 74, 229–30; see also Jankowiak and Li 2017, 146). Taking up a common trope in Chinese society at the time, many people at New Life also described a sensation of being "immature" (不成长 *bu chengzhang*).² Many were also facing a range of distinctly gendered anxieties related to simultaneously internal and external pressures to be good men, good women, and good citizens (Fincher 2016, 2019, 2021; J. Yang 2018b; Wong 2020; L. Zhang 2020; Xie 2021).

As detailed in chapter 1, nearly all who showed up at New Life had also suffered some kind of a *rupture* or "breach of life plan" (Myers 2016): a specific incident or series of incidents that had fractured their relationship(s) with their spouse, child, or parents or which had transformed the relational environment at home or work. Having struggled to resolve their suffering on their own, newcomers to New Life often poured their energy into trying to figure out *what*, exactly, had happened, *when* it had happened, *who* was to blame, and—of course—how to fix it. Here, their narratives often oriented toward hegemonic cultural ideologies of gender, family, and the self that, over the course of their life, had become deeply intimate (e.g., filial piety), but which no longer seemed to offer a solid sense of direction, belonging, or purpose. The confusion and sense of imbalance that newcomers to the center were experiencing was thus also often framed as a feeling of having lost—or having never successfully found—their "home" (家 *jia*). The *desire* that motivated their participation in psychospiritual development, accordingly, was often described as a persistent feeling of nostalgia or longing for one's "home-place," whether one had ever existed or not (Joniak-Lüthi 2015). The sense of longing here was rarely focused on a specific place, but rather pointed to the illusive feeling of relationally situated *agency* and *connection* that anthropologist Michael Jackson (1995) frames as "being-at-home-in-the-world."³

Following the title of John Bradshaw's 1990 bestseller—Homecoming: Reclaiming and Championing Your Inner Child—learning to love was thus frequently cast as a "homecoming" centered in the individual body-self. Situating agency somewhere between individual action and passive discovery, New Life exercises like the one described above often involved a form of embodied inquiry through which our body-selves were mapped spatio-temporally vis-à-vis the past (where we had been, who had contributed to shaping us); the present (who we had become, what our current struggles were); and future (what we wanted to contribute to the world in our relationships, our work, and our presence). Drawing on a common psychoanalytic frame for understanding human development over time and within various spaces, such effort was often cast as a kind of "house-cleaning" that required us to discover, face, and *feel* what Teacher Jo sometimes referred to as the "mess" inside. The mess, here, referred to the accumulation of the unconscious, implicit, and embodied memories, both positive and negative, that had shaped us in the world.

"The work" of learning to love at New Life did not always or only mean facing darkness and pain, however. It also involved a great deal of *play*, within which we were encouraged to viscerally remember the curiosity and joy of an innocent and uninhibited child. On the afternoon described in the opening vignette, for example, we were roused after about ten minutes of meditation. Teacher Johan's demeanor shifted suddenly, and he excitedly told us to clear away the tissues, teacups, and other debris scattered about the room. He then told us to pick up a pillow as he moved to the large stereo system. We were going to have a pillow fight, he told us enthusiastically as the familiar sound of "Gangam Style" began to reverberate throughout the large room. For the next fifteen minutes or so, we thus ran around the room bopping one another with pillows and laughing hysterically.

As evident in the meditation described above, in which Teacher Jo guided us to interrogate "the I" beyond emotion and image, learning to love was likewise often framed as an opportunity to encounter one's "True Self" (真我 *zhenwo*), a simultaneously individual and collective as well as *connective* entity that, like in many spiritual practices, extended far beyond the individual body-self (Satir 1988, as cited in Akça Koca 2017; Albanese 1999; Heelas 2008). In this sense, learning to love at New Life often took shape as a relationally situated process of "collective development" (共同成长 *gongtong chengzhang*), as a participant once put it toward the end of a workshop. Whether done alone or with a partner/group, finally, exercises thus also often involved a form of "time travel" in which we became able to interact directly with our parents, teachers, and other authoritative figures, who were embodied by other participants. Learning to love here involved a complex, (inter)corporeal, and socially engaged process of healing the extended, embodied familial body-self, which pointed both backwards and forwards in time. In inner child workshops, for example, there were several exercises that involved tuning into an embodied current of love that flowed through our ancestors' bodies. These visualizations and meditations often constituted a novel opportunity to experience ourselves as occupying a rightful "position" or "status" (位置 *weizhi*) within an embodied, moral, and relational ancestral lineage stretching both backwards and forwards in space and time. Family constellation therapy or *jiapai*, on the other hand, involved an intensive process within which participants served as "representatives" for the non-co-present relatives and ancestors of a "focal participant," who then observed the "constellation." In a collaborative but mostly unspoken interaction that I refer to as "wrangling with ghosts," learning to love here meant coming to "know" the unspoken dynamics of the recent or distant intergenerational past and thus restoring the "hidden symmetry" of love within the extended family body-self (Hellinger 1998, 2001). In a twist on Derrida's (1994) framing of "learning to live" as a relational process within which one learns "only from the other and by death," learning to love—across workshops and events at New Life—thus often took shape as a collaboratively enacted process of "turning our ghosts into ancestors" (Wolynn 2016, 49).

As I discuss throughout the following chapters, such encounters did not refer only to *personal* histories, however, as the ghosts and ancestors in question also scaled outward, often quite rapidly, even instantaneously, toward a vast relational, sociocultural past in which multiple forms of suffering had affected (and were continuing to affect) most (if not all) of the families of the largely ethnically homogenous population. As I discuss throughout the following chapters, the horizoned promise of learning to love was, in this sense, often a simultaneously intimate and *scalar* process pointing both backwards and forwards in time, inward to the most intimate, private experiences and outward to the most broadly public encounters. Though often centered around participants' most intimate relationships with parents, partners, and children, learning to love at New Life, in other words, often constituted an inherently collective endeavor that extended "love's promise," as bell hooks writes, from the most intimate relationships to the most broadly social, spiritual, and even political realms (2000, 27). Healing imbalances that had persisted across multiple generations was here often framed as a strategy to enact *justice* (公平 *gongping* or 正义 *zhengyi*) in the present as well as for *future* generations. Learning to love, from this perspective, emerged as a form of "being-with specters," in Derrida's terms, that offered a pathway toward learning to *live* both "better" and "more justly" (1994, xvii–xviii).

To return, then, to the question of why these relatively normative, privileged, and materially successful participants were pounding their fists at pillows and yelling at their "parents," it might be said that they were *not*, actually, yelling at or hitting their mothers and fathers (or were not frozen in place at the thought of doing so) but were, rather, enacting an intimate and relationally situated rage and despair about past forms of injustice as well as cultivating their capacity for an embodied, relational, and collective form of justice. Though arguably emphasizing the kinds of "low justice" that, in China, focuses on interpersonal rather than higher, political realms (Lin 2017; Lee 2023), I make the case in this book that the absolute line between "high" and "low" was often blurred at New Life. This was not least because most participants—like the majority of Chinese citizens—were well aware of the limitations that exist for enacting any form of large-scale social transformation. The kinds of justice engaged, discussed, desired, and debated by participants at New Life nevertheless often emerged in a collaborative *anticipatory mode* (Sumartojo and Pink 2019) within which learning to love consisted of numerous forms of interrogation, theory-building, and *dreaming* (Loizidou 2016) that engaged with multiple scales of the simultaneously personal, social, cultural, and political past at the same time as it oriented toward possible collective futures in which "love," rather than fakery, violence, and other forms of oppressive governance, might prevail.

ENTANGLING DIFFERENTLY

New Life, it is important to note—I cannot be clearer about this—*did not have any intentions of politicizing or otherwise developing participants' social or political engagement.* As in most settings where psychology was and is implemented in China, there was very little explicitly politicized analysis of anything in any of the workshops (see, e.g., Y. Zhang 2007, 2018; J. Yang 2015, 2018a-b; L. Zhang 2015, 2017, 2018, 2020; Hizi 2018). In a statement I revisit throughout the book, in fact, the director of New Life once emphatically suggested that all the center offered was brief space-time of "comfort" to people whose lives were otherwise chaotic and overstressed. As I discuss throughout this book, however, the kind of stress people at New Life were facing did not relate *only* to the increasingly fast-paced and competitive conditions prevailing in urban China at the time. It also derived from the sense of mismatch people were experiencing, in their intimate relationships and everyday lives, between the moral and relational discourses they had previously held as absolute "goods" and the realities of their situations.

When people came to the center, I show, they were often struggling—similar to Europeans engaged with what Heelas (2008) refers to as "inner-life spirituality"—within a *circumscribed* set of horizons. The courses and textual materials offered by New Life offered *hope*, as well as a kind of relational moral compass or promise that participants might regain or simply find a better sense of spatiotemporal, relational, and affective orientation in the world. New Life thus offered participants a range of novel "vistas of significance" (Heelas 2008), at the center of which lay the "horizoned promise" of finding "a good life beyond material success" in a society that had become increasingly centered around the competitive pursuit (and display) of status through wealth (L. Zhang 2020, 133; see also I. Johnson 2017). The horizons offered at the center, from this vantage point, often pointed simultaneously inward and outward and encompassed multiple scales of both "private" and "public" experience. This book thus examines how interactions and relational experiences at New Life invited participants, at least *implicitly*, to interrogate the ways in which social, cultural, and historical systems of power existing in the past had become entrenched within their relational body-selves; how such systems continued in the present; and how they might be transformed in the future.

Such interrogation, it is critical to note, only applied to *some* participants *some of the time*. This book is therefore *not* a study of genre or the translation of genre (e.g., psychology in China). Nor is it a study of some kind of generalizable middle-class Chinese response to group psychotherapy. It is not even a study of how "most people" at New Life engaged in the project of learning to love. I offer this book, rather, as a study of the communicative, ethical, and environmental possibilities or *affordances* presented by the theories, practices, aesthetics, and physical environment of the center (Gibson 1979; Keane 2014, 2016; Ramstead et al. 2016). Implicit conversations about governance, justice, and the future of Chinese society here *afforded* but did not guarantee that all participants took them up—as did others—in what I frame as an embodied, collaborative, and interrogative project related to *political subjectivity*, if not necessarily social action (Loizidou 2016).

This may come as a surprise to many readers, as psychology in China is often approached as a "technology of the self" (Foucault 1988) or a form of "therapeutic governance" (Polsky 1991; Szasz 1974). Both conclusions suggest that psychotherapeutic interventions seem inherently designed to direct the attention of citizens away from social, historical, or political concerns (see, e.g., Lin 2012; Ma 2012; Hendriks 2016; Hizi 2018; Hird 2018; J. Yang 2015, 2018a-b, 2020; Wielander 2018a-b). By attending to how (some) participants at New Life turned *more* rather than *less* toward the social, this book does not seek to undermine or even contest these observations. In addition to being a study of affordances or possibilities, it is thus also a study of the kinds of *perplexing particulars* defined by Cheryl Mattingly as singular experiences, encounters, or events that themselves serve to *unsettle* existing categories and characterizations (2019, 427). In this sense, my analysis aligns with a range of ethnographic scholarship beyond China that shows how—at least *sometimes*, for at least *some* participants—engagement in psychotherapeutic group practice opens up the space for a more broadly social and even political understanding of self, other, and society (Wright 2011; Duncan 2017, 2018; Matza 2018, Pritzker and Liang 2018; Pritzker and Duncan 2019). It is further grounded in the work of anthropologists who have variably engaged with the notion of ethical subjectivity and moral agency, in China and elsewhere, as a situated and emergent relational process of interrogation (Zigon 2009; Stafford 2013; Mattingly 2014; Kuan 2015) as well as recent historical work demonstrating a lineage of scholars and practitioners in psychoanalysis who, beginning with Sigmund Freud himself, developed psychotherapy as an intervention that was as much oriented toward the social and political as it was toward the personal (Gaztambide 2019, 177). Perhaps more than anything, however, my analysis is specifically grounded in the theories and methods of linguistic anthropology (Duranti 2009; Farnell and Graham 2015; Perrino and Pritzker 2021).

But *how*, one might justifiably ask, does a linguistic anthropologist go about conducting what might be framed as an "ethnography of the implicit"? The short answer is that my analyses are thoroughly grounded in the reality that linguistic anthropology, in Constantine Nakassis's famous framing, is "not about language" (2016, 331) but rather constitutes the study of culture and meaning as continually *communicative* processes that emerge through spoken and written language as well as (more frequently) through unspoken communications grounded in body language, gaze shifts, prosody or rhythm of speech, overlapping speech, self-corrections, grammatical phrasing, and so on.[4] Meaning, from this perspective, often emerges as a result not of direct or semantic meaning but through *indexicality*.

An "index," according to Charles Peirce, *points* to other things within specific social, historical, and economic contexts. Depending on context, then, precise meaning shifts are based on the "senses or memory of the person for whom it serves as a sign" (1992 [1955], 107). It is thus only within specific interactive situations that we might be able to apprehend the meaning and impact of specific forms of spoken or embodied language. This view of language-as-interaction underscores the ways in which language is far from being simply a form of reference—a set of words and symbols that freeze or "murder the thing," as Jacques Lacan might say (1988, 174). As noted by Elinor Ochs (2012, 148), the "indexical capacity of language" is precisely what allows it to function in interaction in ways that complement or compensate for its referential limitations. Such an approach centers the apprehension of meaning *in* and *as* interaction *over* time, *within* institutions, and *across* bodies.

The analyses I offer throughout this book are thus grounded in the close study of historically, relationally, and spaciotemporally situated interaction or "co-operative action" as a series of continually unfolding "horizon of constrained, but open-ended, possibilities" (C. Goodwin 2018, 445–46). In defining co-operative action, Charles Goodwin takes care to distinguish his notion of "co-operation" from the related but distinct idea of "cooperation." Co-operative action, he notes,

> ... is not the same as what evolutionary biologists, anthropologists, and psychologists investigate as cooperation. It does not require benefit to the recipient of the action; nor need it incur a cost for the party performing the action. It is central to the organization of aggressive as well as helpful action. (2018, 432)

By centering the ways in which interaction at New Life emerged as co-operative action, I thus attend closely to the ways in which encounters at the center were often challenging for participants, as much as they "helped" them.

My analyses further center the *chronotopes* people use to situate themselves in time and space. Chronotopes were originally developed by Mikhail Bakhtin (1981) as an analytical tool for discussing the ways in which novelists depict characters' relation to space over time. "Without such temporal-spatial expression," writes Bakhtin, "even abstract thought is impossible" (1981, 256). While Bakhtin's focus was restricted to artistic writing, a growing body of literature foregrounds the ways in which people, in their everyday lives, also regularly draw upon dominant *cultural chronotopes* in order to orient themselves in space and time as well as vis-à-vis various moral "person-types" (Agha 2007). I engaged the cultural chronotopes discussed throughout this book are, further, inherently *scalar* in the sense that they always work to imagine and instantiate *contrast* (Agha 2007; Lempert and Perrino 2007; Divita 2019). As narrative frameworks that knit time, space, and moral, embodied forms of relationality and possibility together in even the most mundane everyday terms—words like *here*, *there*, *home*, or *hope*, for example—cultural chronotopes map the world in a set of interconnected scalar processes that precede and shape bodies as well as their experience in space and time. Indeed, (cultural) chronotopes "shape our *experience* and thus subjective *feel* for history and place" (Wirtz 2016, 344, italics in original). In concert with linguistic anthropology, my analyses thus further take up the theories and methods of psychological anthropology and person-centered ethnography (Levy and Hollan 1998; Hollan 2001, 2005) to offer a refinement or expansion of existing literature on cultural chronotopes by attending specifically to chronotopes as embodied, phenomenological *orienting devices* (Ahmed 2007).The following discussions of experiences and encounters at New Life are thus further grounded in a detailed investigation of the paired processes of *scalar intimacy* (Pritzker and Perrino 2020) and *scalar inquiry* (Pritzker 2023). Scalar intimacy, specifically, refers to the participatory, relationally situated, discursive process by which people position or *scale* themselves in relation to intimate others as well as dominant ideologies, concepts, and ideals (Pritzker and Perrino 2020).

Underscoring the deeply felt experience and discursive enactment of what Roseneil et al. (2020) frame as *intimate citizenship regimes*, scalar intimacy in this book likewise engages the ways in which emotion, imagination, and desire emerge at the intersection of the personal and national. In this sense, it is inspired by Kevin Carrico's (2017) assertion of the importance and relevance of paying closer attention to investigating the contours of the relationship that Chinese citizens have with the Chinese nation itself. Though always agentive in the sense that it "does things with words" (Austin [1962]

2023), moreover, the enactment of scalar intimacy often reproduces institutionally entrenched scales that precede any interaction and are often upheld *in* interaction (Carr and Lempert 2016, 3; see also Delfino 2021; Wong et al. 2021). Scalar *inquiry*, on the other hand, points to the equally dialogic process through which speakers variably interrogate these forms, their relationship with them, and their participation in reproducing them (Pritzker 2023). The following chapters thus engage with how both spoken and unspoken interactions and relational, embodied experiences at New Life invited participants, at least *implicitly*, to adjust or rescale their interrogations of their "personal" experience in relation to a range of both past and present hegemonic ideologies and structures of power in Chinese sociopolitical history. To the extent that it involves the deconstructing of hegemonic ideologies, scalar inquiry, I show, sometimes emerged as a form of what Hannah Arendt termed "defrosting," a fundamentally *ethical* process in which frozen thought-forms are interrogated in ways that afford sometimes dramatic and sometimes subtle interventions (Arendt 1971, 433–44; see also Mattingly 2019). Such interventions, as I discuss in multiple chapters, sometimes emerge as the kind of *rechronotopization* that Karimzad and Catedral (2018, 2021) define as a process through which established chronotopes are reformulated in and across interactions and in relation to speakers' experience over time in different spaces (2021, 8). Pointing to the kind of "tiny agency" implied in Judith Butler's theory of performativity, this perspective on rechronotopization underscores how, in enacting scalar intimacy *differently*, people sometimes reposition or experiment with repositioning themselves vis-à-vis dominant cultural chronotopes, even if only for a moment.

Throughout this book, then, I attend closely to the ways that, in the context of New life, scalar inquiry often constituted a cultural, embodied, and intimate hermeneutic process that often took shape as an "adventure" into *uncertainty* (Gadamer 1981). The strange reconfigurations of space, time, and embodied relationality occurring within exercises and encounters at New Life, I show, often instantiated a form of radical uncertainty, within which "something queer" (J. Butler 2016, 18) sometimes took shape, at least temporarily, in the ways that participants engaged with, embodied, or resisted social norms that felt oppressive. Scalar intimacy and scalar inquiry, I thus demonstrate, serve as theoretical and methodological interventions that afford insight into the implicit ways in which people, within situated interactions, variably position themselves in relation to hegemonic cultural chronotopes or norms, ideologies, and experiences.

In the application of chronotopic analysis, as well as attention to both scalar intimacy and scalar inquiry in the narratives and group encounters included in the following chapters, I take up Li Zhang's engagement with the ways in which the social took shape, within and in the "inner revolution" (内心的革命 *neixin de geming*) sweeping across China, as a paired process of "disentangling" and "re-embedding" (2020, 18). Enacted within workshops, retreats, and private clinical encounters that variably combine psychology (心理学 *xinli xue*) and spirituality (灵性 *lingxing*) in practices that emphasize embodied experience (体验 *tiyan*) and an often-unspoken "dialogue with images" (意象 *yixiang*), Zhang suggests that spaces where the inner revolution takes place present the opportunity "to detach one's self temporarily and mentally from the familial and social nexus in which one is deeply embedded in everyday life so as to create a space for contemplation" (2020, 18). The complementary notion of "re-embedding," wherein people "return to the social once certain therapeutic self-work is done," underscores both distance and proximity as people move out of the social world to enter the therapeutic space, but always—at least in some capacity— return to the social (2020, 18). Overall, I concur with Zhang's description of disentangling and re-embedding, particularly in terms of the ways in which these concepts underscore the numerous pathways by which the "work" done at New Life "traveled out" beyond the space. Throughout this book, however, I emphasize rather the ways in which scalar intimacy and scalar inquiry, as they took shape in interactions, embodied experiences, and intimate encounters at New Life, might also be considered a lived experience of *entangling differently*.

In the context of New Life, my analyses throughout the following thus emphasize how New Life participants engaged with or *experimented* with making slight adjustments in their positioning vis-à-vis scalar, chronotopic norms that have structured their experience in the world over the course of their lives (e.g., boy/girl, man/woman, citizen/foreigner, good citizen/ dissident). Returning to the opening scene, for example, there were numerous culturally salient scalar distinctions that were invoked in the exercise, including piety/betrayal, harmony/chaos, success/failure, justice/injustice, and past/present/future to name just a few. Dominant chronotopes associated with these scales were also inverted or adjusted in multiple, provocative ways in the very enactment of an exercise that required expressing anger toward one's parents. When Teacher Jo explicitly noted how participants who struggled to access anger, rage, or grief might feel that they are "doing it wrong" in comparison to others who seemed able to express emotion more readily, for example, he seemed attuned to the salience of the chronotope of *competition* in Chinese educational contexts. And yet his invitation to express negative emotion "publicly" (or at least among others) arguably constituted an inversion of the more salient cultural chronotope of harmony and emotional restraint (Yan 2013). In this sense, within the collaboratively enacted chronotope of learning to love, participants were thus invited to explore, examine, or interrogate their relationship to a range of dominant cultural chronotopes, often simultaneously and intimately. Their inquiries, importantly, were not directed only at the pillows, nor even simply at "injustice" in the past, but also vis-à-vis their proximity to one another. Engaging the ways in which these dynamic relationships are configured and sometimes reconfigured in interaction, entangling differently through both scalar intimacy and inquiry thus attends to both the reproduction of normative discourses and to the ways in which speakers sometimes reposition or experiment with repositioning themselves vis-à-vis these discourses.

IMPLICIT JUSTICE?

Although conditions are vastly different in China, it is relevant, here, to briefly review the ways in which scholars have engaged with the politics of psycho/spiritual communities throughout the world. Although Paul Heelas identifies what he calls a "spiritually grounded politics of well-being" (2008, 206) among practitioners of holistic spirituality in Europe, for example, such communities have also been critiqued for embracing a range of radical political, economic, and social ideologies without necessarily acting on them. Critical scholarship has thus questioned the ways in which participants in this broad milieu often orient to the idea of "being the change"—a notion derived from the oft-cited guidance, frequently attributed to Gandhi, to "be the change you want to see in the world"[5]—without necessarily participating in explicitly politicized movements (Heelas 2008; Wood 2008; Jain 2020; Lucia 2020). Wood (2008), for instance, interrogates how the founders of Esalen, a well-known psychospiritual center in California, embraced a "hopeful, even utopian" orientation that was "always eager to harness science and faith to bring about a progressive political agenda and democratic ideals" (2008, 487). In practice, however, she notes how "specifics on how to change society" were (at least historically) scarce at Esalen, which "operated more as a think tank, a form for cross-cultural dialogue, and greenhouse for individual growth" (2008, 464–65). Paul Farrelly identifies a similar ethic within early Taiwanese renditions of the New Age. C. C. Wang (王季庆 Wang Jiqing), who translated Kahlil Gibran's *The Prophet* (1970) and Jane Roberts's *Seth* series (1982, 1984, 1987) into Chinese, for example, oriented to the notion that "the accumulation of many individual transformations" would lead to a so-called social paradigm shift (Farrelly 2017, 311). Later proponents of New Age/Body-Mind-Spirit, importantly, such as Terry Hu (胡因梦) and Tiffany Chang (张德芬 Zhang Defen), have taken slightly more explicit political stances. Terry Hu, for example, who became well-known in Taiwan for "her promotion of the New Age as a feminist instrument of empowerment is significant in this climate of growing awareness of, and political engagement with, women's rights" (Farrelly 2019a, 67). As Jie Yang observes, Tiffany Chang's emphasis on the cultivation of one's inner child, on the other hand, can be read as "an implicit criticism . . . of the Chinese government's failure to protect its people" (Yang 2018a, 188). The notion that Taiwanese psychospiritual authors have used their writing to directly comment on social issues as well as to develop *implicit* critiques of the state is important to keep in mind for interpreting the ways in which, as I suggest throughout this book, New Life practitioners similarly tentatively engaged with "the social" beyond their immediate circle of friends and family.

Again, it is important to keep in mind the fact that New Life was not designed as a space for social organization or even civic engagement—and, indeed, would unlikely be allowed to continue operating if it was. Here, then, I might take up critiques from the emerging literature on "embodied social justice" (see, e.g., williams et al. 2016; brown 2017; R. Johnson 2018, 2023; Haines 2019; Magee 2019; Fikes 2021a–b; Ndefo 2021; King 2021). The absence of "broader conversations of how we are shaped by social conditions, about oppression and privilege, about our individual and collective survival strategies that come from these conditions," notes Haines (2019, 5), is one of the primary ways in which purportedly "transformational" or "spiritual" practices, or both, reproduce and perpetuate systemic inequality in the U.S. as well as globally. The application of such an argument to China is complicated, however, most obviously because people who speak out directly on social justice in China are often subject to "disappearances," and their family members are equally at risk (I. Johnson 2017; B. Xu 2017; Chen 2019).

Another major reason why so much conversation at New Life was implicit, however, was that much of the past was either unknown or only vaguely known. It often pointed, I suggest throughout the following chapters, to the kinds of *public secrecy* that Margaret Hillenbrand describes as "like the ghost ... a thing that hovers between the visible and the occluded, the known and the unsayable" (2020, 37). Drawing on Michael Taussig's definition of public secrecy as "that which is generally known, but cannot be articulated" (Taussig 1999, 5, as cited in Hillenbrand 2020, 2), Hillenbrand notes that public secrecy functions as a collaborative social process in the "cryptocracy" of Chinese society (2020, 8). The specifics of public secrecy change over time, but—as Hillenbrand notes—variably include details about the massive famine that killed millions during the Great Leap Forward (1958–62); the violence enacted as well as endured during the Great Cultural Revolution (1965–75); and the massacre of student protestors during the 1989 protests at Tiananmen Square. Hillebrand observes, however, that the silence surrounding these public secrets does not necessarily point to the kind of "amnesia" or "forgetting" often identified in China, but rather might be considered as an agentive process that is both "protective" and "pragmatic" (2020, 3). "Knowing what not to know" here points less to knowing what not to remember or even what not to know, however, and more with knowing what not to *say*. This makes public secrecy incredibly difficult to track, let alone document, but Hillenbrand makes the case that researchers can study public secrecy by attending to "aesthetic forms" such as the kinds of adapted or *coded* photographs that often circulate anonymously online and which she calls "photo-forms." These images, she suggests, afford insight into how "the shared consensus to stay quiet" is betrayed, at least indirectly, in the circulation of aesthetic forms that evoke a sense of *revelation* among viewers (Hillenbrand 2020, 143). Public secrecy, in this sense, might be said to emerge as a form of *cultural intimacy* or "social poetics" that binds citizens together in a shared project of knowing when to speak and when to remain silent (Herzfeld 2016, 21). Stretching across bodies, moving rapidly between the sociopolitical world and the individual body, and structuring society from the most intimate relationships to the most public, public secrecy is nevertheless often intimately felt.

Although Hillenbrand argues that language is "where secrets go to hide" (2020, 95), in this book I engage with the ways in which public secrecy is constantly communicated *indexically* within the kinds of mundane everyday interactions that suggest but do not directly refer to the complex emotions and experiences in the past. Rather than invoking a firm line between "those who know and those who have no idea," in Hillenbrand's terms—or between the past and present—attention to both scalar intimacy and scalar inquiry in conversations where participants speak but do not *refer* centers the unspoken ways in which public secrecy is communicated across the bodies of those who know from firsthand experience and those who *feel* or know "intuitively" (Feuchtwang 2013). Public secrecy, from this perspective, itself constitutes a form of scalar intimacy through which the *public* past persists in *personal* embodied, relational, affective, indexical, and scalar memories, many of which are unclear and indistinct process of indexicality wherein interactions, both spoken and unspoken, often come together as a collaborative "wrangling with ghosts."

Such dialogue is often turned toward a nuanced interrogation of the shared present, within which many secrets continued to exist. Learning to love at New Life—in addition to being a personal project focused on self-development—thus also consisted of a collaborative interrogation of many past and present and public "secrets." To name just a few, these included the rapid development of the economy and the fast-paced, competitive tenor of everyday life in a society increasingly focused on the accumulation of wealth (Farquhar and Zhang 2012; Kuan 2015; Dai 2018; R. Johnson 2018; L. Zhang 2020). It also encompassed the state's increasingly hegemonic insistence on the consistent performance of "happiness" (幸福 *xingfu*), and "positive energy" (正能量 *zheng nengliang*) as an expression of moral-political personhood (Wielander and Hird 2018; J. Yang 2018a-b; Karl 2020) as well as the collective coenactment of a "harmonious society" (和谐社会 *hexie shehui*), held in place through the inculcation of fear of difference or "chaos" (乱 *luan*), or both (Fu 2020). It included, finally, reimagined ideologies of Chineseness and "tradition" that have reinstated and reinvented a range of gendered and intergenerational patriarchal norms (Evans 2012; Yan 2016, 2018; Santos and Harrell 2017; Fincher 2016, 2019; Z. Yang 2017; J. Yang 2018b; Karl 2020; Wong 2020; Xie 2021).

Though such investigations are often considered inconsequential in terms of instigating meaningful social change, in her examination of photo-forms that indicate public secrecy in China, Hillenbrand (2020) emphasizes the ways in which acknowledgment in and of itself constitutes a kind of action. "In an economy of secrecy, asserting the affirmative powers of the clandestine can be a strong countermove," she writes (153). I thus consider the ways in which attendees, staff, and instructors often seemed to form what Hillenbrand frames as "coalitions of shadowboxers" made up of people "willing to experiment together with being more candid about those things that are broadly known but seldom said aloud" (2020, 21). My analysis also attends to how "the remembering present"—as opposed to "the remembered past" (J. Li 2020, 7)—here emerged as a distinctly therapeutic mode in which "the anticipated future" also constantly loomed.

At no point in this book do I suggest that these conversations were *enacting* justice per se. Indeed, most participants were acutely aware of the severe constraints that made conversations about justice, universal rights, and freedom particularly dreamlike in China. They were also largely aware, importantly, of the ways in which most state propaganda constituted the kind of "bullshit" that, notes Haiyan Lee, "obfuscates, overwhelms, and mystifies more than it deceives" (2023, 78). Indexicality and public secrecy—while they suggest how indirect reference can be incredibly effective for addressing unknown or unacknowledged forms of oppression—are, in this sense, entirely unreliable for organizing people into any form of active resistance. I turn back here, however, to the work of numerous practitioner-activists writing in the fields of liberation psychology and embodied social justice. Liberation psychology, for example, traces to a lineage that began with Freud and developed in the work of practitioners such as Sandor Ferenczi, Otto Fenischel, Frantz Fanon, and Erich Fromm as well as overlapping with civil rights activists and scholars such as Richard Wright, Ralph Ellison, and Paulo Friere (Gaztambide 2019). What Daniel Gaztambide refers to as the "the spirit of social justice" within psychoanalysis, though repeatedly "displaced, exiled, killed, and repressed time and again" in institutionalized forms of therapy, eschews the notion that self-inquiry always constitutes a turn "away" from the social (2019, 176). Gaztambide repeatedly emphasizes, however, the central role that *explicit* and *guided* "political mentalization" plays in supporting people to recognize what Martín-Baró (1976) called "the truth of the lie" (as cited in Gaztambide 2019, 173). Gaztambide thus argues that, to enact the political potential of therapy, "it is critical that we actually allow ourselves with our patients to actually mentalize politically about this world of interlocking systems and structures, in order to imagine a different world, a different set of relationships" (2019, 200). Multiple authors writing in the area of embodied social justice—also sometimes referred to as "politicized somatics" (Haines 2019) or "embodied activism" (R. Johnson 2023)—further embrace the perspective that an embodied form of interrogation and healing is necessary in order to promote substantive, long-term social change (see, e.g., williams et al. 2016; brown 2017; R. Johnson 2018, 2023; Haines 2019; Magee 2019; Fikes 2021a-b; Ndefo 2021; King 2021).

Given the real and severe constraints on having explicit conversations about social justice (let alone engaging in revolutions) in China, this book does not therefore condemn implicitness. Indeed, "knowing how to refer without saying" is a vastly important skill in China that points to far more than public secrecy and, in fact, is often drawn upon in the kinds of "non-confrontational activism" examined by Jing Wang (2019). Without explicit dialogue, however, the central question becomes how the shifts made among people engaging in psychospiritual self-development or "learning to love" eventually "scales up" (or does not) or "travels out" (or does not) into the world. Heelas, for example, makes the case that the kinds of small changes that people make in the way they relate to others because of their participation in self-development often "[flow] from the person into the relational" as they begin to permeate public settings in Europe (2008, 7). The argument here is that even small shifts in relationality might have what could be framed as a butterfly effect as they "travel outward" and are carried forth in everyday interaction across sites. In highlighting the ways in which small shifts travels out into the everyday lives of participants as they "re-embed" in the world, Li Zhang makes a similar observation in studying the inner revolution in China. Zhang's conclusion nevertheless interrogates how participants in the inner revolution—like most at New Life—are often concerned primarily with *interpersonal* forms of "low justice" rather than higher forms of justice touching on political realms. She thus concedes that "the social" as it is configured within the inner revolution constitutes "a specific form with its own limits" (2020, 129). With this book's emphasis on the nuanced ways in which scalar intimacy and scalar inquiry extended far beyond both personal and interpersonal realms, however, my analysis engages with the question of the limitations restricting *to whom* and *where* such transformations might travel.

Justice in a Hantopia

In engaging with New Life as a "Hantopia," I turn to the recent work of Amanda Lucia (2020), who conducted an extensive ethnographic analysis of global transformational festivals such as Shaktifest and Burning Man. Lucia's study specifically centers the multiple ways in which the kinds of "communitas" in these "imagined utopian worlds" (2020, 80) has the capacity to be transformative not only within the temporary space of the festival but in a (potentially) enduring way that extends outward into the world (2020, 317). Drawing upon Benjamin's (2009) notion of "Whitopias," however, Lucia underscores the fact that the utopias constructed at transformational festivals are overwhelmingly *white* utopias. She thus interrogates how such ethnic and racial homogeneity not only perpetuates a number of racial, ethnic, and socioeconomic injustices but also constrains the potential of the "transformations" experienced in a space of racial comfort to effect real change in society. Indeed, my analysis of New life is directly inspired by Lucia's observations, and—in framing New Life as a "Hantopia"—similarly embraces Benjamin's dissection of the ways in which the sociocultural emergence of "Whitopias," no matter how well-intentioned, ultimately "imperils a collective commitment to the common good" (2009, loc. 4242). My main critical inquiry throughout this book thus centers on the ways in which Han-ness at New Life came to implicitly represent Chineseness in an essentialist fashion that underlies the kinds of "mundane racism" that permeate Chinese society (Cheng 2019, 17).

Indeed, even while they questioned numerous forms of injustice and interrogated a range of public secrets, New Life participants and teachers alike often seemed to accept and perpetuate what Cheng and Qin describe as "a racialized concept about 'who we are' [that] especially helps Han people to find a common belonging in order to overcome discrepancies generated by economic, political, regional, provincial, and ethnic distinctions" (2019, 21). The Han-centrism at New Life was arguably vastly distinct from the kinds of *Huanghan* discourses that overlap with extreme nationalism in China, which "conveys a meaning of a racially and socially superior group" (Cheng 2019, 273; see also Friend and Thayer 2017). The kind of Han-centricity that prevailed at New Life, rather, often unwittingly placed ethnic minorities—whose art, clothing, and spiritual practices were often admired, adorned, and embraced at the center—in what Michel-Rolph Trouillot famously called "the savage slot" (2003, 7). At the same time, it often seemd to enact a consumptive desire for the Other that bell hooks observes as enacting an intimate form of "power-over" (1992, 367). Further centering Trouillot's observation (in a different treatise) that "history is to a collectivity as remembrance is to an individual" (1995, 14), my primary inquiry thus engages with the ways in which the imagination of past, present, and future forms of "Chineseness" were imagined as both uniform and *shared* at New Life.

As noted above, given the ethnic homogeneity of the clientele at the center and the nearly forty years in which China was largely closed to the outside world, it is true that much of the *past* here *was* at least broadly shared. While it often engaged with public secrecy in ways that challenged dominant narratives—for example, the (false) notion that "everyone was a victim" during the Cultural Revolution (Rofel 2007; Hillenbrand 2020)—it also sometimes seemed to reproduce a range of hegemonic ideologies even as it unsettled them. As is the case in China more broadly, for example, there was no discussion about the ways in which the violence of the past was itself rooted in a narrative of racialized Han supremacy that long preceded the rise of the Chinese communist Party (CCP) (Friend and Thayer 2017, 93; Cheng 2019). The ways in which the shared *present* was imagined, moreover, likewise oriented specifically to a range of sociopolitical, economic, and moral discourses, structures, and tensions and that prevailed in Han, urban, middle-class Chinese society. As noted above, in the sense that many of these discourses and tensions were also formulated as forms of *injustice* (不公平 *bu gongping*), learning to love at New Life also consisted of a collaborative interrogation of many past and present and public "secrets." To this end, the process of learning to love, for most participants, also involved an acute awareness of the ways in which their ability to enact love was severely constrained by economic and political forces beyond their control (Kuan 2015; L. Zhang 2017, 2020). There seemed, however, to be only a surface awareness of the ways in which the increasing wealth gap in society separated them from the migrant workers who they passed by daily on their way to work, or who served our meals and provided our nightly foot massages at the hotel. No one (at least at New Life) at the time, arguably, could predict what was in motion in terms of the massively scaled up surveillance, detainment, displacement, and torture of Uyghur and Kazakh citizens in Xinjiang Province (Byler 2018, 2021a-b, 2022; Grose 2019; S. Roberts 2020), and a few participants also admitted, at least privately, that they were also disoriented and confused by the increasingly violent forms of ethnic nationalism in China. There was nevertheless rarely any kind of either explicit or implicit questioning about whether or how the "Chineseness" that was often scrutinized itself constituted an exclusionary discourse that reproduced both class and ethnic disparities.

In returning to the question, as noted above, of where (and to whom) the "love" in learning to love ultimately "travels out," I thus maintain a certain skepticism, throughout the following chapters, with regard to the ways in which learning to love may or may not have contributed to participants' ability to envision a more broadly inclusive form of justice in China. In distinguishing political subjectivity from social action, however, I turn back to liberation psychology's emphasis on how "decoding the implicit realities of one's world [and becoming] aware of oppressive mechanisms" constitutes a relational, cognitive, and affective process that "opens up the horizon for new possibilities for action" (Martín-Baró 1994, 40, as cited in Gaztambide 2019, xxxi). Given that I did not conduct a longitudinal study that followed individuals over time, I strive to maintain an analytic openness with regard to the possible ways in which learning to love *might*, under some circumstances, constitute the kind of groundwork or first step in contributing to the process of becoming aware, but also *becoming vulnerable* in the context of dialogues across difference that do—as I discuss in the conclusion—sometimes occur in China. In this sense, this book engages with the notion of justice in terms of what somatics practitioner and social activist Staci K. Haines describes as the "unbounded terrain" that exists "between known ways of interacting or coordinating" and a range of as-yet *unknown* possible alternatives (2019, 25; see also Fikes 2021a).

SITUATING THE RESEARCH

This book is informed by nearly twenty years of experience living, studying, and conducting research on psychology and healing in China. Beginning in 1995, for example, I began to track the emergence of the so-called psycho-boom among Chinese citizens struggling with relationships, mental health, and everyday social stress (see, e.g., Kleinman et al. 2011; H-Y. Huang 2014). After focusing on the clinical study of Chinese medicine and becoming a licensed practitioner myself, this was followed by a more focused ethnographic study on the diagnosis and treatment of mood disorders in several integrative departments of "Chinese medical psychology" (Pritzker 2003, 2007). Though I diverted my attention to focus on the translation of Chinese medicine for my dissertation and first book (Pritzker 2011, 2012, 2014), I continued to track the explosion of psychological services in China as many of my close friends became increasingly drawn to engage with the kinds of holistic, spiritual psychology examined in this book.

I formally returned to the topic in 2014 when I was funded by the Wenner-Gren Foundation to conduct the present study. Originally, the project included research at a large Chinese medical hospital where one prominent physician practiced a unique form of Chinese medical psychology (Pritzker and Liang 2018) as well as with an independent practitioner who saw patients at New Life. I had heard about the center from friends beginning as early as 2008, and became increasingly intrigued with the workshops, texts, and retreats that they offered. Between 2014 and 2016, I thus expanded the research to include observation at multiple New Life events, especially workshops, salons, and retreats focused on inner child and family constellation therapies. Over the course of the research, I also spent many whole days "hanging out" at New Life and conducted open-ended interviews with about twenty-five staff members, instructors, interns, and clinicians and over forty participants.

Upon initiating research beyond the clinic at New Life, I was immediately faced with a significant challenge, however. My training and previous research in linguistic anthropology, specifically, emphasized the importance of video recording naturally occurring interaction in order to track the emergence of meaning in interactants' gaze, prosody, gesture, pauses, overlapping speech, self-corrections, grammatical phrasing, and so on. This method, as Sabina Perrino and I have noted in our recent volume on research methods in linguistic anthropology, "allow[s] researchers to repeatedly return to the data in order to analyze nuanced layers of particular interactions that might not be captured in the moment" (Clemente 2013; Farnell and Graham 2015, as cited in Pritzker and Perrino 2022, 140). It also allows researchers to generate detailed transcriptions that take care to mark a range of nuances and discourse features such as pauses, interjections, and overlapping speech, gesture, gaze, and so on (see, e.g., Ochs 1979; Jefferson 2004; Bucholtz 2007; Shohet and Loyd 2022).

In our chapter on participant observation, however, Perrino and I also underscore the importance of not relying on video recordings. This ethic proved vital when I arrived at New Life to conduct this research and was told that I would be welcome but would not be allowed to record any group interaction at the center. Indeed, "This unexpected shift forced [me] into more of a mixed-methods approach than originally planned" (Pritzker and Perrino 2022, 148). Methodologically, the research was different from any kind of fieldwork I had ever done because I couldn't record. But it was also unique because it required me to participate alongside New Lifers in the often emotionally intense exercises that we would do in the workshops. I was expected to follow the exercises myself, to draw, for example, my childhood home, to dance wildly in the darkness while allowing myself to feel any anger or resentment or nostalgia for what I may have felt was missing in my childhood, to pretend to be a mother re-birthing another woman, who I then held and looked upon while she cried. Even without the benefit of video, it also motivated me to reconsider the ways in which my training in linguistic anthropology served as a "lens" for observing interaction as well as recording it in my fieldnotes. The inability to video record ended up providing a kind of freedom, however, as I was able to fully immerse myself in the workshops without the encumbrance of unwieldy cameras and equipment. Perhaps most relevant to the current analysis, the inability to video record, finally, allowed me to pay more attention to the kinds of unspoken exchanges that I examine throughout this text. As a result of this methodological shift, however, it is important to note that all interactions described in the following chapters are based on fieldnotes and, in some cases, brief, consented audio-recordings that were destroyed after being anonymized. All data from interviews is extracted from audio recordings with consented participants, and all data is anonymized via the use of pseudonyms and slight changes in identifying details.

Learning to Love, importantly, engages primarily with the stories of women at New Life. As mentioned above, this bias accurately reflects the population at the center, where far more women than men were present at events. It also reflects the ways in which my own embodied identity as a thirty-something-year-old, white, cis-gendered and het-presenting woman afforded far more intimacy with the women of New Life. The book, finally, focuses on a very specific period (2008–18) in China, with most of the research focusing on events and encounters occurring between 2014 and 2016. Though China has always been a context in which studying social justice (or social action) requires researchers to attend to the unspoken or unsaid, or both, it is nevertheless important to center the ways in which the time period covered in the following chapters represents a time of relative opening. In contrast, restrictions on what is permissible to say or write in China have exponentially increased, especially since the outset of the COVID-19 pandemic in 2020. This shift is addressed more explicitly in my final conclusion, which nevertheless argues that the kinds of scalar inquiries that I examine throughout this book are still worth considering, even if they fall far short of inciting a revolution.

OVERVIEW OF CHAPTERS

This book begins, in chapter 1, with an investigation of the ways in which newcomers to New Life described their suffering. Though their stories differ in detail, newcomers frequently engaged in a tentative narrative mode that

also to *entangle differently* with one another as well as numerous culturally salient ideologies.

Chapter 3 offers a complementary discussion of the affective, embodied, and moral geography of New Life as it took shape during events, for example, in the space-time between opening and closing circles. Emphasizing the ways in which, as Marjorie Goodwin and Asta Cekaite write, within interaction "the body becomes a field of experience" (Goodwin and Cekaite 2018, 14), the discussion here investigates the embodied rhythm of interactions and movements as participants *attuned* to one another in a variety of exercises that *distributed* the bodies of individual participants across the bodies of others in the space. Demonstrating how multichanneled embodied displays of (inter)subjectivity involving silence, gaze, language, and *touch* (Goodwin and Cekaite 2018) contributed to the development and maintenance of a "mysterious atmosphere" at New Life, I further examine the ways in which the kinds of intense, affective, discursive, and embodied encounters at New Life invited participants to begin to rescale themselves in relation to intimate others in their lives as well as to fundamental concepts such as "the self" and "love." The chapter thus engages with the ways in which embodied encounters at New Life at least sometimes had the capacity to challenge and contest participants' deeply entrenched ways of experiencing the self, others, and the world more broadly. Focusing on the emergence of an extended body-self in mirroring, enactment, movement, and "time travel" exercises, I go as far as to suggest that this relational process often invited participants' to interrogate, if not reformulate, a number of culturally salient ideologies, including the very notion of the "Great Self," or *dawo* (大我) in China, though only within certain bounds.

In chapter 4, I foreground the ways in which participants at the center, along with instructors, engaged in a collaborative mapping of history, memory, and *Chineseness*. Throughout the chapter, I thus adopt an ethnographic perspective that embraces such everyday dialogue as a key form of *theory-building* (Rosa 2019) through which participants, as "amateur historians with various degrees of awareness about [their] production," in Trouillot's terms (1995, 20), interrogated at least a *shared* history both in interaction and narrative. Emphasizing the ways in which such conversations emerged as a kind of *dreaming* (Loizidou 2016) or "anticipatory mode" (Sumartojo and Pink 2019), I show how interlocutors drew variably upon both historically available ideologies as well as specific components of previous talk in order to interrogate "Chinese culture" in intimate ways that link shared histories to personal experiences in the present and desires for the future. The presumed "sharedness" of such histories, I argue, afforded a broad form of cultural affinity within which implicit messages could be intuitively "translated" across bodies. Contributing to the shaping of the atmosphere at New Life as what I call a "Hantopia," I also nevertheless foreground ways in which learning to love at New Life constituted a kind of collaboratively enacted form of *political subjectivity*.

Chapter 5 focuses on family constellation therapy (*jiapai*), which is often publicly framed as a practice that corresponds to the state-mandated discourse on maintaining a harmonious family. This chapter proposes, however, that in addition to this correspondence with hegemonic state narratives—or perhaps *because* of this overlap—*jiapai* is also immensely successful in China because it offers participants an opportunity to "wrangle with ghosts" in an intimate, embodied relational as well as anticipatory register that requires very little explicit communication. Constellations, within which participants enacted the living and deceased ancestors of a focal participant who sat observing the interaction, here took shape as complex conversations in which *epistemic authority* was granted to our ghosts and ancestors, who then replied to us through other participants' bodies. Positing that constellations emerged as old family photographs coming to life in a space-time that felt "out of time," the chapter thus engages with the "agency of images" to affect and *move* participants toward broader considerations of history, culture, and in/justice. Continuing my discussion of the ways in which the center constituted a "Hantopia" in which histories were imagined and experienced as shared, the chapter then examines how constellations often indexically pointed to events and historical trajectories beyond the familial past of particular participants. Suggesting how even indirect or "small acts of speech" sometimes offer a "vital relief" to the burden of silence in China (Hillenbrand 2020, 223), the chapter, finally, examines how group conversations about *jiapai* often subtly challenging dominant forms of "historical forgetting" (Rofel 2007) that prevail in China. Indeed, learning to love here frequently involved a collaborative interrogation of "what really happened" in the past. I conclude with a discussion of the ways in which collaborative wrangling here offered participants a revelatory experience of engaging with the so-called "elephant in the room" (Hillenbrand 2020, xx) as a form of collective scalar inquiry.

Chapter 6 examines the ways in which experiences of what I call *embodied defrosting* contributed to multistage embodied, affective, relational process of transformation described by multiple people who I met at New Life. Whether occurring over time or instantaneously, participants often described a kind of *melting* of that which had previously been or remained "frozen" in their bodies. Such experiences furthermore often afforded movement out of what was variably described as a physical and social "frozenness." As I discuss throughout the chapter, however, these experiences also often guided particular participants to become more aware or *attuned* to the fact that their suffering is indeed both their "own" in a personal sense and something more "collective." Emphasizing the ways in which participants described embodied defrosting as a more or less "spontaneous" or "mysterious" experience of self-driven "political education" (Haines 2019), I focus on how embodied defrosting, as a form of *embodied political subjectivity* in which participants questioned the past in an anticipatory mode that looked forward to the possible future, was often situated as the "spark" or "opening" that afforded explicit, ongoing forms of moral interrogation or scalar inquiry.

Chapter 7, finally, draws upon the notion of "tinkering" to engage with the gradual, situated process of attempting (and sometimes succeeding) to shift long-standing patriarchal relational patterns, within both generational and gendered relationships, at New Life. As a continuous dialogic process of interrogating and experimenting with particular relationships and cultural ideologies of both intergenerational and gendered hierarchy, I show how the process of what Santos and Harell (2017) frame as "transforming the patriarchy" in China was a project that involved a near-constant form of scalar inquiry within which participants, including both men and women, experimented with repositioning themselves vis-à-vis dominant cultural chronotopes. In a detailed examination of the ways in which particular participants variably proposed or enacted reformulated understandings of lineage, temporality, and authoritative classical texts, I entertain the notion that co-constructed interaction at New Life at least sometimes pointed to scalar inquiry as an *alchemical* process that consisted not only of personal transformation but, rather, pointed to the transformation of entrenched forms of scalar intimacy that contributed to perpetuating relational patriarchy in dominant/Han Chinese society.

I conclude with a brief review of the main perspectives offered in the book. This summary is complemented by remote research that I have been conducting in various online public spaces in China since 2020. I offer insight, here, into the enactment of scalar intimacy and scalar inquiry on the public Weibo page of Li Wenliang, a physician in Wuhan who was sanctioned for sending warnings of a potential new virus to friends and colleagues in late 2019, and later died of COVID-19 in February 2020. I further center a nearly-eleven-hour interaction involving upward of 4,000 Uyghur, Kazakh, and Han Chinese citizens, among others, that spontaneously emerged on Clubhouse, a social media app. Examining how the conversation took shape in and as an intimate participation framework in which Uyghur and Kazakh participants were positioned as "speakers," I discuss how Han participants thus became "hearers" or "recipients." As an encounter across difference that referenced many of the same "ghosts" and more-or-less-public "secrets" invoked at New Life, I further propose that it also afforded a spontaneous form of *extimacy* that "allow[ed] conceptual space for the outside to affect and move one's inner world in intimate ways" (Fikes 2021a, n.p.; see also Lacan 1959–60; Pavón-Cuéllar 2014). I further discuss how this encounter—as a *rupture* in the everyday discursive enactment of scalar intimacy—encouraged a collaborative process of scalar inquiry that situated both Han and non-Han participants in the same spatiotemporal "zone" without collapsing difference. While this research did not document the long-term "outcomes," the Clubhouse conversation nevertheless suggests at least the possibility that the kinds of embodied political subjectivity that were collaboratively constructed at New Life might, under some circumstances for at least some participants, afford the kinds of alliances across difference that perhaps, far down the line, make possible more collective forms of social action. This directs me to at least preliminarily conclude with an intimate, anticipatory, and scalar form of inquiry that engages with the ways in which *learning to love*, while not "social action" per se, might serve as the embodied foundation for broader forms of collaboration and social transformation in the future.

1

Suffering/Desire

I think desire isn't lack, it's surplus energy—a claustrophobia inside your skin.
—CHRIS KRAUSS

I met Ken, a quiet man in his forties, at a 2016 weekend salon on family constellation therapy (家庭系统排列 *jiating xitong pailie* or simply "*jiapai*"as I refer to it throughout this book). When I met up with him at a downtown coffee shop for an interview about a week later, he told me that he was relatively new to the practice, having only experienced one other weekend workshop at another site. He had tried various other groups, including a program for "life coaching" and an accountability program for aspiring leaders. He was still searching, however, for something that might help him overcome what he described as a persistent feeling of ambivalence about his career. Having pursued master's in business administration after college, he had started working at an international technology firm immediately after graduating. He had quickly progressed within the company and was soon earning a comfortable income, he explained, but the work had never felt fulfilling. It did not, for example, seem important or even "real" most of the time.

As we spoke, the ambivalence Ken described felt palpable. To be honest, it felt like he was even ambivalent about the interview itself, as if he was partly present and partly somewhere else. As I became aware of this, I noticed my own ethnographic desire to pull him into a dialogue, as well as my fear that the rest of our conversation would be tense and difficult. I asked to hear more about his feelings about specific aspects of his career that were troubling. He shrugged in response, mumbling something about how

/ 31 /

he had begun to think that he might have been better suited to an academic career. He might have had more time to reflect upon society if that were the case, he said, rather than being forced to participate in it.

When I asked for more specifics, however, Ken changed the subject. As if he had just remembered, he told me he had also come to New Life because he was struggling with relationship issues.

"Like what?," I asked.

Rather than offering a description of his personal experience, Ken began talking about his friends and colleagues who he had witnessed getting married and starting their own families or "homes" (家 *jia*). He described how he often observed them with a sense of curiosity as they worked tirelessly to maintain their marriages, to nurture their growing families, and to achieve success at work.

"I guess I kind of want to have a home," he said, "but I don't know—maybe I just don't want the responsibility." Ken went on to explain that it was not so much that he was overly picky or even particularly resistant to the idea of marriage.

"Every time I begin to get close to settling down, I just push it away," he said, as if confessing. He then admitted that he was currently entangled in not just one but two long-term, intimate relationships with women, unknown to one another, who were both pressuring him to marry.

"I don't know, though," Ken said, telling me that he was having trouble making the choice between one woman or the other. "I like one for certain reasons, and the other for other reasons," he said, shrugging his shoulders. He then mused that perhaps he just liked having multiple relationships. "Or perhaps I just like being alone," he finally said, his eyes drifting off to somewhere in the middle distance.

Still trying to engage him, I asked if he felt mature.

"I think I'm very immature, actually—in my heart, I'm very young." There was a long pause. "But I would like to grow up," he said, finally.

"Has *any* of the self-development stuff been helpful?," I asked.

"Not that much. It hasn't solved any of my problems," he responded, pausing again for what felt like a long time. When he finally spoke, he admitted that he *had* begun to understand his emotions a bit better. He had begun to understand, for example, that a lot of his problems related to the environment in which he grew up. I asked him if he could say more. This is when he told me that the instructor in his first *jiapai* group had suggested that his problems seemed directly related to what his parents experienced during his youth in the 1970s, for example, during the Cultural Revolution.

"Maybe it's because my mother endured a lot of criticism and denunciation (批斗 pidou) during that time," he said. "Because of that, I've become numb (麻木 mamu). I just can't find the feelings." He went on to tell me that the teacher had suggested that he find videos from the Cultural Revolution to watch to better understand and process his numbness.

"But I haven't looked for any yet," he concluded.

THE TENTATIVENESS OF DESIRE

As we spoke, I couldn't help but note how Ken positioned himself in relation to multiple moral and socio-spatial norms that prevailed in urban, Han Chinese society at the time, including "home" (家 jia), "maturity" (成长 chengzhang), and "success" (成功 chenggong), to name just a few. He repeatedly placed himself at a distance from these ideals, however, positioning himself as alienated from a sense of purpose in either his work or his personal relationships.

In relation to his friends and colleagues, Ken likewise situated himself as an outside observer who had watched them curiously as, one by one, they married and established homes. In what may have been his only certain statement throughout our entire conversation, he also situated himself far from a recognized state of maturity. Describing how, in his *heart*, he was both "very immature" and "very young," Ken offered a description centered in an embodied, chronotopic formulation of his inner self. Specifically, within the space of his heart, he felt like he was "off-time" with his desired state of development, and thus his place in the world.

Most of Ken's other descriptions, notably, included qualifiers like "maybe/possibly" (可能 keneng), "I don't know" (不知道 bu zhidao), and "kind of/a little bit" (有一点 you di dian). As he spoke, in fact, Ken seemed to discursively enact the very ambivalence that he described as the problem. Telling me that he guessed that he "kind of" wanted to have a home/family, for example, he went on to describe his lack of certainty about settling down with either of his two girlfriends. Casting his ambivalence as a long-term pattern of "pushing people away," he also seemed to be conducting an ongoing, spatiotemporally situated investigation of why he did this, and where he had developed this tendency.

Although not particularly optimistic, Ken nevertheless seemed to narratively enact a spatiotemporally situated *desire* that oriented toward an investigation of both the cause(s) of or reasons for his suffering and multiple possible "solutions." He proposed, for example, that *maybe* he just did not want the responsibility of maintaining a relationship or home, or both. He also tentatively formulated alternative possible futures in which he might settle in some other-than-standard way, such as by remaining alone or embracing a more explicit form of polyamory (e.g., having multiple intimate relationships at once). Here, however—both in relation to my specific questions and his previous experience in a *jiapai* (family constellation therapy) workshop—he also contemplated the ways in which his persistent sense of "numbness" and inability "to find the feelings" might relate to a past that was simultaneously personal and more broadly collective. Ken questioned, for example, how the kinds of "criticism and denunciation" (批斗 *pidou*) that his mother had been subjected to during the Cultural Revolution had (perhaps) given rise to his enduring sense of numbness. The details were still unclear, however. And although he articulated his desire to "grow up," he had not yet made the effort to try to unearth the kinds of videos that the instructor had told him might provide clues.

Though the intensity of his ambivalence was unique, Ken's inquiries here demonstrate how the process of "telling suffering" among newcomers to the center often took shape in open-ended, tentative narratives within which they concurrently examined multiple, often-conflicting explanations and possible solutions to what they framed as "the problem" and its possible solutions (Good and Good 1994; Shohet 2017; Samuels 2018). Often described as a complex "knot" that needed to be untied or a puzzle that needed to be solved, the exact problem was nevertheless often unclear. Though sometimes associated with a particular incident or relational rupture, their narratives, like Ken's, depicted a feeling of being "distant" or "off-time" in relation to their previous lives or with the people and broader social structures they occupied. Indeed, it often seemed like they were "stuck" in what I have called a "chronotopal dilemma" within which they struggled to make sense of themselves in both space and time, as well as in relation to others (Pritzker 2018; Pritzker and Duncan 2019). As described in the introduction, the lived experience of spatiotemporal disjuncture is commonly observed to be one of the most widespread forms of suffering facing Chinese citizens from all class backgrounds in the twenty-first century.

As I discuss throughout this chapter, the kind of suffering that brought people to the center suggested an ongoing, embodied, relational, and moral as well as spatiotemporal sense of not quite feeling "at-home-in-the-world" (Jackson 1995). Newcomers' narratives also often took shape, as Ken's did, as *investigations* into "what it takes to live well" and what it might feel like "to know what *home* means" (Akomolafe 2017, 26; emphasis added). Shaped by the kind of *desire* that Chris Krauss frames as "a claustrophobia inside your skin" (2016, 223), newcomers' investigations also variably invoked a sense of *hope* for possible resolution. Though readers familiar with Krauss know she is unambiguously referring to sexual desire, her inversion of the Lacanian understanding of desire as *lack* by reframing it as a simultaneously spatial and temporal *relief of pressure* is apt. Underscoring the ways in which suffering is often an "active, forceful presence" (Parish 2008, 127), even ambivalent newcomers like Ken thus demonstrated a desire to examine the present in relation to the past in the formulation of possible futures in which they might become able to find or reestablish their *place* in the world.

Telling Suffering

Telling suffering among New Life participants—in private conversations with me as well as in more public settings at workshops and events—points to the situated process that Sabina Perrino and I refer to as *scalar intimacy*. The concept of scalar intimacy builds on the observations of linguistic anthropologists who have noted the ways in which people, in any social setting, continuously engage in "scaling projects" that "anchor and (re) orient" them in the world (Carr and Lempert 2016, 3). The *scaling* involved in scalar intimacy thus attends to the scalar distinctions that people make, for example, "between relatively and relationally emergent realms of experience like size (e.g., big-small), time (e.g., past-present-future), place (e.g., town-city-global society), and socially or politically meaningful categories (e.g., private-public)" (Pritzker and Perrino 2020, 366). Often enacted through the deployment of proximal and distal pronouns (e.g., *here* and *there*), the deployment of identifiable rhetorical structures (e.g., parallelism, hyperbole), or shifts in prosodic intonation (e.g., rhythm, speed, voice quality), scalar intimacy is also observable in the body movements, gaze shifts, gestures, and facial expressions that people deploy in order to discursively position themselves within, alongside, or apart from people, ideologies, or concepts with varying degrees of cultural salience. Tracking scalar intimacy in interaction, Perrino and I further argue, demands an attention toward the ongoing embodied, discursive, affective, and relational process through which people situate themselves as cultural beings in space and time. Highlighting the ways in which *cultural chronotopes*—recognized ways of narrat-

liberally deployed what Good and Good (1994) call "tactics of subjunctivity" to pose numerous possible interpretations for their suffering as well as the ways in which it might be addressed or even "solved" (see also Shohet 2017; Samuels 2018). Often framed an experience of having lost—or never successfully having found—their "home," I examine how newcomers also described a sense of feeling "off-time" with their previous lives or with the people and broader society around them. I also center the ways in which their narratives were frequently driven by a powerful form of *desire* that moved people to interrogate the situation (e.g., *what* had happened, *when* it had happened, and *who* was to blame, and how to "fix" it). Centering the dialogic, relational context as an affordance for engaging with uncertainty, the chapter thus demonstrates the nuanced ways in which newcomers enacted scalar intimacy as a continual process of a highly circumscribed form of scalar inquiry that variably interrogated a range of hegemonic cultural ideologies yet also often generated *more* rather than less uncertainty. While Li Zhang (2020, 130) highlights the remaking of the self in sites where the inner revolution takes place, this chapter thus draws attention to the far less ambitious goal of simply making sense of suffering. For newcomers, the narrative process of formulating a new self, I show, was often more like an experimental scaling project that had the *potential* to generate new meanings, new self-interpretations, and even new selves.

Drawing on Shanti Sumartojo and Sarah Pink's discussion of the indeterminacy of "atmosphere" (2019), chapter 2 focuses on how the intimate geography of New Life emerged as an aesthetic "mode of experience" (Taylor 1989, 374). My analysis includes a description of the ways in which objects, lighting, and specific interactions all functioned in tandem to map the center, especially in "opening" and "closing" rituals, as a space and time that was both distant and distinct from the outside or "default world." Pronouns and deictic forms such as "this place" or "in here," for example, once uttered and heard, contributed to the constitution of the immediate spatiotemporal context of New Life vis-à-vis what I identify as "home" and "horizon" chronotopes. Together, I show, the home and horizon chronotopes generated a rich moral, affective, and embodied relational geography that simultaneously invoked dominant ideas of homefulness at the same time as instigating participants' desires for a relationally situated form of "collective development" that interrogated dominant chronotopes of home, relationality, and possibility. This chapter thus examines how learning to love at New Life invited participants not only to "disentangle" (L. Zhang 2020) but

ing space and time as well as moral personhood (Agha 2007)—constitute intimate *orienting devices* in the world (Ahmed 2007), scalar intimacy thus attends to how such chronotopes become entrenched *within* and *as* the body, including affective, cognitive, and sensory "states" (Seligman 2018).

In examining the enactment of scalar intimacy within situated narratives, it thus becomes essential to attend closely to the ways in which people "'zoom in' and 'pan out' of both time and space" (Pritzker and Perrino 2020, 367). Scalar intimacy likewise demands a close investigation of the *chronotopes* that speakers draw upon to narratively configure themselves, though not necessarily using words, in relation to variably scaled spatial and temporal trajectories. As described in the introduction, chronotopes are constantly invoked in interactions between speakers orienting toward, within, or away from recognized places and times such as "home," "school," or "work," for example, all of which are also, importantly, *moral spaces* where belonging is often mediated by expectations of "good" behavior. Cultural chronotopes here contribute to the collaborative imagining of the kinds of moral and relational emotions and behaviors considered "normal" or "appropriate" within such spaces (Agha 2007, 324–25; see also Leander 2004; Lempert and Perrino 2007; Perrino 2007; Wirtz 2016; Divita 2019; Karimzad 2020; Karimzad and Catedral 2018, 2021; Pritzker and Hu 2022; Pritzker 2023).

Scalar intimacy further constitutes one of the primary ways that people experience and enact their *political subjectivity* as "a relationally co-emergent understanding of one's affective-relational body-self in relation to real or imagined social, spatial, or temporal trajectories" (Pritzker 2023, 2). Scalar intimacy therefore also centers embodied intimacy or felt experience articulated or indexed by a speaker, underscoring how particular chronotopes feel or what biocultural anthropologist Rebecca Seligman describes as "the sensory-motor or experiential state associated with a concept" (2018, 401). Specifically attending to the ways in which other people as well as moral norms and cultural ideals serve as phenomenological *orienting devices* that precede interactions (Ahmed 2007), Perrino and I have thus noted that speakers often relate to cultural ideas and ideologies as if they comprise or are located *inside* of their own bodies (Pritzker and Perrino 2020, 368). As such, scalar intimacy must be understood as a deeply intimate and embodied sense of orientation or positioning vis-à-vis other people as well as social structures such that they derive a sense of *value* or a feeling of *belonging* (or do not). The close study of scalar intimacy in co-constructed narratives, I demonstrate here, offers a novel view into the instantaneous, felt linkages that inhere between scales of spatiotemporal, moral, and embodied experience.

Scalar inquiry, on the other hand, constitutes a related process that is far more experimental and thus often tentative and preliminary. Scalar inquiry, specifically, points to the chronotopic ways that people begin to become curious about cultural forms, practices, and ideologies that have otherwise been held in place through scalar intimacy throughout their lives. Underscoring how "morality is . . . *more* than simply reproducing social norms and conventions" (Shohet 2017, 557), scalar inquiry constitutes an inquisitive and agentive type of *reflection*. Reflection, according to anthropologist Xiang Biao, is necessary in order for one to shift the *direction* one takes in life: "The meaning of reflection is that I want to stop myself, hold myself back, and not keep moving forward in the same direction" (Xiang and Wu 2022, 231–32). Scalar inquiry can likewise be considered a form of "defrosting," to borrow Hannah Arendt's term, wherein one becomes willing to interrogate or "unfreeze" culturally dominant ways of knowing (1971, 433–34; see also Mattingly 2019). Scalar inquiry, finally, further constitutes a relationally situated "ethics of trying" (Kuan 2015) in which people try to make at least tentative sense of themselves as moral, relational beings in time and space (Taylor 1989; Bruner 2002; Capps and Ochs 1995; Ochs 2004; Mattingly 2014).

The following sections thus foreground the often-sublte and implicit ways in which people at New Life scaled themselves in relation to a range of dominant cultural chronotopes, including filiality, motherhood, marriage, and education, among others. Speaking from a place of simultaneous suffering and desire, participants often attempted to make sense of *what* had happened, *when* it had happened, *who* was to blame, and how to "fix it." As Ken did so, for example, he scaled himself in relation to numerous established and entrenched cultural chronotopes, including chronotopes related to family, home-place, and gender. Such configurations served, here, as touchpoints or guardrails of sorts, as participants made efforts to regain a sense of being "on-time" with their lives and the world around them. This kind of scalar inquiry, importantly, does not always or even often generate stable or definitive answers. In this sense, instances of scalar inquiry present as distinct from the uptake of discourses that offer easy answers, often embracing rigid divisions between self and other or contrasting the disordered present with a romanticized (and often fictional) past, or both (Carrico 2017; Bloom and Moskalenko 2021). Within the Han clothing movement, for example, traditional Han clothing frequently functions as a potent index pointing to multiple discourses, including narratives of imagined "racial purity" and historical glory. Accordingly, Han clothing is likewise engaged as a form of resistance against the imagined hegemony of barbarian leaders, especially the Manchu, who are—in one prominent conspiracy theory—intent on destroying the Han (Carrico 2017, 140).

The kind of scalar inquiry I discuss in this chapter, rather, often moves rapidly back and forth between self and world in search of explanations, causes, and possible solutions. In Ken's case, however, such investigations seemed to further entrench the embodied, affective feelings of "distance" from ideals that he oriented to as normative for others. Indeed, as I discuss throughout this chapter, newcomers often initiated scalar inquiry within the "relatively circumscribed frame[s] of reference" described by Heelas (2008, 121). Circumscription here contributes to a frequent sense of going endlessly in circles wherein the imagination of possible solutions often contributed to furthering the experience of distance and isolation.

Telling-in-Relation

The relational context in which stories are told matters deeply, as Perrino and I note (2020). People thus enact scalar intimacy in slightly different ways, depending on the setting and interlocutors, both present and remembered or invoked. In circumstances where one party is confused or uncertain about fundamental life trajectory issues, for example, interaction sometimes acts as a *constraint* upon engaging in anything but the most superficial scalar inquiry. In many conversations, it is important to remember here, speakers are refused the opportunity to engage productively with uncertainty, with the unknown, or with possible futures that drastically differ from the present. Speakers may not be taken seriously, for example, or they may feel or be judged or even excluded outright. In such cases, people often experience an affective, moral, and relational feeling of *disavowal* (Butler, Gambetti, and Sabsay 2016b). Here, it is not just their inclination to question that is dismissed, but also their basic value as a vulnerable person engaged in a mutually affecting relationship with both specific interlocutors and the world more broadly.

Conversations characterized by the kind of intimacy that Samuels (2018) characterizes as "being-with," on the other hand, afford the ability for speakers to engage within a broader expanse of interrogation. "More than a mostly retrospective effort to make sense of experience, narratives effect a present 'being-with' others and thereby actively make and remake the world," writes Samuels (2018, 98). Interaction, as a form of "co-operative action" (C. Goodwin 2018) involving the bodies of speakers and a variably shared present and historical contexts and systems of power (social, political, economic, and so forth), can thus also be framed as a kind of "peopled opportunity" within which one is "recognized as [a] good, accountable person by others" (Myers 2016, 430; see also Fisher 2014). One might go as far as to say that such moral inclusion is, indeed, a relational prerequisite for enacting scalar inquiry as a form of moral experimentation (Mattingly 2014, 1; see also Zigon 2008; Throop 2014).

Ethnographic interviews, while not necessarily intimate in a physical or even temporal sense, nevertheless often take shape within a space that is chronotopically and experientially removed from the everyday space-times within which interviewees operate. In this research, for example, they often afforded slightly more investigative latitude, especially for those presently navigating difficult decisions or facing challenging circumstances, than conversations with friends, family members, and colleagues. As I discuss in the latter part of the chapter, group interaction at New Life often provided a similar "container," so to speak, for an intimate, open-ended form of scalar inquiry. In both sections of the chapter, however, I underscore the ways in which the investigative latitude afforded by such encounters often generated *more* rather than less uncertainty. I nevertheless suggest that these interactions offer insight into a nuanced, relationally situated process that, over time, has been demonstrated to result in the reconfiguration of "a new self" (see, e.g., Duncan 2018; Matza 2018; Zhang 2020).

THE FEELING OF HOME

Before proceeding to introduce specific New Life participants and their narratives, it is worthwhile to linger on what was perhaps the most common and ubiquitous—as well as expansive—concept at the heart of newcomers' narratives of suffering and desire: the notion and ideal of "home" or *jia* (家). As a normative moral mode of being in the world to which people orient within particular interactions (Agha 2007; Karimzad 2020), the notion and ideal of home here arguably constitutes a specific cultural chronotope, or way of narrating space and time with often conflicting affective, visceral, and relational as well as moral meanings. For Ken and nearly every other participant who I engaged with as part of this research, moreover, home chronotopes functioned as a central narrative touchpoint simultaneously indexing both loss and desire.

This section, accordingly, offers a brief overview of the texture, meaning, and influence of the home chronotope in China, which often instantaneously scales from the most intimate, personal spheres to the most broadly social or national. First, it is critical to recognize that home in China, instead of existing as a single concept, place, or ideological configuration, points also to intimate experiences of the self *in* and *in relation to* space, time, and other persons. On one hand, then, it points to the deeply affective and relational experience of "spatial kinship" (Joniak-Lüthi 2015, 72), embodied by the notion of *jiaxiang* (家乡) or what Joniak-Lüthi (2015) translates as "home-place." Alongside its association with intimate homeplaces, however, the home chronotope in China also points to broad, collective spaces as well as forms of governance (Xie 2021). The word for nation is, for example, *guojia* (国家 country-home). Relatedly, the notion of home likewise serves as one of the most central concepts in contemporary state-generated discourses of "Chinese values" (中国价值观 *zhongguo jiazhiguan*) (Wielander 2018a). Here, home is often framed in public service announcements, advertisements, and television programs as the ultimate fulfillment of "the China Dream" (中国梦 *zhongguo meng*). As the foundation and core of "harmonious society" (和谐社会 *hexie shehui*)—another state-promoted cultural chronotope that holds a great deal of influence in China (see, e.g., Carrico 2017; J. Yang 2018a; Lin 2017)—conversations that directly or indexically invoke the notion of home in China are thus always deeply entangled with the "emotionally charged ideological discourse" set forth by the state (Xie 2021, 211)

The spatiotemporal representation of home in early twenty-first-century China thus frequently situates a stable home as the very basis for a harmonious society at increasingly vast scales. At the same time, home is also frequently formulated as an idealized space of refuge *from* society. The notion of home as a protected space-time, full of nourishment and intimacy, further carries important moral connotations in early twenty-first-century popular and political discourse. "Homemaking," for example, is increasingly seen as the ethical imperative of *women*, particular, who are tasked with staving off social chaos through their enactment of "good family values" (家风 *jiafeng*) (Fincher 2021; Xie 2021). Here, what Xiao (2014, 20) describes as the "middle class dream of a 'private paradise'"—attainable only through home ownership—serves as an imaginary retreat from the pervasive sense of *dis*harmony that actually prevails in contemporary society. As several scholars have highlighted, however, such discourses often elide the fact that the chronotopic imaginary of "home as refuge" is itself driven by powerful market forces that work through moralistic forms of control. Jie Yang, for example, suggests how politics invades the home through the formulation of home as a place of feminine contentment within which middle-class "happy housewives" can achieve and maintain happiness simply by buying "the right things" (2018b, 135). In Yang's research with housewives, however, middle-class Chinese women are largely *not* happy with the "comforts" of domestic life (2018b, 135). The reality that home is not, indeed, a place of happy refuge for both women and men despite vigorous advertising campaigns is further highlighted by Huang (2020), who notes that images of the home in China are so often entangled with discourses of material wealth and consumption that they give rise to persistent, felt tensions between prevalent moral ideals regarding the "warmth" and "harmony" of home and the "cold" consumerism of public spaces.

The hegemonic moral idea and ideology of the home is thus an embodied moral orientation that commands power over cis-gendered, heterosexual men and women as well as queer Chinese citizens of all genders. For those who identify as male, for example, there is immense pressure to enact the hegemonic ideal of what Wong (2020) calls "the able-responsible man." This ideal man, as the name implies, is expected to embody a responsible, capable provider who dutifully enacts the role of "son/son-in-law, father, and husband" within their families/homes and beyond (2020, 84). Wong thus examines how able-responsible manhood, far from being an abstract set of ideas or standards, constitutes an embodied, affective, and relational ideal—held in place by both men and women—that encompasses everything from the mediated expression of emotion in interaction to reliable embodied performance and even sexual prowess (see also E. Zhang 2015). For women, on the other hand, heteronormative "homemaking" is increasingly seen as an ethical imperative held in place by a form of scalar intimacy linking women's enactment of "good family values" (家风 *jiafeng*) to the sociopolitical goal of staving off chaos through the collaborative enactment of a so-called harmonious society (J. Yang 2018a; Fincher 2021; Xie 2021). Meanwhile, the socioeconomic security of owning a home is a right largely reserved for men (Fincher 2021). Despite such increasingly stringent castings of appropriate gendered behavior within Chinese discourses of the home, John Wei likewise observes the centrality of the home chronotope in the desire and aspirations of queer Chinese citizens of all genders. The significance of peoples' ability to establish and maintain nourishing homes, in this case, is amplified by the sheer fortitude required to be able to preserve a queer home within the kinds of "compulsory heterosexuality and familism" that prevail in contemporary China (Wei 2020, 112).

In this environment—even for the many citizens who are aware of the kinds of "fakery" inherent within such discourses (see Wielander 2018)—having and maintaining a heteronormative "home" in terms of being married, having children, and caring for elderly parents constitutes a marker of *moral personhood*. A long-term participant named Sulin once drew upon a potent set of chronotopes linking the home to the self to describe the circumstances that originally pushed her, out of sheer desperation, to check out the psychospiritual self-development scene and what it had to offer. At the time, her husband had quite suddenly and unexpectedly filed for divorce, she explained. The effect was profound.

"I felt like I just didn't have a self anymore (没有我自己了 *meiyou wo ziji*)," Sulin said, pausing and reframing her sense of disorientation in the world, at the time, as a *question*: "Without a home (家 *jia*), who am I?"

Underscoring how what Michael Jackson (1995) frames as "being-at-home-in-the-world" constitutes a feeling of being situated in time and space, Sulin's loss of her home generated the kind of world-shattering "disorientation, discomfort and distress" that, as Renos Papadopoulos notes, often accompanies people's loss of their home (2018, 59). Indeed, losing her home affected Sulin to such an extent that she had begun to doubt her own value and her innate sense, as she put it, that she was "worthy of love" (指的爱 *zhide ai*). Sulin's experience further demonstrates how the home chronotope stretches to encompass a range of affective, visceral, and relational as well as moral meanings in China. This is especially true for women, who are frequently marked as "abnormal," "deviant," and even "pathological" if they do not remain married or never marry (Xie 2021, 108; see also Fincher 2016, 2021). Women who remain unmarried even as early as their late twenties are referred to as "leftover women," for example, a term that Fincher (2016) demonstrates as deeply tied to increasingly stringent forms of patriarchal dominance in twenty-first-century China. Under these circumstances, even the professionally powerful, feminist-leaning Sulin experienced a sense of disorientation and devaluation upon the breakup of her marriage. It should come as no surprise, then, that the phenomenological experience of being or *not* being at-home-in-the-world is deeply entangled, simultaneously, with the deepest aspects of the embodied, relational, and moral self as well as a vast array of politicized, gendered, and economic chronotopizations of home as a space, a time, and a way of being-in-relation in China.

No matter what the circumstances, New Life participants thus rarely spoke of their loss of home or their search for home in terms divorced from embodied, affective, and relational experience. Another striking example of this intimate link between the social, emotional, and embodied self relates to the ways in which New Life participants frequently spoke of the feeling and experience of home as if it existed simultaneously in the world and in their own bodies. As I discuss in detail in chapter 7, for example, an administrator at New Life named Gracie once remarked that, prior to coming to New Life, she never understood the meaning of home. Nor did she think that she would ever become capable of successfully enacting it, of "being home" for herself or others.

"I mean that home in your subconscious (潜意识的家 *qian yishi de jia*)," Gracie clarified, placing her hands on her chest, "that home in your inner heart (内心那个家 *neixin nage jia*)."

Invoking the home chronotope as an index of intimacy, warmth, nourishment, and care, this comment—and many others like it at the center—suggests the ways in which participants in this research engaged with the very notion of home as an intimate, embodied sense of place in the world. Invoking home also as a kind of capability or practice, this comment likewise underscores how being-at-home-in-the-world, Jackson notes, might best be considered a "mode of activity" (1995, 149) rather than a stable and enduring feeling. Home as a mode of being-in-the-world, Jackson highlights, often relates to a situated sense of *efficacy* or agency vis-à-vis other humans within particular structures and institutions. Home as a mode also points, others have noted, to experiences of feeling *open* and *expansive* in terms of one's ability to affect and be affected by the world (Rapport 2018, 17). Scholarship on home as a relationally situated practice, finally, calls the temporal boundaries of home/being-at-home into question. Papadopoulos (2018, 55) thus argues that the spatiality and temporality of home is fundamentally fluid and open-ended. Gracie's comment, however, underscores the ways in which the capacity to have such an experience in *any* setting is always embodied, not necessarily in the form of memories but also in the organic and functional makeup of one's muscles, tissues, and cells. As I demonstrate below, such embodied chronotopizations of home—whether in terms of past feelings of being-at-home-in-the-world that had been destabilized or whether in terms of the desire to find that feeling for the first time—were ubiquitous at New Life. This was especially true for newcomers, who frequently presented with the kinds of impossible "knots" described by Ken in the short vignette above.

SPACE INVASION

I met Ping, a thirty-three-year-old professional woman, at one of New Life's five-day inner child workshops, where we danced together, cried together, and chatted over a few meals. We never had the chance to talk privately, however, beyond her telling me that it was her first time ever doing anything like this. She was eager to talk more with me after the workshop. When we met at a bus stop near my apartment in the heart of the old city about a week later, however, we laughed at how strange it felt to be together in the world outside of New Life. After awkwardly navigating the crowded streets to my tiny apartment, we finally settled on the couch in my living room.

Ping's affect began to shift immediately. Her brows furrowed and her shoulders seemed to drop several inches as she set down her tea and reached for a box of tissues on the coffee table.

"May I?," she asked, and I nodded quickly in response.

Like many of the people I spoke with and witnessed at the beginning of their "journey" to becoming mature, Ping was in the midst of immense suffering that was both deeply confusing and difficult to explain. Indeed, throughout our interview it felt like Ping's bewilderment was in the room with us, constantly taking on new narrative shapes as we spoke.

Ping then launched into her story, beginning by explaining that she had always been someone who was "on the right track" in her life. Originally hailing from a nondescript, midsized city in a neighboring province, for example, she nonchalantly described how she had tested into a prominent, top-tier university. She had always been successful at school, and this continued throughout her college education as well as her graduate study. She had effortlessly found a well-paid, executive position in a prestigious international company, moreover, immediately upon completing her master's degree. Shortly after beginning work, finally, Ping met the man who would become her husband and the father of her young son. Everything in Ping's life had thus always proceeded successfully in the right direction. She had moved steadily toward the right goals and easefully through the potentially treacherous challenges of getting a respectable college degree, navigating an advanced degree program, finding a job, getting married, and giving birth.

Recently, however, she had been experiencing a persistent sense of feeling "off," out of balance with her life. It had begun about six years into her marriage, when the couple had decided to have a baby and thereby became an official "household" (家庭 *jiating*). Prior to that decision, Ping recounted, her relationship with her husband had been characterized by a great deal of fun, as if—in Ping's words—the two of them had been kids playing together. Over time, however, the couple had developed a stronger sense of responsibility. "But maybe we weren't really that ready," Ping reflected. "I still felt very young."

In suggesting the possibility that neither she nor her husband had been "ready" to become parents, Ping highlighted her felt experience of being young, playful, and carefree during the first years of their marriage. Positing a possible reason—or set of reasons—for the trouble that later emerged, Ping's expressed tentativeness here (e.g., "maybe we weren't really that ready"). This indicated to me that she might not yet have a well-formed story about what had happened or, rather, what *was* happening in her life. It also suggested, however, that despite lacking a coherent explanation, Ping's desire had motivated an active search for narrative resolution.

After a pause, I asked Ping if this feeling of being "off" had been what motivated her to come to the inner child workshop. In response, she elaborated on the temporal framework she had established thus far, posing a (rhetorical) question to me: "I came because after I went to college, I didn't live with my parents anymore, right?" The question was arguably a simple discursive effort to confirm my recall of her previous narrative. In reporting how long it had been since she had lived with her parents, however, Ping also introduced a complex chronotopic casting that situated both the previous and following narrative. In so doing, Ping emphasized the temporal and spatial as well as *relational* distance between the past, when she had lived with her parents, and the present, which consisted of over a decade living in a city far from her natal home. I nodded.

"And then now," she continued, "I've been in the city about fourteen years. Then last year, when I was pregnant, my mother came to take care of me, to help me cook and stuff. Then once I had my son, my father came. They helped me—together—to take care of the baby. Then there were a lot of problems that came up," Ping detailed.

Continuing to emphasize the distance between the past and present, Ping thus situated the "problems" that had begun to arise in her home as a simultaneously spatial, temporal, and relational tension that had taken shape once her parents had moved in with her and her young family. This, Ping stated in no uncertain terms, was when the "breach" (Myers 2016) occurred, the time when and where things had begun to go wrong. As such, Ping centered her narrative around a specific time-space, as occupied by specific characters, that demarcated the present from the past and which had seemingly changed everything. From the outset of her story, Ping thus scaled herself in relation to multiple physical spaces and times but also vis-à-vis multiple intimate others, including her husband, her parents, and her baby. As such, even just the beginning of Ping's story demonstrates how scalar intimacy is continually enacted as individuals *place* themselves in relation not just to other people but also to multiple dominant discourses in society, including education, maturity, and the very notions of "home" or "family."

Underscoring how suffering, in this case, emerged as a complex experience of disjuncture and disorientation as well as desire, Ping remained silent for an extended time here. In the novel context of our conversation, it seemed that she was taking a moment to "process," to let it sink in that these relationships and concepts, which had always seemed like anchors in her life, felt somehow *wrong* in the present. Noting this, I chose not to push for further explanation, at least not yet.

"Oh, is that so?," I asked.

"Yes, a lot of problems between my parents . . . and with my mother-in-law."

More silence.

"Like what?," I asked cautiously.

"It was—I know they were good to me," Ping said quickly, looking up at me as if to ensure that I was well aware that she appreciated her own and her husband's parents. Lack of gratitude—especially for one's own parents or in-laws—is, after all, a serious transgression in China, where filial piety mandates "unconditional respect and obedience of the junior generation to the senior generation" (Yan 2016, 219). It made perfect sense to me that Ping was taking care to make absolutely sure that I knew that she knew that she should be grateful, and that she was.

"But it was, like, *awkward*," she continued. "I just didn't want my parents to care for me (管我 *guan wo*)."

She went on, here, to elaborate on the tension that had arisen in her home once her parents moved in. "I just couldn't accept their help," she said. "For example, my mom might say to me, 'Oh, you are very exhausted, I'll help you. I'll watch the baby, you eat first.' And then after I would eat she would say 'you go rest, go rest, or take a shower.' In all kinds of ways she would give me orders (规定 *guiding*). 'Go do this, go do this, go do this.'"

Ping's voice began to grow progressively louder and more abrupt as she voiced her mother's orders. "Reported speech," writes Xochitl Marsilli-Vargas, "is very useful for the analysis of how alterity is brought to light. . . . It points to *how* listeners listen to each other's words" (2022, 97). The tension accumulating in Ping's voice here, accordingly, offers insight into how she was hearing her mother. Indeed, she switched to speak in her own voice, in the present tense here, emphatically articulating her own desires vis-à-vis her mother as well as the space of her home.

"I don't want her controlling me!," she said. "I want my own space! I just really can't accept it." Ping was silent for a moment before she spoke further, this time in a still-stern but slightly milder tone.

"And then my mother and father," she added, "some of the methods they use to educate my son (教育方法 *jiaoyu fangfa*)—I don't approve (赞同 *zantong*). It is just not very pleasant. I've begun not wanting to interact with them at all."

Underscoring the ways in which parental "education" in China continues throughout the life span, readers familiar with what it means to *guan* another person in China will not, perhaps, notice anything out of the ordinary in Ping's representation of her mother's care. After all, as Bregnbæk (2016, 4) notes, the word Ping uses for "care" (管 *guan*) is indeed a mix between "care and control." Paired with other words, moreover, *guan* references the idea of teaching (*guanjiao*), managing (*guanli*), or keeping under control (*guanzhu*). In explaining the concept of teaching, for example, Jing Xu (2017) thus describes how the term *guanjiao*, which might more aptly be translated as "care-mediated teaching," "integrates the meanings of both discipline and care" (2017, 5; see also Pritzker and Liang 2018). Ping's narrative therefore made immediate sense to me, especially in terms of the complex ways that being cared for or "managed" by her mother felt less like *care* and more like *control*. Alongside her assertion of appropriate feelings of gratitude and respect to her parents, Ping's story further felt like a confession of sorts, as if she had done something deeply wrong and was now trying to come clean.

Ping's additional, specific reference to her distaste for the methods that her parents had been using with her son, moreover, further points to the entangled ways in which care is entangled with "education" as a form of discipline as well as governance in China. Indeed, discourse about education constitutes a form of *cultural intimacy* (Herzfeld 2016) through which "education is both a metaphor for governing and a tool of governing" in China (Kipnis 2011, 7; see also Lin and Trevaskes 2019). Ping's disapproval, however, also indexes an intimate and ongoing challenge facing many young mothers (and some fathers) in early twenty-first-century China. There is a profound tension, here, between perceptions of traditional and contemporary modes of education. In twenty-first-century Chinese discourses of education, specifically, traditional modes and methods are formulated as autocratic and stern, fostering compliance without initiative. In contrast, modern or contemporary modes and methods of education emphasize a softer style that supports children's personal growth as well as their individuality, thus fostering the kind of "personality, initiative, and creative potential" considered necessary in the (possible) Chinese economic future (Kuan 2015, 6–7). Ping's frustration with her parents suggests just such a tension but does so in a way that demands recognition for the ways in which the tension, for Ping, is far more than a mere philosophical distinction or pedagogical preference. Nor does it make sense within a simplistic binary of tradition and modernity. Reflecting the kinds of ambivalence expressed by Chinese mothers struggling with a combination of gratitude and blame with regard to their parents' "help" with child-rearing (Mason 2020), the tension for Ping, rather, exists as a phenomenological series of encounters through which culturally salient chronotopes are embodied and enacted within the context of particular relationships and particular intimate spaces.

For Ping, I want to take care to stress, none of this came together in any kind of coherent narrative. It emerged more in alignment with the kind of open-ended narrative that is still *in the making* and is not (yet) coherent, but which nevertheless aspires to understanding (Ochs 2004). Ping's ongoing narrative project, rather, involved a continuous and constantly shifting investigation of the *why* behind the when, where, and who of the world-altering rupture that had occurred in her life. Ping's story at times therefore seemed to circle around an open-ended and inconclusive examination of her own role in creating the problems. Earlier in her narrative, she positioned herself as the possible culprit, for example, tentatively situating her and her husband's previous naiveté and ongoing immaturity as well as her own apparent inability to tolerate her mother's care as the underlying (possible) cause. Here, on the other hand, Ping's presentation of her mother's "orders" (规定 *guiding*) framed them as a serious, ongoing set of transgressions within the most intimate spaces of her home and her body-self. This latter framing positioned Ping, notably, more as a *victim* than a culprit.

Discussing the ways in which conflicts had begun to reverberate throughout the family in recent weeks, Ping continued by invoking what Mason (2020) calls the "mother-in-law script" in order to offer more insight into the extent of the problems in her home. The mother-in-law script, Mason explains, constitutes a culturally salient, "socially acceptable" narrative that allows—even expects—problems to emerge between women and their mothers-in-law in China.

"Normally in China," Ping thus said, "the relationship between a wife and her mother-in-law is strained." While the mother-in-law script is frequently considered as an affordance for women to deflect or avoid discussing any tensions they might have with their *own* mothers (2020, 17), Ping very quickly turned away from what she here situated as the norm in China.

"But my mother-in-law is good," she protested, speaking in the present tense, "she cares for me (关心我 *guanxin wo*)."

Ping then switched suddenly to speaking in the past tense. "I felt honestly like I was her daughter," she reminisced. "We would chat all the time and we would go for walks together." Thus taking care to scale her previous relationship with her mother-in-law as different from and immensely better than the norm in China, Ping then proceeded to describe the ways in which her mother-in-law had "changed" since the birth of the baby.

"Once my mother came," she said, "my mother-in-law maybe felt like our relationship wasn't as good, and she felt hurt. At the time—maybe her reaction was a bit—it wasn't good. Then once I had the baby, she also started to *guan* me. It was like suddenly it was her son's house—that feeling. But she didn't feel welcome, she thought we didn't want her and felt like she was wasting her time. Forget it (算了 *suanle*). She was tired. We were tired. The communication when she would come over was strained, not very smooth (不顺利 *bu shunli*). She felt like it wasn't her house anymore."

This portion of Ping's narrative arguably aligned more thoroughly with what might be expected from the mother-in-law script in China. It is worth noting, however, that Ping here took care to adopt a temporal, spatial, and relational investigation in which she exhibited a kind of curiosity as well as compassion with regard to her mother-in-law's reaction to her own mother's appearance in their home. This effected an important chronotopic as well as scalar shift, as Ping distanced herself and her family from the normal, expected Chinese family. Ping embraced, rather, a temporal frame in which any tension between her and *her* mother-in-law, in contrast to the norm, had emerged as a relationally situated process that could be traced back to the arrival of the baby and her own parents. The unfortunate result, however, was that it had repositioned her mother-in-law in the standard role of "oppressive mother-in-law" whose management and control, alongside that of her own parents, had seemed to exclude Ping from her own home. Ping thus experimented, again, with occupying the position of the "victim" of a complex assemblage of ongoing relationships and cultural narratives that had come together to cause intense strife in her home.

I asked Ping, at this point, if she had had problems with her own parents in the past.

"No big problems," she said immediately. "They would support me in whatever."

"There were no conflicts with them until recently?"

"Right," she replied, pausing to think for a moment before continuing.

"Maybe this is how I feel," she posited, "maybe when I was little and they would *guan* me I would feel, ah, this is—my parents *guan* me, and I would like them to *guan* me. And then if they wouldn't, I would feel that they weren't concerned about me (不关心我 *bu guanxin wo*). But after I grew up, I felt like I should have my own space. And then it had already been more than ten years of not living together. And then suddenly living together, I wasn't used to it."

Demonstrating a nuanced and tentative form of scalar inquiry, Ping here offered an additional possible explanation for her inability to accept her parents' care in the present. Narratively situating her parents' care as having remained consistent over time, she drew here on a temporal framework to highlight how such care had, at least *previously*, always felt like genuine concern or love (关心 *guanxin*). In this framing, however, the temporal as well as spatial distance separating Ping from her childhood provided a coherent chronotopic structure for making sense of her current challenges *without* attributing absolute blame to any party.

Ping paused briefly again before adding an additional reflection: "And also a lot of our habits (习惯 *xiguan*) are different," she said, "so living together is really awkward.... I really don't want to live with them anymore. I want to run away."

The moral, affective, and relational geography of Ping's home was clearly quite complex, and involved her feeling simultaneously grateful, responsible, guilty, and harassed. I soon learned that this guilt and, indeed, desire to run away, had been exacerbated by the ways in which her close friends had responded when Ping had turned to them for advice. After she had confessed to her friends, Ping detailed, they had only scolded her, repeatedly reminding her how lucky she was that she had any help at all. They had also suggested countless ways for her to be "more accommodating" to her parents. Her voice cracking with emotion, Ping thus described how it felt like her friends completely discounted her suffering. Ping's experience with her friends thus underscores the ways in which the intimate work of scalar inquiry often requires, as I discuss in more detail in the next chapter, what Myers (2016) describes as distinct "peopled opportunities" or encounters in which one is valued as a morally valid person. Their response, in other words, (re)positioned Ping in the role of (immoral) culprit whose feelings of persecution were invalid.

Despite this disavowal, Ping nevertheless persisted in engaging in what might be framed, following Teresa Kuan, as "an ethics of trying" within which individuals are constantly assessing the intricacies of particular relational situations or *qing* (情). Situations demand a response, Kuan emphasizes. Indeed, if nothing else, Ping's narrative demonstrated a continuous commitment to investigating the problem, her own role in creating it, and importantly, her own (possible) role in resolving it. After another poignant pause, Ping thus offered up a simple possible solution: "Maybe if everyone was further from the city, it would be better," she suggested hopefully, looking up and offering what may be a more neutral explanation.

Ping soon began to look very distressed, however, and was quiet for a long time.

"You're feeling something now," I said. "You are crying?"

"Yes—bringing it up, I feel a lot."

We were quiet for a moment while Ping continued to weep, telling me about her guilt over a fight that she had had with her mother the day before the workshop.

"You are still feeling a lot of emotion about that," I observed.

"Yes," she said. "Guilt (內疚 *neijiu*), a lot of guilt... maybe it is because I haven't been understanding to my parents. Or my attitude hasn't been good to them."

Circling back to positioning herself as the (possibly) guilty party, Ping nevertheless went on to detail how she had begun to feel small but significant glimmers of *hope* after attending the inner child workshop at New Life. She related it, in particular, to an experience in which she saw herself, at the age of six, in a family photograph from long ago. This vision, Ping noted, moved her to entertain the notion that her parents really *did* love her. In that instant, she further reported, "the knot in my heart (心结 *xinjie*) just opened."

The recent revelation had not—in the week since she had returned home from her first New Life workshop—proffered any quick (or easy) "solutions." Ping did note, however, that there had been a slight shift in the way she related to her mother. Centered primarily around her own patterned responses—specifically her tendency to become irritable and even angry when she felt controlled by her mother—Ping had begun to feel more willing to meet her mother's suggestions with calmer, more relationally connected forms of refusal.

One week had not by any stretch of the imagination, however, "solved" Ping's problems. The relational, moral, and affective geography of Ping's home was, indeed, incredibly complex. This geography consisted of an intricate assemblage of intimate relationships (with her husband, her son, her parents, her friends, and her mother-in-law) as well as culturally salient concepts or cultural chronotopes for understanding the ways in which time, space, and personhood *should* be (e.g., care, control, education, filial piety, motherhood, desire, and home or household, to name just a few).

Even though all of these problems persisted, Ping reflected, she also noted how the workshop had encouraged her to see how—regardless of who was to blame—her previous behavior may have impeded the very possibility of initiating an honest dialogue with her parents. This awareness alone, Ping noted, afforded an ever-so-slight but noticeable shift in the dynamic at home. If only in her own attention to being calmer and more compassionate in refusing her mother's care, this, importantly, offered Ping a vague sense of hope, a feeling that change was possible in the future.

It is worthwhile to note how even here, however, Ping drew on a vast range of narrative scaling strategies as her narrative bounced back and forth between perspectives and temporalities in an effort to make sense of the situation and craft visions of a possible future. Ping's uncertainty and mixed feelings of anger and guilt lingered, for example, even as she engaged a more hopeful anticipatory mode. The constant scaling that Ping enacted throughout her interview nonetheless suggests how telling suffering, specially within discursive contexts that afford openness and subjunctivity, often leads not to resolution but to *further inquiry*. Ping's story, in other words, underscores the ways in which experimental enactments of scalar intimacy, as an "ethics of trying" (Kuan 2015, 18) or scalar inquiry, also point to both desire and *hope* as a strategy for orienting toward possible futures within which such tensions would be resolved, a future where she might be able to find her way back to a feeling of being-at-home in her own home.

THE TIMID AND WEAK TYPE

Hua Hua was my twenty-five-year-old roommate during one of the extended inner child retreats at the suburban hotel. After several days of laughing and crying and dancing together in the larger group, eating meals together, and staying up late talking in the dark, we finally found the time to conduct an official interview in the evening before the final day of the event. We were sitting comfortably, both in our hotel bathrobes, on her bed.

"So why did you come to this workshop?," I asked to start us off.

"I plan to have a child with my husband," she replied matter-of-factly, repeating an explanation she had referred to multiple times over the previous days.

"I wanted to do some psychological treatment (心理治疗 *xinli zhiliao*) because it will have benefits for the baby," she explained. "I want to become mature. I want to realize myself (实现自我 *shixian ziwo*), like I want to have a bit more belief in myself, a little less timidity and be more courageous."

"Really?" I asked, "You feel you—"

"I am the type of person who is intensely fearful and easily anxious. I really am that kind, " she said, going on to tell me that she had barely left the house for more than a year. Here, Hua Hua distinguished herself from what she perceived to be normal, scaling herself in relation to the (imagined) ordinary housewife, who chooses to stay home. In contrast, she claimed, there was a distinct pathology to her confinement. Indeed, Hua Hua described how, whenever she "encountered society" (接触社会 *jiechu shehui*), she experienced a deep-seated sense of terror. She had tried to work at several jobs, she told me, but she would soon become overwhelmed with anxiety and would have to quit. After this had occurred in her most recent position, her family had encouraged her to stay home and rest so that her anxiety would not affect the desired pregnancy.

Unlike Ping, Hua Hua did not remember ever having a sense of "being-at-home-in-the-world." She nevertheless had several well-developed theories about what had happened to cause her timidity as well as her terror. Rather than a single rupture, however, Hua Hua described how it had emerged over the course of many years and many encounters.

"Because in childhood I went through a lot," she explained, "I had no way of controlling a few very stressful situations (压抑的事 yayi de shiqing) and, at the time, I had no way to escape."

Her family had moved from the countryside to the city when she was in elementary school. Her uncle, who had loose ties to the military, had secured her a spot in an elite, specialized school focused on the performing arts. Hua Hua, however, was a clumsy, awkward child, and hated everything about performing in front of an audience. Her self-confidence, she explained somberly, immediately plummeted.

Over the next hour, Hua Hua further told me multiple, detailed stories about how both the teachers and her peers would frequently humiliate her in front of everyone. She was ridiculed for being clumsy at dance and incompetent at music, for example, but also doing poorly in academics. Her classmates constantly reminded her, moreover, that she was only part of the elite program because of her family's connections (关系 guanxi) rather than her aptitudes and skills. These experiences had impacted her young heart-mind, Hua Hua explained, causing her to become increasingly fearful, timid, and constantly anxious as well as frequently depressed.

To illustrate, Huan Hua shared the memory of being called up to the front of the classroom by her math teacher only because she had been crying in the back of the room. The teacher made her into an example for other children, calling her a disgrace and a range of other insulting names.

"The whole class was watching," Hua Hua tells me, her eyes growing larger. "It was extremely painful."

As she related horror stories from her childhood to me, one after the other, I began to get the sense that Hua Hua seemed to put a great deal of effort into formulating her personal history as rooted in the kinds of interpersonal violence that index broader cultural and structural injustices. At one point, I thus asked her if she thought that the kind of cruelty she had endured was common in China. She nodded emphatically, replying that she thought that her experience was extremely common, especially within elite urban schools.

"Couldn't you have switched schools?," I asked, perhaps naively.

She shook her head vigorously. "I would never have been allowed to switch schools! My parents would have never even considered it," she explained, adding that "they didn't know how much pain I was in. But even if they had, they would have said 'it just has to be like this.'" Her parents, Hua Hua further explained, both relied primarily on the strategies of tolerance, compromise, and endurance or "forbearance" (忍 ren).

"It is their answer for *everything*," she explained. "My whole family is like this. It's always 'wait, compromise, do not express anything,' at least when they are out in the world. Things were very different at home. It would all come out," Hua Hua said, describing the home she had grown up in as a constant war zone in which her father, especially, would frequently become violent. Returning to the question of whether she could have switched schools, however, she noted that even *she* would have never thought of it. Her so-called happiness—something that is now on the top of many peoples' minds in contemporary China (e.g., Wielander 2018a-b; J. Yang 2018b; Zhang 2020)—was simply never a concern.

"I didn't have *any* ideas at the time, really. I just felt like 'uh, this is really painful'," she explained. Hua Hua had thus suffered quietly all the way through middle school. She couldn't talk to anyone, she said, because they would just think she was being ungrateful. There was too much shame, Hua Hua elaborated.

"You can't talk about this pain with other students. You have to conceal it. Because this is a situation that you can't share with other people, and then so I was in terrible, terrible pain."

Though she did her best to conceal her feelings, she became more and more depressed over the years. Her tendency to withdraw had continued to grow worse all the way through high school. Even in university, she told me, she only had one friend and had never had a boyfriend until she met her husband. She was still far from well, she concluded, but she returned to her desire for her imagined future child.

"Because actually me—I'm just this way. I want my child's future to be bright, however. I don't want them to be like me, to experience this kind of pain, to feel so much pain when memories come up. I want them to be strong in their inner heart and not to be like me, like timid and afraid of everything."

Unlike Ping, whose narrative emerged in a highly subjunctive mode of inquiry, Hua Hua seemed to scale herself in relation to her own past as well as a range of ideologies and "norms" prevailing in Chinese society with considerable certainty, at least initially. She spoke confidently to the fact that she "was" a timid and weak person, for example. She also presented multiple, consistent stories of bullying and even abuse that moved rapidly between specific encounters and a range of culturally salient moral-relational notions such as *guanxi* (connections), forbearance, shame, and performance.

As she spoke, Hua Hua likewise engaged a nuanced chronotopic contrast between urban and rural Chinese society. Based on her own experience, specifically, she formulated rural education as a more humanistic, moral sphere compared to the city. After they had moved from the countryside to the city, for example, she had longed for the experience that she had had at her rural school, where, in her words, "they take care of you more" and "don't hurt your self-esteem." Even though she had only limited experience in such spaces prior to moving to the city at age ten, in other words, Hua Hua situated her experience as taking shape in relation to an absolute contrast between urban and rural, within which urban equated to immoral, deceitful, and cruel and rural indexed caring, nurturing, and moral. Hua Hua's story here also notably often made vast temporal and spatial leaps, zipping back and forth from the past to the present to a desired future in which her baby might not inherit her weakness and timidity.

Extending this scale over time throughout her life, Hua Hua thus also enacted a fairly intense and negative outlook toward anyone who had been able to succeed in an urban environment. Such success—whether financial or social—was, in Hua Hua's formulation, inevitably gained at the expense of the family. Anyone who had "become rich" in the city, according to Hua Hua, thus reflected the kind of hypocrisy and fakery that had prevailed in her own family. Indeed, she had been terrified of coming to the New Life workshop, she explained, because of her fear that it would be populated entirely by "people with money" (有钱人 *you qian ren*) who lacked the kind of moral compass that she associated with rural environments.

Even though she and her husband would arguably be perceived as "having money" by others, she protested, she had nevertheless been confident that she was fundamentally *different* from such people.

"I thought that they didn't have the same kind of problems as us, that they were absolutely self-confident in any setting. I thought that they were different from us. So when I started, I didn't feel good at all."

Hua Hua had, however, been pleasantly surprised by the experience she had had over the previous several days, especially after a series of intense movement exercises. A more tentative story in which Hua Hua seemed to be experimenting with reformulating herself thus seemed to be emerging as she spoke. She increasingly began to end sentences with a rising tone, for example, seemingly asking me to confirm that she had, indeed, been successful and competent in the kind of social ituateion that previously would have terrified her.

"The first day of class, when we were told we had to speak from her hearts, I laughed. I could not accept. I didn't want to laugh, but I felt so *awkward*, ah? I felt like I just couldn't get in the right frame of mind. So [in the exercises] I would just stand back. I felt like I was locked in a kind of ironclad awkwardness." Hua Hua here explained how, during one movement exercise where Teacher Jo had encouraged us to dance as if we were in a madhouse (疯子院 *fengzi yuan*) (see chapter 3), she had stood frozen in place, watching others and wondering at their apparent comfort with the exercise. Hua Hua couldn't move, she explained, because she felt far too self-conscious and was too concerned with "losing face." "I really felt I couldn't possibly stand it—because I didn't want to laugh, but I felt so strange," she said. *Something* had happened to her as she watched others participating, however.

As she watched, Hua Hua described a feeling of something beginning to open up within her. She did not yet fully understand what, but she noted a distinct shift that had occurred afterwards. Indeed, Hua Hua's experience of *witnessing* others in the movement exercise had seemed to open something up within her such that she was able, upon waking the following morning, to be "more open," "more cheerful" with people.

"I felt like I *changed*, I started opening up—I was still uncomfortable and I was always thinking about whether other people were looking at me, whether I might look shameful (丢人 *diuren*)—but I felt like I opened up, or opened up a bit. It was like I was expressing my inner self for the first time—Really!" We both laughed.

Her experiences over the past few days during the workshop, Hua Hua explained, had moved her to begin to question some of the "facts" upon which she had based her previous fears. While she had initially scaled herself definitively in relation to multiple (perceived) "norms" in Chinese society, in other words, Hua Hua had begun to engage in a tentative kind of scalar inquiry. She was, accordingly, beginning to at least catch glimpses of a new framework for understanding herself and her possible future. At several points in our conversation, in fact, Hua Hua was downright giddy about the implications of this new way of being in the world. She understood this process as far from complete, however.

"I'm sure it will take a much longer time to progress," Hua Hua noted toward the end of our interview, "but I already feel like it is much better."

Overall, then, Hua Hua's narrative underscores how relational contexts in which people are granted enough embodied, affective, and moral agency to be "awkward and uncomfortable" offer a discursive opportunity to begin to interrogate and even revise formerly entrenched narratives.

AWKWARD INTRODUCTIONS

The previous sections have focused on narratives that were collaboratively developed in private interviews with me, outside the immediate space of New Life. Focusing on the participation of two newcomers during the introductory circle of a summer evening salon in 2014, this section demonstrates how the kinds of scalar inquiry that I have been examining thus far also often emerged in group interactions at the center.

The evening began with about twenty of us arranged in a circle, seated on cushions. The ritual process of introductions began with several regulars, who, as per the usual format, discussed their experience in self-development at New Life and beyond, the classes they had attended at New Life and adjacent sites, and the books they had read. Some mentioned their reasons for attending that evening, briefly describing any interpersonal, emotional, or spiritual issues that they had been struggling with. Others focused on their desired goals and intentions for the evening, or a question related to their recent reading or encounters with center teachers.

About halfway through the circle, it was time for a newcomer, who I will call Sophie, to introduce herself. She laughed awkwardly. The room was silent as she spoke, but all eyes focused on her in a kind of collective encouragement through which regular clients, as well as our instructor for the evening, seemed to convey our acceptance of her clear lack of familiarity with and discomfort within the space.

When she began, Sophie spoke quickly and articulately in a standard northern Chinese accent. From the outset of her introduction, however, she entered into a somewhat rambling narrative as she attempted to describe her struggle. She thought that she may take work too seriously, she told us at first. She may also bring her feelings about work home too often, she added, since her husband has told her that he feels like her "punching bag." She desperately wanted to resolve what she referred to as "the problem," she then admitted, but she was unclear about what was even happening.

"I'm not sure if this is emotional or psychological or what," she said, going on to tell us that she was really nervous when she had first arrived. She hadn't wanted to speak because she didn't know how to express the issue clearly. After hearing others introduce themselves, however, she had decided that it was worth a try, even if she was not able to be completely coherent.

Sophie's brief introduction, like many offered by newcomers at the center, demonstrates the kind of confusion that I discussed above in terms of a chronotopic disorientation—an embodied, spatiotemporal, and relational disjuncture, often of unknown or unexpected origins, provoking a desperate search for answers and possible solutions. Sophie was thus confused not only in her experience but was also clearly discomfited by the effort to narratively structure her story in a way that she expected we could understand. Pointing to the ways in which newcomers' narratives are often framed in open-ended terms that lack coherence (Ochs 2004), her final comments also show how such framings pragmatically implicate or *recruit* co-present interlocutors, who thus become co-participants in the speakers' narrative sense-making project (Ochs 2004; Shohet 2017, 2021). Indeed, although introductory circles are premised on a participation framework in which a single speaker addresses a group of listeners, there are also often brief responses from the teacher as well as the group.

Here, Teacher Du—our facilitator for the evening—responded to Sophie immediately once she signaled that she was finished. Specifically, Du lightly praised Sophie, commenting on her quick mind and rapid speech.

"It's because I sell luxury goods," Sophie responded, not missing a beat. Everyone in the room laughed, including both Du and Sophie.

"I would certainly buy anything after listening to you," Teacher Du joked back, generating another wave of chuckles from the group. Suddenly becoming more somber, however, Du continued.

"I think, though, that we all want to tell you that in this kind of event (场合 changhe)," he said, "no matter what you say, no matter how fast or slow you say it, no matter if it is right or wrong, we are all willing to listen, we will all be very patient to listen." There were multiple nods of agreement from the group, and Sophie's shoulders seemed to visibly relax.

In this portion of the segment, one begins to see the ways in which "co-operative action" (C. Goodwin 2018) at New Life was a constant and collaborative process that "moved" interlocutors, in multiple ways. By "moving" here, I am referring to the kinds of affective shifts that occurred, often quite rapidly, during interactions such as this one. As just one moment within an ongoing interaction taking place during the opening circle that evening, moreover, it further points to the ways in which interaction at New Life constituted a constant, collaborative, process within which "new action [was] built by decomposing, and reusing . . . resources made available by the earlier actions of others" (C. Goodwin 2018, 1). While Du's response here seemed, at least initially, to downgrade or even disavow Sophie's suffering by invoking a casual, joking atmosphere, for example, a co-operative approach eschews the notion that we could discern the meaning, intent, or impact of any statement without investigating both prior and following talk. Indeed, in combination with the latter, more somber portion of Du's response, I suggest below, Du's initial playfulness arguably contributed to a kind of *normalization* of Sophie's confusion. By commenting on Sophie's verbal prowess rather than the content of her narrative, specifically, Du successfully set the stage for his more serious following comment.

Thus avowing her position as a moral being within the space, he then shifted to presence Sophie's suffering as something that did not require interpretive clarity in order to garner compassion. Drawing on collective pronouns to imagine a shared desire, spoken in a shared voice ("we all want to tell you"), he also notably crafted a nuanced chronotopic formulation of the "kind" of event that was occurring ("this kind"). Framing it as a certain kind of *relational* space, Du thus conveyed that "in here" (as opposed to out there) the collective "we" was not only willing to listen to her, but would undoubtedly also be patient with her, regardless of whether or how capable she was of enacting either coherence or confidence. Rather than considering whether all participants agreed with such a statement, his comment might be approached as a *suggestion* that afforded the opportunity for several participants to glance and nod toward Sophie. As a simultaneous ratification of Du's comment and endorsement of the normality of Sophie's suffering, this collaboratively enacted meaning or sentiment, finally, moved Sophie herself to smile and relax.

Overall, Sophie's value as a speaker, regardless of her coherence, was, indeed, positioned as normal here, so much so that it afforded an in-kind humorous response to Du's comment about her "quick mind and rapid speech." Scaling herself here in relation to a shared cultural orientation toward luxury goods and the positionality often occupied by those who are good at selling them, Sophie's retort here moved the feeling in the room toward a mirthful—if also ironic—engagement with the tension inherent between her present state of confusion and her normative mode of "self-assured and confident salesperson." Du here built upon the shared joke, conveying his confidence in *any* product she was selling based on her presentation of self. By declining to engage with the specifics of Sophie's circumscribed and inconclusive narrative, in other words, Du's overall response, rather, enacted an acknowledgment or *avowal* that endorsed Sophie's position, regardless of her confusion, as a moral being within the space. This positioning, moreover, was largely ratified by other group members who had laughed, nodded, and held intimate eye contact throughout both Sophie's introduction and Du's response. Interactions like these, I detail in the following chapter, contributed to the co-creation of a distinct affective, moral, and relational geography at New Life as a simultaneous space of comfort *and* possibility.

We moved on, here, directly to another newcomer, who I will call Luli. Unlike Sophie, Luli began speaking tentatively, in a quiet voice. She spoke slowly as well and paused frequently. Her voice began to waver with emotion, moreover, almost as soon as she started talking.

"I've attended some events, and encountered a little bit of this kind of thing, but only very shallowly (浅薄的 *qianbo de*)," she said, drawing on a chronotopic formulation of herself in relation to the content and customs of the genre represented by New Life. Luli's opening comment thus served as a chronotopic marker of her own embodied experience in relation to the context in which she imagined that she was currently participating in. She went on, however, to tell us that she had come to "solve" a particular problem.

"The problem I want to solve (解决 *jiejue*) today is an emotional one," she said, going on to give us a sense of how she experienced the world, as well as herself, in generalized emotional and relational terms. "My emotions, they can be characterized as pretty strong (强 *qiang*)," she said. "I have many misgivings/suspicions (猜疑 *caiyi*) and heart-heaviness (心重 *xinzhong*). Also I am timid (胆小 *danxiao*) and feel inferior (自卑 *zibei*), this kind of thing."

After offering a general description signaling why she had come to New Life that evening, Luli began to zoom in on a particular situation in her life.

"I've been wanting to resign recently," she said, "and I feel certain that I am the reason."

Beginning with an expression of desire, Luli's framing here was also tentative, for example, despite expressing "certainty" with regard to the truth of whether she was or was not the underlying reason for whatever problem was making her want to resign from her job. Before we were able to get a sense of what kind of situation she saw herself as having (possibly) caused, however, Luli zoomed out again, offering us a spatiotemporal context with regard to her workplace. Here, she emphasized the durative nature of her work, telling us that she had worked at this particular "firm" for six years "already." Alongside her tone and rate of speech as well as her largely negative self-description, this seemed to highlight a possible tension between her commitment to the job and her professed plan to (possibly) resign. It also, importantly, situated her as a person living in a certain socio-professional milieu (a *firm*).

At this point, Luli zoomed back in to the specifics of her story, telling us about how, "a while ago," a "young girl" (女孩儿 *nuhaier*) had arrived to work in her firm. She interjected her narrative to assure us—after calling her new coworker a term often used to describe female children and—that "she's very young." This chronotopic formulation of age seemed to serve as an index of comparison with which we might interpret her following utterance, in which she told us that she felt as if the girl had gradually come to "replace" her at work. Though not her "home" per se, Luli's grief here pointed to the disjuncture of feeling no longer at home in one's place of work. Indeed, her young colleague had seemingly caused Luli not only to feel obsolete in the firm where she had already spent six years but had moved her to reevaluate her very worth as a person.

Luli thus returned, at this point, to the logic that she first presented regarding her assessment that *she* (not the girl) was the problem, "And—because you could characterize me as the kind of person who likes expressing myself, but I am also afraid to express myself," she said, "like I'm relatively low-key (低调 *didiao*), that type of person. I want to make the boss acknowledge me, but I don't have that kind of self-confidence (自信 *zixin*)."

This portion of Luli's narrative revealed to us a little more about how, in the context of her profession at least, Luli valued the socio-moral quality of "self-expression" and, indeed, *was* or *would have been* more expressive if she were not always, in her words, so intimidated by others or the world, or both. She did not offer a specific definition of what she meant by "self-expression," however it seemed to suggest the chronotopic quality of persons who are appropriately assertive within the competitive professional marketplace. Luli further contrasted it with her fearfulness as well as the fact that she was a relatively "low-key" (低调 didiao) type of person. Also translatable as "low-profile," low-key here indexed another culturally salient type of moral personhood, specifically invoking the ideal Confucian "gentleman" (君子 junzi) who "is dignified but does not wrangle" (Analects 15.22, as cited in Z. Li 2010, 61). As opposed to the achievements of "the petty man," the successes of a junzi, importantly, arise not out of aggressive self-promotion but through hard work and recognition by others. Luli's choice of terms to describe herself thus indexed a number of relational cultural chronotopes related to ethical behavior in time and space. Luli's anxiety about being "low profile"—a part of her timid "nature," in her framing—here began to take on a gendered, culturally, and spatiotemporally situated shape. Indeed, women in China are often tasked with the dual and conflicting obligation to be feminine and "low-key" in the home and outgoing and "self-expressive" in business (see Osburg 2013), all the while maintaining a "soft" (温顺 wen shun) demeanor that is "non-threatening and compliant" with men in general (Xie 2021, 158). The conflicting demands Luli articulated, in other words, constitute a well-known moral dilemma that likely felt deeply recognizable and familiar, at least to the women in the room.

Luli's low-key nature had become visible in direct contrast, we soon learned, with that of her younger colleague. "And then this young girl came," she said, "and over time, she started going on business trips with the boss, gradually replacing me."

Without mentioning the gender of the boss, Luli here located the girl's rise to a position of power within the firm specifically because she frequently went on trips with "the boss." This stood out, immediately, as a further index of the gendered aspects of Luli's dilemma. Was Luli suggesting that this young colleague had begun to sleep with the boss? Why else would she so easily replace someone who had clearly devoted a great deal of her life to the firm? I place these questions here because, as is often the case in conversation, the "full story" was not entirely accessible. Perhaps Luli herself did not know for sure, but I would surmise that many of us in the room—the women at least—had suspicions.

Luli returned to describing her emotional experience here, however, making it clear to us how *personally* she had felt the sensation of being replaced. "And then so now I feel like I have no purpose at the firm," she told us, her voice straining even more. "And so I feel very wounded (伤心 shangxin), and very sad (难过 nanguo). I feel wronged (委屈 weiqu). Actually, there are so many aspects to it. And I have no way to really explain it—once I start talking about it, I feel really awkward, but this is just how I'm thinking." She was crying softly at this point.

Luli concluded, telling us that she felt wounded, sad, and wronged but also deeply confused. Drawing upon a series of indexical connotations that pointed to multiple unspoken and conflicting gendered, economic, and social chronotopes in Chinese society, Luli's invocation of what could broadly be glossed as "the social" was conveyed as her *personal* dilemma, a dilemma in which her body no longer seemed to belong in her own workplace. There was, moreover, a continuous search for possible explanations lying at the heart of Luli's storytelling efforts—and, like with Ping and Sophie as well as Hua Hua, an active and agentive search for the culprit, even if that meant condemning her own behavior or "nature." A fundamental sense of uncertainty was explicitly centered in her concluding remarks, where she admitted that she was struggling to understand the situation, was indeed engaging multiple possible answers to the question of what, exactly, had happened at her previously comfortable workplace.

There was long pause before Teacher Du responded to Luli. "I hope that you can pay attention to—actually what you just said about yourself—so many of the words were negative," he said. "But at the very least, what you just expressed (表出来 biaochulai) was a very, very sincere way of being (真诚的一种状态 zhencheng de zhuangtai). Everyone here perhaps noticed, because others among us have spoken with a lot of pretense (虚假 xujia). You were the only one who directly connected (接上 jieshang) to the problems in your inner heart. But when you were speaking, I believe we could all feel your sincerity. You've done this very, very well. Thank you. Keep it up."

Du's praise evoked a slight nod from Luli, who was now seated with her head down, her hands covering her face. Her tears seemed to flow more freely with his words, however, and her shoulders began to drop as if a great tension had been released in her back. The moment Du framed her expression of authentic confusion in *positive* terms, the shift in Luli, in other words, wass subtle but noticeable. It was as if Du's acknowledgment of what he framed as her *achievement* began to offer her a sense of relief, or at least an opening for further inquiry. As he was speaking, furthermore, many of us gazed at Luli compassionately and nodded, as if ratifying his encouragement. When she began to look up, several long-time clients of the center smiled at her knowingly, and she even began to smile back as we proceeded to the next introduction.

In his initial response, Du thus seemed—as he had done with Sophie—to discount the negative content of Luli's story, instead attending to its "sincerity" as perceived by himself as well as the others for whom he, again, spoke. Although he arguably evaded a direct engagement with the kinds of systemic and structural gendered inequalities indexed within her introduction, he also notably resisted providing any kind of explanation or recommendation that would have normalized such inequities. This kind of avoidance, I suggest later in this book, sometimes functioned as an unspoken yet pragmatic and arguably strategic way of communicating that inspired many participants not to turn away from the social—as is often assumed when therapeutic contexts are deemed inherently "apolitical"—but instead as an *invitation* to further interrogate the historical, political, and social dynamics contributing to suffering. Here, however, I want to focus on the ways in which Du's response to Luli served the function of "format tying" (M. H. Goodwin 1990, 177–85). His comments here thus mirror the ways in which, we recall, Du had articulated a chronotopic casting of New Life as *different* from other settings. In that response, specifically, he had authoritatively invoked a distinct form of relationality in the present and future vis-à-vis a specific kind of authoritative and collectively framed speech act (a *promise*) (Austin [1962] 2003). In this case, similarly, by highlighting the ways in which other participants likely also "noticed" and could all feel her sincerity, Du recruited those of us who were co-present to acknowledge this observation. His utterances here, like his response to Sophie, thus situated the *value* of Luli's expression as lying within emotional sincerity rather than coherence or accuracy. Finally, it served to recruit Luli to attend to the way she was *seen* as worthy and possibly even *more* successful than others within the relational space.

"Listening orders and orients our attention," writes Marsilli-Vargas (2022, 28), as well as generating a kind of *directionality* in terms of relational possibilities (91). Learning to love, in this instance, equated to learning how to *listen* as well as—for Sophie and Luli—learning how to be listened *to*. Either alone or in combination, I therefore suggest, Du recruited participants to coenact a distinctly *moral* stance, enacted here not so much through the competent production of language, but rather through its reception (Stivers et al. 2011; Marsilli-Vargas 2022). By discursively invoking multiple language ideologies—ideas about what language is and what language does

(Silverstein 1979)—Du moreover successfully modeled an inversion of the normative notion that narratives should be coherent. His responses to both Sophie and Luli, rather, enacted a dual ideology of language and *ideology of listening* in which the point of communication (rather than to convey preestablished forms of coherence or precise content) is to express affect as well as selfhood and desire. This moral stance and ideology of language, I suggest, collaboratively contributed to the emergence of New Life as a space within which interactions take on different shapes from those that occur within other spaces in contemporary China.

CONCLUDING REFLECTIONS

Narratives developed within therapeutic settings, as Li Zhang details, are often seen as supporting people in a constructive process of "scaffolding and guiding a new self" (2020, 130). In emphasizing the experience of newcomers throughout this chapter, however, my aim was to draw attention away from this constructive dimension of therapeutic talk. Instead, I emphasized how, especially among newcomers to the space, the process of developing "a new self" at New Life often began with the far less ambitious goal of finding a way out of suffering. Newcomers, I demonstrated, were variably entrenched within complex experiences of rupture, disorientation, and disjuncture that caused them to feel "off-time" with themselves and their loved ones, here often wanting nothing more than to "get back on time" with their lives. Despite the differences in their individual situations, their narratives here, it is important to highlight, reflected a range of issues facing individuals—especially middle-class Han individuals—in twenty-first-century China.

In analyzing their narratives, both in the context of interviews and group interaction, however, I thus drew specific attention to the ways in which Ken, Ping, Hua Hua, Sophie, and Luli each drew upon various "subjunctivizing tactics" in order to formulate multiple, often competing explanations of their suffering. Often though not always organized as an effort to discover who was to blame, and articulated in tentative statements that moved quickly between self-blame and the attribution of blame to others and then back, without resolution, the narratives I have shared here demonstrate the ways in which newcomers lived, to a large degree, within what Paul Heelas describes as "relatively circumscribed frame[s] of reference" (2008, 121). I have suggested, however, that both interviews and group interactions served as "peopled opportunities" within which newcomers were "recognized as good, accountable person[s] by others" (Myers 2016, 430). Drawing on Samuels (2018), I noted how this intimate "participation framework," in contrast to other professional or familial settings, afforded them the opportunity to tell incomplete stories, contradict themselves, and express confusion in ways that did not undermine their personhood. While such encounters often worked to avow newcomers' vulnerability, however, they did not, arguably, provide much *specific* scaffolding in terms of the project of "building a new self."

Nor did they offer many—or *any*—concrete solutions for newcomers' particular dilemmas. Indeed, interactions within the space often seemed to purposefully generate a sense of *more* rather than less uncertainty. In addition to validation, however, they did provide an opportunity for newcomers to engage with the various forms of scalar intimacy through which culturally salient or dominant norms, ideas, and practices or *cultural chronotopes* had become entrenched within them as the kinds of orienting devices through which, in Sara Ahmed's words, "the world unfolds" (Ahmed 2007). The interrogation of such chronotopes, I further suggested, emerged as an intimate form of *scalar inquiry*. Showing how narrative practices emerged dialogically in ways that simultaneously invoke personal and shared as well as temporally present and past experiences, ideologies, and possibilities, telling suffering here took shape as an experimental scaling with the *potential* to generate new meanings, new self-interpretations, and even new selves. This was true, I suggested, even when no "solution" or reformulated sense of certainty or "self" resulted.

It is important to note, here, that such interactions alone do not tell us much about the ultimate "efficacy" of the encounters. The narrative, dialogically situated telling of suffering among newcomers at New Life as I witnessed it, however, did call into question the oft-accepted notion that therapeutic encounters, through their emphasis on the individualized self, foreclose the opportunity for participants to engage with more broadly political, sociohistorical, and economic histories, structures, and events. Scalar inquiry, as I have presented it here, rather demonstrated how therapeutically (or ethnographically) scaffolded conversations provided opportunities for people to experiment *more* rather than *less* with rescaling their relationships to the past, to navigate the uncertainty of the present, and to formulate visions of the future. In this sense, the nuanced interactions that emerged between me and New Life participants, as well as between participants at New Life events, constituted an opportunity for people to at least *begin* the work of learning to love and "reshaping the self" as a situated process of *theorizing* that, as I detail in chapters 4 through 7. The following two chapters, however, turn toward a description of the complex, multimodal emergence of the ways in which learning to love took shape in the embodied, affective geography of New Life.

2

Home/Horizons

In this loose assembly of bodies, manifested in the media, in the ways we govern ourselves, in the ways we name things and educate our children, we are desperately trying to investigate our circumstances, to ask what it takes to live well, to struggle with aging and dying, to know when to be wary of the other and when to be hospitable. To know what home means.
—BAYO AKOMOLAFE

Viewed from afar, horizons hint at, perhaps express, perhaps even reveal, the allure, the "gravitational pull" of what lies within them or beyond.
—PAUL HEELAS

One evening in 2014, people began filing into New Life for a free weeknight salon. The space was brightly yet softly lit, and straw mats had been arranged in a large circle on the light-stained laminate wood floors. Wearing loose, hemp clothing in reimagined traditional Indian and Chinese styles, several regular New Life clients embraced in extended bear hugs. Krishna Das, a widely recognized American musician famous for his adaptation of Hindu devotional kirtan music, was playing softly on the ceiling-mounted speakers. As I wrote in my field notebook, I overheard an interaction between Julie—one of the lead administrators at the time—and a participant. They were standing at the edge of the room having an in-depth conversation about how to love oneself (爱自己 *ai ziji*). Others were involved in intense conversations of some kind, holding each other's gaze and nodding.

There were also several newcomers who were easy to spot in their street clothes. Looking wide-eyed around them, their eyes moved quickly from the people to the shelves of books to the flyers. They looked, in fact, as if they were trying to figure out what to do, where to sit, and how to behave.

Gracie, a New Life administrator at the time, went over and began chatting amicably with them. She welcomed them into the space and led them to mats that, I noted, were positioned in the middle of the circle rather than directly to the left or right of the teacher's cushion.

When the chatter died down, Teacher Du, who was adorned all in pink, traditional Indian pants and top with a long loose scarf draped across his shoulders, welcomed us and guided us to sit. There were roughly twenty people total, about five presenting as men. The rest were women.

Du began speaking, his voice calmly telling us to come into our bodies and settle in our experience. "Can you turn off the lights?," he asked Julie. She jumped up and hit the switch. We then sat quietly listening to the music for several minutes before several participants began chanting softly along with Krishna Das. Julie's voice stood out, loud and enthusiastic. The light was dim, but I was still able to observe her making eye contact with newcomers, seemingly beckoning them to join in. This continued for about five minutes. When the song came to an end, it was quiet for a moment.

Teacher Du rang a small bell and told us to take a deep breath, into our bellies.

When he finally began speaking, it was in a soft, gentle voice. He told us that he had been with the center since 2008, when he and his wife had started attending the center's evening reading groups.

"But the reason why I am sitting here today," he said, "is because from the moment I took that first course, the impact in my life has been profound, and I can honestly say that his whole realm (领域 *lingyu*)"—he waved his hands across the room—"is just really very important. It has taught me so many things that I never, in my whole life, understood."

He then invited us to go around the circle introducing ourselves. The second participant in the circle, who appeared to be in her early thirties, began by telling us that she had attended several other inner child events at the center.

"I really like this atmosphere (环境 *huanjing*)," she then said, "it is a feeling of returning home (回家 *huijia*)."

The room seemed to shift as she said this. Bodies softened, gentle smiles appeared on faces, gazes moved around the circle, making eye contact and resting for a moment longer than usual. It was almost as if the regular participants in the room actually experienced the feeling of "returning home" in concert with the speaker.

Others—newcomers to the center—seemed unsure. New Life was clearly not "home" for them, at least not yet.

ATMOSPHERES

In their recent book on methodological approaches to studying *atmosphere*, Sumartojo and Pink (2019) note the importance of attending to the multiple ways in which atmospheres emerge over time, drawing objects, affects, and interactions together in a complex and ongoing process that continually lands upon and within bodies in the space. New Life, from this vantage point, might be considered in terms of a continuously unfolding aesthetics consisting of texts and other objects, lighting, and, importantly, interaction, all of which might be seen as functioning together—in Charles Taylor's framing of aesthetics—as "a mode of experience" (1989, 374). Taking an atmospheric approach to New Life, I suggest in this chapter, affords appreciation of the ways in which context or atmosphere collaboratively emerged within the space as a situated—but not necessarily uniform—experience of time and space.

Though ineffable in terms of the ways in which it centers affect, an atmospheric approach, I further suggest, need not exclude a specific focus on language-in-interaction. Interaction, in Charles Goodwin's (2018) reframing of it as *co-operative action,* emerges as a collaboratively co-constructed intersubjective affective experience that is inclusive of other bodies, objects, and the overall space (Goodwin 2018; see also Wilce 2009; Shohet 2018; Pritzker 2020). Language, importantly, is considered here not just in terms of semantic meaning but in terms of its multiple indexicalities within an interaction as well as the ways in which conversations emerge over and within time and space, invariably drawing upon rhythm, prosody, objects, gaze, and body positioning to (co)create context or atmosphere. As discussed in the previous chapter, *listening* here also creates atmosphere as "a particular scenario, a setting, a possibility" (Marsilli-Vargas 2022, 93), as well as a generic practice that *"shape[s] the listener's orientation at the moment of reception"* (2022, 38; italics in original).

This chapter, accordingly, focuses on the ways in which the atmosphere or "context" at New Life was continually constructed or *mapped* as a "space apart." The boundary between New Life and the outside world was constructed, I demonstrate, through emergent co-operative action (C. Goodwin 2018) as participants engaged with objects, texts, ideas, and each other. In the scene described above, for example, a noticeable distinction inhered in the extended embraces and intense conversations among regular participants prior to the start of the salon, as well as the ways in which their attire marked them—at least to one newcomer—as "different." It also cohered when Du, in introducing himself and the center, waved his hands across the room, pointing to the books and other materials and noting the ways in which the whole "realm" (领域 *lingyu*) had offered him an appreciation of "things" that he had never, in his whole life, understood before.

Du's comment here served as a suggestion—as did his responses in the previous chapter—that New Life was distinct from the outside world, so to speak. It also, however, invoked what Paul Heelas calls a "horizoned promise" (2008, 128). "Horizons," Heelas writes in the epigraph above, "hint at, perhaps express, perhaps even reveal, the allure, the 'gravitational pull' of what lies within them or beyond" (2008, 121). Instructors and other leaders in the holistic milieu, Heelas thus argues, often offer horizons to participants, who, at least at the outset of their journeys in self-development—as described in the previous chapter—are often operating within "a relatively circumscribed frame of reference" (2008, 121). Horizons here "open up *vistas of significance*; to bring more into view" (121–22, italics in original), while teachers act "as beacons, signaling, pointing or directing the way to more distant horizons" (122). Du's comment here arguably functioned in precisely this way in indicating an uncommon horizon of possibility affording new potential worlds at the same time as offering what the speaker in the opening circle described as a feeling of "returning home."

"People reach for the label of atmosphere to express not only their experiences, but also how these experiences feel sensorially *and* how they feel about them," write Sumartojo and Pink (2019, 16). As she spoke, the return participant thus offered her interlocutors insight into the ways in which her immediate sensorial and affective experience of the atmosphere landed upon her as a feeling of being-at-home-in-the-world (Jackson 1995). Making a simultaneously spatial and *moral* distinction between the spaces she occupied on a daily basis and the space of New Life, this participant thus contributed to the mapping of the center as an intimate "space apart" from the chaos and disorientation that, as discussed in the previous chapter, prevails not just in Chinese society broadly but in the particular dilemmas that participants faced in their lives. She further situated herself *temporally*, however, indicating how her *past* experience in the space shaped her present experience, in temporal terms, as a *return*. Finally, one might also argue that she was also *anticipating* the ways in which the rest of the event that evening would emerge as a continuation of that feeling.

"Talk itself both *invokes context* and *provides context*," write Duranti and Goodwin (1992, 7, italics mine). I suggest that the notion of "returning home" here served as a chronotopic orienting device that contributed to generating, rather than simply reflecting, what is often referred to as "context." Her utterance undoubtedly landed differently upon various others who were co-present in the space at the time, however. For some people—including myself as well as other regular participants—the atmosphere seemed to *settle* in response to suggestions that New Life was "home" or at least was "homelike." Indeed, many people began to relax immediately once she had spoken, as if they had also suddenly returned home. Others, especially newcomers, looked around curiously, perhaps trying to imagine how they might someday experience the unfamiliar space as home. For newcomers, we might therefore situate the participant's comment alongside Du's, as another kind of "horizoned promise" that pointed to the moral-relational possibilities that existed within the space. Throughout this chapter, I thus emphasize the affective, moral, and relational geography of New Life as a continual, emergent process that oriented, in particular, to the culturally salient "home" chronotope, as described in the previous chapter, worked alongside (and often in tension *with*) what I formulate as the horizon chronotope.

The home chronotope, I demonstrate, was thus frequently invoked to construct the center as a space of intimacy and nourishment as well as connective recognition. The horizon chronotope, on the other hand, oriented the body-selves of participants within an atmosphere of possibility. It also, importantly, situated interlocutors along a temporal trajectory consisting of progress along a pathway of development that was eminently intimate and personal as well as social. Home and horizon chronotopes served as "locatives," in other words—terms that locate the bodies of both speakers and listeners within space and time (Gal 2002, 81)—with both simultaneously affective, relational, and moral connotations. Alongside the books and objects in the room, pronouns and deictic forms such as "this place" or "in here" thus worked as orienting devices that constituted New Life simultaneously as a space apart and a space of possibility.

Underscoring the persistent tension that often exists between *nostalgia* and *longing*, the home and horizon chronotopes at New Life further pointed to the ways in which "home is always lived as relationship, a tension" (Jackson 1995, 4). The home and horizon chronotopes here drew upon and even amplified the tension between the experience of "home" in reality and the search or desire for the felt experience of being-at-home-in-the-world (as horizon or "future homecoming"). Contributing to the crafting of the relational atmosphere at New Life as an intimate social space not unlike other psychotherapeutic group contexts (Duncan 2018; Matza 2018; L. Zhang 2020), they also contributed to the mapping of the space, as I show below, as a space of what one participant framed as "collective development" (共同成长 *gongtong chengzhang*).

The mapping of New Life as a space apart, a space of possibility, and a space of connection, I further argue, served as at least an invitation to participants to engage in an embodied, affective, and dialogic process of scalar inquiry or interrogation of their relationship(s) to powerful cultural orientations. Participants here were thus invited, though not required, to reexamine their past and present experience in light of the horizons of possibility that were invoked in the space. As such, I suggest, New Life became a space for "disentangling" (L. Zhang 2020) as well as *entangling differently* with the relational worlds, ideologies, and practices that were continually indexed in particular interactions. New Life could not, in other words, actually be considered a space apart from the social, political, and economic realities that constituted the everyday lives of participants. It was, rather, a place to reflect upon them, rescale oneself in relation to them, and sometimes even challenge them. This chapter thus considers how chronotopic formulations invoking the home and horizon chronotopes constituted one of the primary ways in which participants were invited to enact scalar intimacy and scalar inquiry as they formulated and sometimes even interrogated their relationship to dominant cultural chronotopes such as "home," "progress," and "collectivity." Pointing not to an enduring "culture" or way of being in the world but rather emerging as an *anticipatory* mode, moreover, the temporality of the space emerged here not only in terms of *duration*, as Sumartojo and Pink note, "but also in terms of the ways that the past and the *future* [was] folded into, perceived and understood in the present" (2019, 24; italics mine). Learning to love was thus deeply entangled with participants' yearning for the moral-relational and agentive experience of "being-with" both in the space and beyond.

Skeptical readers may point, here, to the ways in which New Life itself existed as a distinctly commodified space that was arguably selling a "home for the soul" in spurious ways that variably "flattened" the rich meanings inherent in the kinds of religious and spiritual traditions with which participants often engaged with as a kind of *style* or consumptive practice—in their purchase of clothing or CDs, for example (Kockelman 2006; Lyons and Karimzad 2019). While I do not deny the role that commodification played in the space, my analysis rather foregrounds the ways in which the atmosphere at the center took shape not just as an aspect of the products or statements uttered by instructors but by participants themselves as they engaged with objects, ideas, and each other. "Atmospheres cannot *make* people feel particular things," Sumartojo and Pink observe (2019, 5), underscoring the fundamental *indeterminacy* of atmospheres, which often emerge in and through the "moments when they do not take hold" (2019, 122). The atmospheres that emerged at New Life might be considered, I thus argue in the following sections, in terms of the ways in which utterances, feelings, memories, and bodies are scaled and rescaled in ways that exceed and overflow the semantic or even ideological meaning of the texts and other teachings offered at the center. Scaffolding participants' embodied experience of the "new kinds of social" that Zhang (2020) discusses as well as offering visions of a new kind of future, the home and horizon chronotopes, I thus suggest, contributed to the formulation of the atmosphere of New Life as affording distinctly intimate as well as scalar *anticipatory modes* that, as I discuss in more detail in chapter 4, often included critical considerations of "culture" and "Chineseness."

TEXTUALITY AND THE AGENCY OF ATMOSPHERES

New Life, at the time I was doing this research, was located at the northwestern outskirts of the old city in a converted apartment on the eighteenth floor of a large complex. Even though most of the units were by then occupied by businesses, the courtyard at the base of the building still had a nostalgic domestic feel. There were guard stations at both entrances, and there always seemed to be doting grandparents and young nannies watching children playing ball or riding tricycles around the large cement space serving as the courtyard. It was a high-traffic building, however, and there was also always a steady stream of people passing through, in the midst of busy days moving to and from work, running errands, or escorting children to activities.

When I visited New Life, I would ride up one of the six elevators with eight or nine other people moving quickly through their busy day. We would sometimes stop at what felt like every floor before the bright red "eighteen" would light up. When the doors would finally slide open, they revealed a landing that invoked memories of the many apartment complexes built in the late 1990s and early 2000s: cement floors, a bouquet of drywall, a darkness that hovered until I stomped on the floor to turn on the lights. Around the corner, the door to New Life would quickly come into focus, however, the soft light of the center peeking out from behind a soft cloth door hanging, a classic Bai-style tie-dye that brushed soothingly across my shoulders as I entered the space.

On most days, the sound of voices speaking softly or quiet music playing would fill my ears upon entering the small makeshift entryway, a transitional space created with bookshelves and a small antique table placed a few paces to the left of the doorway. The smells and sounds of cooking from the small kitchen, located to the right of the doorway, often accompanied my arrival as well. Depending on the time of day, this was where the young woman who we called *Ayi* ("Aunty")—a standard name for nannies and service workers as well as a term of respect for older women in China—might be preparing the vegetarian meals that the New Life staff enjoyed together once and sometimes twice per day. When I would arrive, I would also be greeted by whomever was seated at the small table set at the end of the entryway, opposite the kitchen.

During the first two years of my fieldwork, this was most often Gracie, an administrator at the time, who would sit greeting visitors and engaging in lively conversations that moved fluidly between the mundane and the profound. Beyond the entryway, the sparsely furnished room itself was covered in light wood flooring, the walls sparsely decorated with a few flyers for events advertising courses. Most of these were presented in terms of furthering spiritual growth (心灵成长 *xinling chengzhang*), including welcoming photographs of teachers as well as photos of participants sitting in circles or meditating. Specific courses included various programs in inner child work (内在小孩 *neizai xiaohai*), family constellation therapy (家庭系统排列 *jiating xitong pailie*), or the study of the Enneagram (九型 *jiuxing*). There were also flyers for the center's annual programs in "spiritual travel" (灵魂的旅行 *linghun de luxing*) programs, including a "South India Pilgrimage" (印度南部圣之旅) and trip called "Meeting Himalayan Masters" (与喜马拉雅上师相通). Along one wall at the center, there were three or four sparsely populated traditional Chinese bookshelves, with low piles of thin paperback books. Several were propped up to face outward in artful displays that drew the eye. Consisting of mostly light earth tones and pastels, the cover designs were, as a whole, cohesive and minimalistic, suggested a classical Chinese aesthetic of "unity with nature" (Z. Li 2010, 96). Signaling both spirituality and "difference," an altar with photos of Amma, the Indian guru or "hugging saint," was also propped up behind neatly aligned dishes of crystals next to the books.

Whenever I arrived at the center, day or night, the room was always brightly yet softly lit and the air fresh. It felt cozy and clean, despite the fact that the large window off the balcony—like all windows in the city at the time—looked out upon perpetually gray, pollution-dense skies. The *contrast* this created contributed to the sense that one had entered another world, or at least a unique spatiotemporal atmosphere that was distinct from other urban spaces. This contrast, though slightly different in tone and flavor, persisted when we left the center for longer workshops, which were held at an upscale hotel located in an elite suburban neighborhood roughly an hour outside the old city. For four or five days, New Life would rent a block of rooms and participants (usually between forty and fifty people) would pay a single fee (roughly 5,000 yuan) that included the workshop, a shared room, all meals, and a daily foot massage. This hotel, explained Teacher Jo during one of the workshops, is the destination of choice for New Life events because there are "good vibes" throughout the grounds.

At the hotel, the workshop events themselves took place in the large banquet room. Before the event, the staff would cover the ornate burgundy carpet entirely with pink flat sheets and, in addition to the plush chairs already in the room, would scatter hundreds of pastel throw pillows throughout the space. A few long tables were then placed alongside the inside wall, covered with fabric and used to display a selection of New Life books, CDs, and flyers for upcoming events. There was also always a space set aside for tea, hot water, and snacks that participants could consume throughout the day between meals, which were served in the dining room at special times designated for our group. Opposite the tables, the thick, cream-colored drapes covering the sliding glass doors that comprised the outside wall were drawn closed. During breaks, the drapes and, sometimes, the doors themselves would be opened to let light or a breeze into the space. During retreats, however, one could often hear the sounds of a wedding party or other event taking place beyond the windows or within the other dining area.

Taking meals together, living in rooms together, and spending all day and evening together engaged in exercises seemed to create a barrier between the workshop space and the outside world. Indeed, as we were nearing the close of one multiday inner child workshop in 2016, for example, one participant commented to me that she didn't want it to end. "I don't want to go back to the real world," she said, a drawn-out look of longing on her face. As I discuss further below, these kinds of comments, alongside the aesthetic objects, contributed to the mapping of New Life as "a space apart" as well as a space of intimacy and possibility. For the remainder of this section, however, I want to hover specifically on the ways in which *books*, in particular, served to invoke both home and horizon chronotopes at the center.

Texts occupying a space, Setha Low notes, "can be understood as nonhuman actors or 'actants' that shape actions and outcomes" (2017, 172). Though such outcomes must always be understood as fundamentally indeterminate with regard to how such materials act upon individual bodies in the space-time of specific encounters, it compels the question of the extent to which the books at New Life, as aesthetic/ethical objects that evoked feelings, made promises, and otherwise affected those who encountered them, had *agency* (Gell 1998). The texts that lined the shelves of New Life had at least the potential, in this sense, to *affect* the space as well as the people in the space.

The cover designs, overall, suggested a classical Chinese aesthetic sensibility (Z. Li 2010). The bulk of the books here displayed images of flowers, mountains, rivers, or the rising moon. Some also included a picture of an animal engaged in an activity: a snail gazing into the gap between two wood planks, for example, or a butterfly perched to land above a vibrant flower. The largest characters that stood out on the covers included keywords such as "light"(光 *guang*),"heart" (心 *xin*), "self" (自我 *ziwo*), "life" (生活 *shenghuo*), "love" (爱 *ai*), "spirit" (灵魂 *linghun*), and "understanding" (懂 *dong*). In combination with the soft colors and familiar aesthetic design of their covers, the prominence of these terms, apprehended together, worked together to confer feelings of warmth, comfort, and *homefulness*. Their full titles, including *Journey of the Soul* by Hu Yinmeng;[1] *The Places That Scare You* by Pema Chödrön;[2] and *This Light in Oneself* by Jiddu Krishnamurti[3] (to name just a few) thus invoked the home chronotope as well in the sense that they invoked, or *promised*, that readers might experience a sense of being-at-home-in-the-world. Apprehending them together, the horizon chronotope further came to life in their depiction of a relational body-self on an adventure of sorts, a journey toward a brighter, more loving future, or toward a particularly light-filled, loving, and meaningful experience of being-at-home-in-the-world.

The books—many of them translations of books from Taiwan, India, the United States, and Europe—thus constituted a consistent genre that emerged at the intersections of psychology, spirituality, and the "New Age." Like the collection of texts and practices characterized by Li Zhang as "the inner revolution" (内心的革命 neixin de geming), it was a hybrid genre emphasizing embodied experience (体验 tiyan), spirituality, and a distinctly nonanalytical "dialogue with images" (意象 yixiang) (Zhang 2020). Despite the fact that the books were predominantly translations of books originally written elsewhere, however, the Chinese script—some printed in calligraphic fonts, others in a simple, standard Songti font—tended to appear in larger, darker text on nearly all of the covers. The names of foreign authors here appeared only sometimes in English. Their full names were more frequently spelled out in Romanized letters on the inside cover, while the main cover displayed transliterations such as 梅乐蒂·碧媞 (*Meiledi Biti*: Melodie Beattie) or 艾克哈特·托尔 (*Aikehate Tuoer*, Eckhart Tolle), often displayed in the same sized font alongside the name of the Chinese translator. This symmetry seemed to situate the texts as Chinese, or at most as translations emerging out of a collaborative effort within which the customary hierarchy between author and translator is disrupted.

Contributing to a "linguistic landscape" or *chronotopeography* (Lyons and Karimzad 2019) that functioned as much as an aesthetic experience (Taylor 1989) as an invitation to content (Low 2017), the Chineseness of the texts—at least in terms of their appearance—thus similarly invoked the home chronotope. It also spoke to the process of *bentuhua* (本土化) or indigenization in the "living translation" of psychology in China (L. Zhang 2020; see also Pritzker 2014, 2016). "Bentuhua is not merely a local indigenization of imported Western knowledges and practices," Li Zhang writes, "rather, it is a creative and dialogic course involving bricolage and innovation. Its ultimate goal is not importation or adaptation but transformation by heeding to particular local culture, history, and real societal problems" (2020, 67). The concept of living translation similarly engages translation as a continuous process of inscription, interaction, embodiment, and practice that involves not just leaders but also everyday practitioners (Pritzker 2012, 2014). Here, one must also consider the ways in which most of the texts and practices, at least at the outset of New Life's formation in China, were translations or even adaptations that had not traveled directly from the West. As briefly mentioned in the introduction, they came, instead, through Taiwanese translations of Western and Indian masters. In the process, Taiwanese practitioners and translators had also engaged in an active indigenizing process (Farrelly 2017). From this perspective, the New Life directors, instructors, and staff who contributed to decisions about which texts to display at the center (and how) must also be seen as critical actors who played a key role in enacting *bentuhua*.

It is thus important to attend to the ways in which particular readers were engaged by these texts within particular moments and in relation to the particular circumstances in their everyday lives at the time. Alongside the perspective offered by Louise Woodstock, who comments upon the ways in which self-help books "urge meanings on people by encouraging the adoption of subject positions" (2005, 157), it is here also important to foreground the ways in which particular subjects engage *with* the various texts at various points along their "journey" in self-development. Citing Bakhtin, Elinor Ochs and Lisa Capps note, for example, that "Bakhtin considered readers to be authors and the act of reading to be a dialogue between a text already produced and a reactive text created by a reader" (2001, 3). The framework of living translation—as developed both in the context of translating the theories and practices of Chinese medicine into American settings as well as in the translation of psychology in China—is, indeed, explicitly grounded in such a perspective. Living translation thus emphasizes how "textual material "come[s] alive" (Pritzker 2016, 152) as an embodied, affective experience of both content and atmosphere. In addition to considering the design, formatting, and referential meanings conveyed by particular texts, in other words, one also must consider the way they are encountered within and as *atmosphere* with particular kinds of effects upon different body-selves in and over time. I frequently overheard participants discussing various texts, for example, recommending, evaluating, and debating various approaches to spirituality or psychological self-evaluation promoted by each. Such conversations, I noted, were often held in place by a variably shared orientation toward home and horizon chronotopes as well as the tension between them.

In investigating the historical trajectories of the genre of body-mind-spirit through Taiwan, moreover, it is also relevant to note that many of the prominent author-translators featured at New Life explicitly described their life-changing encounters with specific texts or collections of texts. C. C. Wang, for example, who worked to develop the New Age in Taiwan as early as the 1970s, noted a range of deeply impactful experiences that emerged in response to reading Kahlil Gibran's *The Prophet* in 1968. "Even though she did not understand all of the vocabulary or some of the more obscure passages, she could still feel the beauty of the text," (Farrelly 2017, 305; citing Wang 1969b). Terry Hu, an author and translator who continues to exert an enormous influence on body-mind-spirit in both Taiwan and mainland China, similarly describes how actress Shirley MacLaine's book *Shifting Gears* inspired her "to reassess her life." Simply *seeing* Krishnamurti's face on the cover of his books compelled her, moreover, not only to purchase all of them, but to consume them immediately (Farrelly 2017, 317). Struck by the force of Krishnamurti's wisdom, Hu would later go on to translate many of these same texts into Chinese, first in Taiwan and (even later) in the Chinese mainland.

Texts, it was clear from observing interactions at the center, also played a huge role in the way people engaged with themselves and others in the space as well as beyond the space, for example, at home or at work. Julie—one of the lead staff members of the center during this research—shared a particularly resonant and impactful encounter she had experienced with the texts upon her first visit to New Life. She noted, here, how she had first attended an evening reading group and had been, immediately upon entering, *struck* by the texts in the space.

"I couldn't understand many of them (看不懂 *kanbudong*)," she said, "but I just felt that I really *needed* them. Like they were *my* books."

Julie went on to provide a chronotopic context in terms of where she was "at" in her life at that moment. She was pregnant and feeling extremely anxious all the time. There were tensions at home with her husband and her mother-in-law, who had been on her case for years to have a baby and who had become, once Julie *was* pregnant, even more intolerable and invasive. Despite having attended many trainings in psychology, including a long course that had established her as a professional counselor, she still felt like the books at New Life were mysterious and difficult to understand. Casting a poetic, rhetorically effective contrast between her lack of knowledge and the *feeling* that she not only needed them but that, in fact, they already *belonged* to her (e.g., "these were *my* books"), Julie situated her own agency here somewhere beyond herself, as if instead of the books belonging to her, *she* somehow belonged to the books.

Texts, as philosopher Charles Taylor writes, offer the possibility "of articulating our feelings or our story so as to bring us in contact with sources we have been longing for . . . or through recasting our lives in a new narrative" (1989, 97). The texts at New Life affected Julie in ways that reflect both Wang's and Hu's own initial encounters with the originals. The kind of dialogue that Bakhtin refers to as coemerging between reader and text, presumably referring to the text beyond the cover, was initiated for Julie—as for both Wang and Hu—simply by being in the space and seeing the titles, the covers, and some of the words, however mysterious they seemed. Without understanding them, let alone reading them, Julie thus noted how they seemed to offer her a deeply compelling promise, a new set of horizons that related directly to her current situation within her home. One could thus also say that the books served as an *ethical affordance*, defined specifically by Keane (2014, 7) as anything (objects, other people, the environment, ideas, and so forth) "that [a person] may draw on as they make ethical evaluations and decisions, whether consciously or not." The relationship that Julie instantly formed with the books, in other words, turned them into ethical objects that exerted a moral, affective force upon her. One might even suggest that they offered her a sense of homecoming within which she felt that these were not just any books but were instead *her* books. They also provided her with a new ethical horizon, a sense of *hope* in terms of what they might offer for her particular dilemma.

Here, it is worth revisiting the fact that Julie, at the time, had a great deal of experience in psychology, including much of the massive body of self-help and psychological literature occupying bookstores, magazine stands, and online spaces in China (J. Yang 2018a; L. Zhang 2020) as well as the popular psychological training sessions often run by large companies motivated largely by profit in China (H-Y. Huang 2014), New Life was different for Julie, however, and notably emerged in contrast to the psychotherapeutic genre she had come to know. This contrast, one could argue, may have related to the small, homelike "boutique" environment of New Life. It could have also related to the particular ways they combined psychology with Hindu and Sufi spirituality in an assemblage that distinguished it from other forms of popular therapy at the time, which often tended to integrate more familiar forms of spirituality such as Buddhism, Daoism, and Confucianism (L. Zhang 2020). It is notable, however, that his sense of contrast, of *something different*, offered her an immediate and profound sense that she was, just by being in the space, already beginning to entangle differently in and with the world.

BOUNDARY MAKING

The boundary between New Life and the outside world was often never clearer than in the ritual activities that marked entries into and exits out of the space. In the opening vignette, as discussed above, the music, seating arrangements, lighting, the teacher's remarks, and the introductory circle, both separately and in combination, served to ritually invoke both the home and horizon chronotopes in multiple ways. In a further examination of comments uttered by participants during opening and closing circles, this section examines the ways in which home and horizon chronotopes served to formulate the center as a space apart, a space of possibility, and a space of collectivity or "sameness" across (perceived) difference.

Opening the Space

Importantly, the word "home" was not necessarily always explicitly mentioned within opening circles, as it was in the vignette that opened this chapter. The home chronotope, alongside the horizon chronotope, was nevertheless indexed or "gesturally invoked" (Ochs 2012). Comments during opening circles thus frequently drew on various configurations of the home chronotope, without necessarily using the term, to formulate the center as a space-time of warmth, nourishment, human connection, personal expansiveness, and possibility within which participants might begin to entangle differently with others as well as with self, nation, and memory. During the opening circle at a 2015 free salon, for example, a participant introduced herself as someone with a fairly extensive background in New Life events and products. She then went on to issue a comment about how "this atmosphere (这个氛围 *fenwei*) gives me a feeling of relaxing and setting down (放松和放下的感受 *fangsong he fangxia de ganshou*)."

Here, as in the opening vignette, the participant's reference to "this atmosphere" served as scale-making device that situated the speaker and those who were co-present both affectively and morally in a distinct time and space. Though she did not explicitly use the word "home," she described the feeling that the space conferred upon her as "relaxing and settling down" (放松和放下 *fangsong he fangxia*). Here, she used a melodic phrase that conjured images of "coming home from a long day of work and collapsing on the couch" (Di Luo, personal communication 2020). The "melody," specifically, derives from the parallelistic pairing of the word 放 *fang* (to set down), first with 松 *song* (loose) and then with 下 *xia* (down), leading to *fangsong he fangxia* (放松和放下). The phrase likewise hinges on a deeply familiar syllabic and prosodic patterning (1–2, 1-2-3) known as *wuyan* 五言 ("five speakings") in Chinese (Link 2013). As Perry Link notes, in Chinese text and speech, both parallelism and the five-beat *wuyan* "can produce senses of naturalness, authority, or 'fit'," especially when paired together (103). The phrase is thus grammatically, semantically, and aurally arranged as a kind of metonym or mirror of the sense of homefulness it describes.

In this case, moreover, the descriptor was explicitly tied to the space, thus emphasizing the grammatical positioning of "this atmosphere" as agentive. Specifically, the atmosphere was situated as actively "giving" her a feeling of relaxation. This participant thus actively invoked the space as itself a kind of *agent* that worked *upon* the bodies of those who engage with it and within it. The idea that it was natural and fitting to feel relaxed and settled within and indeed *by* or in response to the space—qualities that corresponds to an ideal home-place—was thus enforced or even *evoked* by this comment.

In yet another example, a participant who spoke during an introductory circle at a weekend event in 2016 likewise began with an articulation of the home chronotope. "I feel so much nourishment (滋养 *ziyang*) here," she said. "Everyone is wide open (敞开 *changkai*). No one wears any kind of mask (面具 *mianju*) and we can all speak openly from our hearts."

In this comment, the speaker chronotopically mapped the space as a space-time of *nourishment* within which people were (or could become) "wide open." Suggesting that, in her experience, the center contrasted with other spaces where people are imagined to be "closed" or where they "wear masks" in order to fulfill others' expectations, this speaker further implied that the space was distinctive. The comment thus emerged as a potential index of the kinds of disorientation and isolation that people were inevitably confronting in their everyday lives in urban China in the mid-2010s. Like the previous examples, this chronotopic formulation of the moral, relational, and affective geography of New Life contributed to the turn-by-turn scaling of the space or context vis-à-vis a constructed contrast between the outside world and the center.

Invocations of home chronotopes at New Life, I thus argue, worked as collaboratively enacted affective-discursive spatializing or "homemaking" (Rapport 2018) projects. These frequently drew, moreover, on past personal as well as shared experiences both inside and outside of the space. Suggesting that the affective geography of the space might work upon others in a similar way, such comments further worked alongside the horizon chronotope in crafting the intimate geography of the space as an anticipatory mode that hinged upon the notions of possibility and collective transformation.

Closing the Space

Closing rituals were likewise rich with ritualistic chronotopic forms marking the boundary between New Life and the outside world. In closing circles, participants also often elaborated specifically on their experience of the preceding event, frequently noting how activities had seemed to help them and sometimes bringing up further questions. Often couched in expressions of gratitude to teachers, staff, and other participants, closing comments were also an opportunity for participants to remark upon their relational experience within the space.

At the close of one evening inner child salon in 2014, for example, one of the men who was attending for the first time told us that he felt like he'd learned a lot over the course of the evening.

"But the most important experience I've had," he finally noted, "is that I feel people really are the same—everyone's emotions are the same." He was surprised and comforted by this, he told us, because he had always assumed that he was fundamentally different from others.

On yet another evening in 2014, a middle-aged newcomer told us that she had similarly felt a sense of recognition throughout the night as she had listened to everyone talk.

"It seemed like I saw myself in so many people's stories. They worry about their mothers or their children—I have all this, too—including the things people said about fear, and also self-denial or self-disapproval."

These comments, and hundreds more like them that I recorded in my field notes over the course of this research, reflect the kinds of intimate "psysociality" (Duncan 2017, 2018) that often emerged as a moral, relational, and affective atmosphere of intimacy and nourishment or "homefulness." They likewise suggest a bit of how this intimacy inhered for many participants who, simply in witnessing *other* participants, were moved in ways that were both surprising and unexpected. After a daylong *jiapai* (family constellation therapy) workshop in 2016, a newcomer noted the ways in which she had seen "her own reflection" in everyone else.

"Even though I didn't get to do a constellation," she said, smiling, "even sitting outside and watching, I had a very deep experience."

During closing circles, newcomers and long-term clients alike also frequently drew either an implicit or explicit chronotopic contrast between their (previously) normative way of being in the world and their lived experience of the atmosphere at New Life. Participants here often suggested that they had always felt isolated and "different" as well as "distant" from others. Indeed, the shift in relational experience that had occurred for many participants contributed to what I discuss later in this book as a deeply embodied, relational sense of "defrosting" that not only indexed the intimacy and relational nourishment of the home chronotope, but was further tied to specific horizons of possibility that had opened up for them, often in relation to specific relationships or other current challenges: "Suddenly, I seemed to understand a little bit about the way my husband is," said the participant who described how she had been able to see herself in others' stories, for example.

The chronotopic contrasts and scalar associations that were crafted during closing comments also, however, afforded the opportunity to (re)consider and experiment with recasting oneself in relation to a range of normative and hegemonic cultural chronotopes and their attendant ideologies, behaviors, and relational practices. During a closing circle in 2014, for example, a return participant offered a commentary on how the events that day had informed her perspective on what she framed as a cultural tendency to deny the self:

"We are often [so hard on] ourselves—at work, there is so much stress, and we can forget ourselves," she began, going on to note how she felt like New Life offered a space in which "we" could, in the future, "remember" to enact various forms of relational self-care.

Notably speaking in the third-person plural, this participant drew upon pronouns to deictically invoke a collective, cultural "we" whose experience was similar to hers. Indeed, the deictic (or pronominal) formulation of a relational "we" during closing circles at the center often worked to (re)instantiate New Life as a distinct space in which participants presumably shared a set of common cultural, even familial experiences, orientations, and histories. This, I suggest, contributed to and amplified the feeling of "being home" for many participants, regulars and newcomers alike. Closing statements thus frequently formulated the kind of "work" we were doing at the center as a *collective* experience. After a *jiapai* workshop in 2016, for example, a relative newcomer observed that *jiapai* seemed to have a kind of "collective usefulness" (集体作用 *jiti zuoyong*) whether or not one had participated in a constellation. On another evening in 2016, a man who had been quiet for much of the daylong event similarly commented on how the class had offered him an experience of "collective development" (共同成长 *gongtong chengzhang*). A male-presenting participant in 2014 likewise noted what he described as the "power" of the collective at New Life.

"What I wanted to say," he noted, "is that the power of the group is actually very, very powerful. This isn't like a person on their own—it isn't something one person can achieve on their own simply by working diligently. Everyone here puts their whole hearts in to work together. So thank you to everyone!"

Drawing upon a chronotopic depiction of the immediate space ("here") as one in which "everyone puts their whole hearts in," this participant notably formulated an *enduring* experience of the center. Underscoring the relational "power of the group" at New Life, this comment also notably mapped the space-time of psychospiritual self-development as a collective project requiring collaborative effort. Thus, by invoking the intimate "home" chronotope as an ongoing relational experience, this participant further highlighted the horizon-like nature of such effort as an ongoing project that he saw as inherently linked to the collaborative contributions of "everyone" present in the space.

Variations on the theme of collaborative, collective power were, in fact, present in some form in the closing circles of nearly every workshop I attended at New Life. Underscoring the co-construction of a perceived "sameness" that contributed to the ways in which, as I argue throughout this book, New Life emerged as a kind of middle-class Hantopia, it raises the question of how intimacy developed in a way that perpetuated broader social differences, for example between Han citizens and ethnic minorities, between relatively wealthy urban residents and poor or rural migrants, or both.

It also, however, begs the question of the ways in which instructors, staff, and other long-time participants seemed sometimes to provoke or "push" the conversation, especially during closing circles, toward a recognition of intimacy and collectivity. Underscoring how co-operative action often takes shape as "new action is built by decomposing and reusing . . . the resources made available by the earlier actions of others" (C. Goodwin 2018, 1), contributions from newcomers and others speaking later in the circle might be seen as a form of mimesis where they were simply following the lead of long-time participants who had been socialized by instructors.

Newcomers also often offered novel insights based on their own experience, however. The following sequence of closing comments thus demonstrates the ways in which we might rather see input from newcomers during closing circles as *building* upon previous utterances rather than simply echoing or mimicking them. The sequence took place at the outset of the closing circle during a family constellation workshop in 2016 when a regular participant began the ritual by offering gratitude all who were co-present.

"Thank you for supporting me (支持我 *zhichi wo*) every time [I come]," he said. Spoken in the context of an embodied configuration in which we were literally supporting one another as we stood holding hands in a large, misshapen circle, this comment notably drew upon a chronotopic formulation of *repetition* ("every time") to map the space-time of the center as consistently homelike. The further implication here, however, was that this participant saw himself as engaged in an ongoing project of moving or living toward an unspoken yet imagined horizon that required consistent support. A newer participant who was returning for the second time spoke next.

"I've been wanting to thank every one of you all along. This is my second time coming," she continued. "Each time, there is a different kind of experience (感受 *ganshou*). It's like every time I can see more things. And this process is also very painful. But I feel like I can face it. This is good."

Formulating her experience in temporal terms that indexed both the duration of the daylong event ("all along") as well as her previous encounter with the center, the participant here highlighted her *return* to the space. As with the previous participant's comments, it also foregrounded her relational experience of New Life specifically with regard to the experience of beginning to see new things and make new connections as a result of her experience within the space. Formulated throughout as a distinctly personal experience—indeed, one that was "painful" but which she nevertheless felt capable of facing—this comment can be seen as building upon and significantly expanding the prior speaker's fairly minimal contribution. An even newer participant went next, beginning to speak softly.

"Everyone is opening their mouths to say thank you. I am no exception," he said, "because today it is my first time attending this salon." Proceeding to describe how he had had a "deep experience" that day, he further recalled a particular lesson in which Teacher Chao had discussed the way memories are sometimes lodged in environments as well as individuals.

"As Teacher Chao explained when he opened the space (开场 *kaichang*) this morning," he said, "every place leaves a record. It's true, I believe it—

I've seen my own reflection in every single person here. This is the greatest reward—thank you all."

Waiting until almost the end of the circle to speak, this participant specifically indicated the ways in which he intended hs comment to work alongside the utterances of those who had spoken previously. Including himself in the group, he thus noted that he was "no exception." Further describing the "depth" of his personal experience, he also tied the particular insights that he had garnered to Teacher Chao's opening lecture. Specifically, he repeated Chao's teaching about the ways in which "every place leaves a record" upon the embodied experience of its occupants. Though in his lecture Chao had in fact been describing the impression left by *past* places upon the bodies of participants, the speaker here notably drew upon the lesson to chronotopically map the ways that *this* place had impacted him. Further pointing to the experience of "collective development," his framing of being able to see his reflection in co-present others as a "reward" or "result" (收获 *shouhuo*) speaks to both home and horizon chronotopes, thus mapping the space-time of New Life as one of both nourishment and promise.

Though not necessarily instituting a *uniform* experience, closing sequences—alongside the sequences of comments offered during opening circles—thus contributed to the co-construction of the center simultaneously as a space apart and a space of possibility, and as a space of collectivity or collaborative experience. Raising multiple questions about the ultimate social impact of New Life and other similar sites, home and horizon chronotopes uttered by participants nevertheless complicate the assessment of the center as (only) a commodified or neoliberal space. Here, what Irvine and Gal (2000) call *fractal recursivity* was thus evident in the moral mapping of home/not-home contrasts and horizoned promises. Defined as "the projection of an opposition, salient at some level of relationship, onto some other level" (2000, 38), fractal recursivity points to the ways in which distinctions such as East/West, inside/outside, public/private, and so on act as "way[s] of bundling qualities into contrast sets and using them to characterize phenomena" (Gal 2016, 91). Fractal recursions, suggest Irvine and Gal, thus work as discursive scaling tools that distinguish spaces, types of people, and many other social processes. As such, they often emerge as chronotopic formulations that situate current interlocutors vis-à-vis dominant ideologies, moral discourses, and patterns of interaction.

It is thus important to attend to the the ways in which chronotopes function to construct the very spaces they describe as distinct *moral* spheres that do not always map easily onto assumed binaries between "public" and "private" as indexical of "incompatible moral principles" (Gal 2002, 79). Gal thus argues how particular instances of such geographic *scalings* or "recursions" point not to stable and distinct spaces but instead work as "tools for arguments about and in that world" that thereby "(re)construct the world" (2002, 86). Pointing to the indeterminacy of atmosphere centered by Sumartojo and Pink (2019), Gal further notes how such reconstructions are "never entirely mimetic" (2002, 86). Recursion, instead, leaves space for a kind of revision or interrogation. This space—even though it was often implicit and "tiny" in terms of the agency it afforded—did often give rise to a collaborative practice of scalar inquiry in which participants collectively interrogated a range of dominant cultural chronotopes and took part in a what I discuss in the following chapters as a kind of cultural "theory-building" (Rosa 2019).

CONCLUDING REFLECTIONS

Throughout this chapter, I have described how the home and horizon chronotopes took shape as *atmosphere* at New Life. They were evident in the aesthetics of the space, including the layout, the lighting, the music, and the linguistic landscape offered by the flyers and texts, for example, as well as within the titles of specific texts. I also provided a detailed account of how these interrelated chronotopes came to life in multiparty interactions involving teachers, students, and staff. Comments offered during opening and closing circles, I noted here, often invoked a chronotopic contrast between New Life and "the outside world." The notion of "home" here facilitated a chronotopic contrast with more broadly societal spaces as consisting of stress, anxiety, chaos, and disorientation as well as the personal lived experiences of participants' private homes. The horizon chronotope, on the other hand, enacted a kind of promise or hope for the possible future.

Especially in opening and closing circles, I have thus shown, the chronotopic invocation of home at New Life provided scaffolding for the continual co-creation of boundaries around the space. I also noted, however, how it afforded the interrogation and (re)scaling of shared discourses of "home" in China, and how spatiotemporally, morally, and relationally emergent "horizons" of possibility opened up the space for participants to consider different ways of thinking about and relating to the very notion of home.

As a spatiotemporal framework that guided interaction, I have suggested the home and horizon chronotopes at New Life, often working in tandem, generated a rich moral, affective, and embodied relational geography that simultaneously invoked dominant ideas of homefulness at the same time as instigating participants' desires for a relationally situated form of development or growth. The promise of concurrently personal, relational, and cultural possibilities for "being-at-home-in-the-world" (Jackson 1995) in new ways thus constituted a central component of the horizon chronotope at New Life. Learning to love, in this sense, constituted a simultaneous experience of intimacy and the possibility of intimacy, both of which were held in place within both aesthetic forms and ritually situated human interactions at the center.

Many studies focusing on therapeutic milieus in China and globally situate individuals trading in horizons or promises as charlatans who capitalize on the suffering of others. Indeed, the promises of various "masters," Li Zhang observes, sometimes "became frail" as they fail to deliver either happiness or fulfillment to clients (2020, 185). "At the same time," she further notes, "one cannot easily dismiss the power of this promissory lure offered by psychological and spiritual practices because they produce tangible effects on shaping people's lived experience" (206). Paul Heelas (2008) likewise notes that the notion of "spiritual horizons" often functions, in other subjective life spirituality settings, to provide *inspirational* rather than *achievable* goals. "Spiritual horizons are meant to serve to inspire; to enable participants to move past their limited frames of reference; to take them out of their 'normal' selves," he thus writes (2008, 123). As I have shown here, the promise or suggestion that participants would find a new framework for understanding their suffering through their engagement with the people and products of New Life was often initiated and maintained in and through interaction among not just teachers and staff but also among participants themselves. Both long-time clients and newcomers were active in co-constructing the atmosphere of the center through both home and horizon chronotopes in any given moment.

The invocation of home/horizon chronotopes at New Life undoubtedly had diverse effects on different bodies in the space, however. One might imagine that newcomers, for example, sometimes found it odd and disconcerting. As suggested by the closing comments described above, many newcomers experienced an enormous sense of relief and a newfound sense of connection on their first visit. In many of these comments, it seemed as if participants felt (or at least reported their experience) as if they *had*, indeed, returned home, or had at least begun to see new horizons of possibility for being-at-home-in-the-world as well as being with others, or both. Home and horizon chronotopes here contributed to the formulation of the atmosphere as a *collective* experience that calls into question the notion of self-development as a necessarily individualizing discourse.

It is critical to observe, however, that the kind of collectivity that took shape here was both ethnically homogenous and socioeconomically exclusive as well as an eminently heteronormative *Han* space. The collaborative co-construction of the center as what I have been calling a "Hantopia"—though it afforded the co-operative emergence of an atmosphere that moved participants to feel less isolated and disconnected—also contributed to the erasure of difference in terms of both culture and ethnicity. In this sense, events at New Life implicitly reproduced the state-sanctioned goal of "social harmony" at the same time as it drew certain aspects of normative everyday experience into question. I have nevertheless suggested how the atmosphere at New Life invited participants to not only "disentangle" (L. Zhang 2020) but also to *entangle differently* with one another as well as with a number of culturally salient ideologies. Such encounters sometimes even afforded an unexpected effect that, Sumartojo and Pink suggest, is possible in any atmosphere and includes "the possibility of unsettling official discourse" (2019, 123). As I suggest in the next chapter, for example, the intimate embodied geography of New Life, within interactions and exercises occurring between the opening and closing circles, seemed to move at least some participants, through the experience of what I discuss as "the expanded self," to reconsider the very notion of the "Great Self," or *dawo* (大我), in China.

3

Great/Small Self

> We cannot talk about a body without knowing what supports that body and what its relation to that support—or lack of support—might be. In this way, the body is less an entity than a relation, and it cannot be fully dissociated from the infrastructural and environmental conditions of its living.
> —JUDITH BUTLER

I met Lina, a forty-five-year-old woman who spoke multiple languages and worked as a high-ranking executive at an international corporation, when I sat next to her at a daylong *jiapai* seminar in 2016. When she introduced herself in the opening circle, she told us that it was her second time coming to New Life. She then immediately commented upon how her previous experience had surprised her. A few days later, during a one-on-one interview we conducted at my apartment, Lina elaborated on the ways in which her first experience at the center had elicited feelings of uncertainty as well as curiosity. What she described as the "mysterious quality" of the center had been apparent to her, she told me, from the moment she walked in. Having expected a lecture format, she had been struck by the organization of the space and the feeling of intimacy during the opening circle.

The first exercise she had participated in, moreover, struck her as especially odd, even shocking. It involved standing face to face with another participant who she was instructed to imagine was someone close to her. They were to remain silent until the instructor rang a bell. Lina described feeling awkward and unsure of herself as the room went quiet and she looked around her to see about ten pairs of participants standing about three feet away from one another, gazing into one other's eyes.

"And so . . . we stand up to each other?," Lina said, describing her experience of standing opposite a stranger, "and she put her hands on my shoulders? And then, so I put my hands on her shoulders and we sort of look at each other, and I don't know *what* to do. And so she just like comes over to me, and she said something just like—I can't even quite remember—she said 'I want to be with you,' she said 'I love you,' and she said, like, 'if you're not happy I'm not happy.' And that's my *son*, actually. I was thinking about my son." Lina referred here to her ten-year-old son, who was living in Japan with his father—Lina's estranged husband—at the time.

"Then she said something," Lina continued, "and I suddenly really, like, *melt*. That moment when she looked at me. It was kind of strange—I, I only spoke with her for a few minutes, and I like I went over there and totally hugged this stranger across the shoulders. I was like 'what the hell'?"

Lina was laughing as she finished telling me her story. Here, she reiterated the sheer oddity and intimacy of this exercise—within which a strange woman seemed to somehow embody her young son—emphasizing how it had struck her body as a force that caused her normative sense of embodied, emotional containment to "melt." This message from her son—that he loved her and wanted to be with her but also wanted to see her happy— had nevertheless stuck with her. Indeed, since that first class just under a month ago, Lina had begun to focus on a question she has never considered before.

"I'm beginning to wonder if I have ever loved my husband," she said. "Actually, I'm wondering if I've ever loved anyone—if I even know *how* to love." The opening up of this new question, Lina explained, was one of the reasons she returned to the center for a second time.

RECONFIGURING THE BODY-SELF

In the previous chapter, I discussed the ways in which the intimate geography or "atmosphere" of the center emerged, within the aesthetics of the space as well as within "co-operative action" (C. Goodwin 2018) between participants, as a space apart as well as a space of (collective) possibility. Both intimacy and the possibility of intimacy, I suggested, were chronotopically held in place physically or aesthetically as well as in ritually formulated interactions that "opened" and "closed" events. I discussed how these contrasts implicated the embodied, affective experience of participants and indexed broader cultural chronotopes.

As a complement to my previous discussion, this chapter further examines the affective, embodied, and moral geography of New Life as it took shape *during* events. My analyses emphasize, for example, how the space-time between opening and closing circles emerged as a kind of "emotion realm" (情境 *qingjing*) (Lam 2018), or atmosphere, within which embodied experience, feelings, movement, and interaction became spatial as well as temporal. As such, I suggest here, we might observe the complex process through which intimate forms of psy/psychosociality emerged at the center (Duncan 2018; Matza 2018; L. Zhang 2020). Emphasizing the ways in which within interactions "the body becomes a field of experience" (Goodwin and Cekaite 2018, 14), I thus investigate the embodied rhythm of interactions and movements as participants *attuned* to one another in various exercises like the one described above. I draw here on the notion that "attunement is neither only verbal/explicit or nonverbal/implicit" but rather "can be imagined as an always-fluid changing wave, interactively constituting a field having emotional significance" (Knoblauch 2021, 90). In addition to aesthetics and interaction, then, the chapter focuses upon how multichanneled embodied displays of (inter)subjectivity involving silence, gaze, language, and *touch* (Goodwin and Cekaite 2018) contributed to the development and maintenance of what Lina described as a "mysterious atmosphere" at New Life.

Underscoring the ways in which the body—as Judith Butler frames it in the epigraph to this chapter—is "less an entity than a relation" (2016, 19), the intercorporeal, multimodal emergence of this atmosphere further points to the kind of "affective, expressive relationality" that Heelas (2008) describes as "feeling-with": a relational mode often central in what he calls spiritualities of life milieus. Throughout this chapter, I thus emphasize the ways in which many participants were guided toward a novel way of "being-emotional-with," which I discuss here as the *enregisterment of intimacy* (Pritzker 2017). Alongside the concept of the "enregisterment of emotion" in explicit verbal forms (Irvine 1990), I suggest that the enregisterment of intimacy took shape in interactions that not only involved the voiced expression of feelings but also included—as in Lina's encounter—embodied position and proximity, sustained eye contact, tears, laughter, and touch.

Importantly, the kind of intercorporeal intimacy I am discussing here, however, existed not as a "given" but rather as an invitation that was taken up differently by particular participants, especially with regard to their shifting intersectional proximity to power in terms of gender, class background, and (sometimes) ethnicity in particular encounters. It also, importantly, took shape in relation to participants' immediate relational predicaments, their relative experience within therapeutic communities, and their habituated and socially constructed embodied capacity for connecting physically with others or tolerating discomfort, or both, as it occurred in a given encounter. Intercorporeal and affective intimacy was nevertheless frequently described by teachers as an important component of events. As described in a translated WeChat article circulated by center staff in 2015, for example, the space itself and the exercises were designed such that "each person's work is everyone's work" and the work is therefore simultaneously "both individual and collective."[1] The goal of many of the exercises and the practices might thus be framed, as prominent inner child therapist Wu Zhihong discusses it (2015),[2] as developing participants' "telepathy" (心灵感应 *xinling ganying*). As a cultivated awareness of the interconnection of different bodies, telepathy here refers to the body's ability to *feel* and sense the world, including other people's experiences. Embodied awareness cultivated in a group setting, writes Staci K. Haines, "can remind us that we are human, connected to a much wider fabric of life" (2019, 18). The "self," in this framing, is neither an individualized self nor a collectively dispersed self. It is, rather, a pathway to interconnection and new forms of intimate relationality. I thus focus, here, on the ways in which the kinds of intense, affective, discursive, and embodied encounters at New Life—like Lina's hug, for example—at times served as an affordance for participants to begin to rescale themselves in relation to intimate others in their lives as well as to fundamental concepts such as "the self" and "love."

This chapter thus engages with the ways in which embodied encounters at New Life at least sometimes had the capacity to challenge and contest participants' deeply entrenched ways of experiencing the self, others, and the world more broadly. As the boundaries of participants' very body-selves sometimes shifted in sometimes profound ways—as they had for Lina with the stranger during her first exercise—people were often invited to question aspects of themselves, society, or both. After her intimate encounter with the stranger, for example, Lina's very capacity to love become fluid and contestable. In my discussion, I therefore go as far as to suggest that this relational process through which the self sometimes seems to expand often invited participants' to interrogate a number of culturally salient ideologies, including the very notion of the "Great Self," or *dawo* (大我), in China.

To be clear, the extended self that I am describing as a new kind of permeable, extended *dawo* might be considered more in terms of the way it emerged as a *potential* rather than a determinable "outcome" of New Life workshops. From this perspective, the examples examined here might best be considered "perplexing particulars" in which something out of the ordinary or unexpected occurred (Mattingly 2019). As a potentiality for disrupting and reconfiguring long-standing notions of the self that relate to dominant discourses and ideologies in China, however, I engage with particular embodied experiences of New Life (including my own) as a foundation for my discussion, in the following several chapters, of the ways in which psysociality in this setting moved some participants not only to reconsider their own selves but also worked to inspire at least some participants to "grapple with the social" as itself a form of self-development (Duncan 2018, 271). Always unfolding in and through interactions that included but were not limited to spoken dialogue, this chapter thus investigates the ways in which the enregisterment of intimacy at New Life afforded intimate forms of scalar inquiry that not only afforded "disentangling" but also *entangling differently* with the self and the worlds that the participants occupied.

BIG SELF, LITTLE SELF

Much ink has been spilled in pursuit of comprehensive and authoritative answers to the question of how the "self" or 自我 (*ziwo*) is constituted in (Han) Chinese society. Scholars focusing on the explication of classical, Confucian ideologies of selfhood, for example, often adopt a durative frame to emphasize the ways in which the private "small self" (小我 *xiaowo*) is always socially "embedded" within the "great" or "big" self (大我 *dawo*) in China (e.g., Tu 1985; J. Yang 2018a; L. Zhang 2020). The *dawo* here constitutes a fundamental moral orientation seen to derive from Confucian ethics, which emphasizes the importance of cultivating and at least aspiring toward what Tu Wei-ming describes as "an ever-expanding network of relationships" that begins with the "small body" (小体 *xiaoti*) and extends to the "big body" (大体 *dati*), including kin, neighbors, and the even the (Han) nation (1994, 180; see also L. Zhang 2020, 166).

Contrasts between the big/small self in China here often adopt a chronotopic framework to construct a geographic, spatialized distinction that opposes "the Chinese self" as a relational (big) self with "the Western self" as an individualized and privatized (small) self. The Western self is depicted here as "self-contained, autonomous, and atomic," for example (Seok 2017, 104). According to philosopher Bongrae Seok, "Asians" raised in "Confucian societies," on the other hand, embody selves who are fundamentally "relational, interactive, and interpersonal [and are] always open to others and the surrounding social environment" (2017, 104). Informed by this perspective on what is imagined as an enduring and consistent "Eastern self," scholarship investigating Chinese selfhood in contemporary society thus also often engages with the very real ways in which economic, social, and political shifts have reformulated and fundamentally reoriented the boundaries of the traditional Chinese body-self. Harriett Evans, for example, argues that ideologies of "the individual self" have increasingly come to replace "a family oriented and collectivist ethics of personal responsibility molded by Confucian as well as socialist principles of personhood" (2012, 119). Such literature provides justified critical commentary on the ways in which capitalism, neoliberalism, and globalized forms of white supremacy, particularly in terms of ethics of normalcy with regard to selfhood and intimacy, disrupt deeply rooted forms of relationality in China. As such, this literature contributes to a further popular chronotopic formulation in which Chinese or more generally "Eastern" conceptualizations of the self become associated with the past, while "Western" notions of selfhood are associated with the present or the future, or both.

Other scholarship, however, interrogates the ways in which the contours of the *dawo* itself have been differently imagined for different actors over the course of Chinese history. In examining the discourse of the *dawo* in China, for example, Li Zhang emphasizes that, at least traditionally, "the moral project" of developing the Great Self "was meant primarily for elite men" (2020, 16). Conducting research in Taiwan in the 1980s, Margery Wolf likewise observes how the *dawo* emerged as a distinctly *gendered* body-self with different implications for men and women. She thus details the ways in which, from a young age, Chinese boys in her fieldsite were taught to embrace a simultaneously binding and expansive sense of themselves as spatiotemporally *continuous* (1994, 261). Girls, on the other hand, became aware from a young age that they "are not a part of anyone's historical past and seem to be irrelevant to anyone's future but their own and, they are told, to some known family in some unknown place" (1994, 261–2). Wolf thus contests the tendency to universalize the so-called Chinese self, questioning the widespread practice of "assum[ing] that what works for men can be applied to women as well, with some modifications for their 'special circumstances'." She thus concludes that, in the case of Chinese women, "the male model doesn't fit" (1994, 261).

Feuchtwang (2013), on the other hand, adopts a more historically specific point of view that encompasses all genders and investigates the ways in which the Great Self was reimagined, especially during the Maoist regime, as consisting of both the "*political* and domestic body" (2013, 225, italics mine). Nationalistic framings of the *dawo* as reflecting a traditional form of fundamental "Chineseness," Wielander (2018a-b) further notes, persist today. Underscoring the changeability of the so-called Chinese self, finally, yet other scholars take a more phenomenological or experiential approach to the fluidity of selfhood in China. Yan (2017), for example, reframes Chinese personhood as "a process of becoming" that is always situated in both space and time (2017, 10). Li Zhang (2020) likewise points to the ways in which both discourses and people's experiences of the self in China are constantly *in motion*. Emphasizing "the constant articulation and re-articulation of the self and the social," she thus examines the variable ways in which people in China actively engage with new ways of thinking about and enacting their "selves" (2020, 18).

Though representing different approaches and emphases, it might nonetheless be argued that, overall, scholarship on Chinese selfhood suggests a certain amount of flexibility in terms of the ways in which the *dawo* is conceived by different individuals at different times and in different social locations in China. The fluidity of the notion of self at the level of the individual, I argue, points to the ways in which culturally salient notions of "individualism" or "collectivism" constitute ideologies that, in everyday lived reality, "may be partial, situational, ad hoc, or inconsistent in nature" (Hollan 1992, 285). It further underscores the ways in which normative modes of enacting scalar intimacy are forged, as dominant cultural chronotopes are reproduced constantly in interactions, institutions, and less formal settings, thereby getting "inside" the body-selves of culturally situated actors (Pritzker and Perrino 2020). Hollan (1992) nevertheless underscores the ways in which, instead of looking for rigid and enduring forms of cultural personhood, anthropologists might rather center the processes through which people continually navigate their relationship to dominant discourses of the self. As a deeply affective and embodied way of enacting scalar intimacy, in other words, individual's ways of relating to and embodying ideologies of selfhood here inform their everyday experience of the self as well as the ways in which they understand their own body-self in relationship to other bodies as well as concepts like "love," "harmony," "order," or the Great Self itself, all of which become phenomenological *orienting devices* in future interactions (Ahmed 2007). Discourses of the self in China, in this sense, are not just about "the self" but also encompass cultural narratives about phenomenological experiences of relationality, filial piety, temporality, nationhood, morality, emotion, and gender, to name just a few.

As Lina's story demonstrates, moreover, this chapter investigates how experiential intimacy at New Life also afforded scalar *inquiry* as people began to interrogate the ways in which their "self" relates to other bodies as well as concepts and ideologies. Notions of selfhood might thus be reconsidered as concepts and benchmarks to which people relate but which are ultimately open to being interrogated and examined. Indeed, an ethnographic approach that appreciates this distinction is capable not only of recognizing cultural norms and ideals, writes Douglas Hollan, but also of observing "dimensions [of personhood] that are disvalued or those that are valued, tolerated, only in narrowly defined contexts" in a particular society (1992, 294). This perspective affords an appreciation of the moment-to-moment ways in which people variably engaged with or *related to* ideas about and prescriptions for enacting the so-called Great Self at New Life. In this sense, I argue, center events and workshops also often became a site for collaborative experiences wherein participants interrogated, examined, and sometimes contested long-standing cultural and moral norms of selfhood and relationality. Such a process was far from "individual," involving group affect and multiple kinds of (inter)corporeal exchange. Many forms of practice at New Life were thus presented as an embodied mode of seeing, listening, and feeling through which our body-selves were guided through encounters that often served as a foundation for the imagination of radically different relational futures.

THE DISTRIBUTED BODY

At New Life, the kinds of "mysterious" intercorporeal encounters like Lina described at the outset of this chapter often took place in concert with or in addition to exercises in which participants' body-selves were literally distributed across other bodies. In *mirroring* exercises, for example, participants acted as a reflection for one another in ways that often exceeded normal expectations of politeness. During the 2016 extended inner child workshop with Teacher Jo, for example, we were broken into groups of nine people. We were then positioned on chairs arranged in a kind of "T" shape, with four chairs facing one another and another positioned at the end facing the others. We were then to take turns in the "hot spot,"[3] remaining quiet while each of our group mates proposed what they observed us transmitting in our "shadow": the negative traits that we kept hidden, under normal circumstances, from ourselves and others.

When he introduced the exercise, Teacher Jo anticipated that it might be a struggle for some participants. He thus provided several examples of what we might say, and how. "I see someone with a lot of shame," he offered. "I see someone who has locked themselves in a castle and thrown away the key. I see someone who lives for others." He then acknowledged that some of the observations might be inaccurate or outright wrong. He suggested, however, that "if several people see the same thing, maybe there is something there."

We then began. A young woman in my group moved to the hot spot, and we proceeded to give her feedback. She was someone who needed others to like her and take her seriously, a group member told her. She was a bit closed and unforgiving toward herself, said another. A man who I had been calling "Harbin" in my notes smiled and said that she seemed to have no shadow, that she was all love.

Harbin said the same for the next participant, a middle-aged woman who was told by others that she lacked confidence and did not want to be seen, that she was anxious and afraid of her own power, that she was continually unable to meet her own expectations, and that she was overinvested in others' opinions of her.

A man was up next, and was told that he was easily nervous, with confidence fluctuating between very high and very low. Harbin again offered only positive feedback.

I was then told that I was too hard on myself, that I tended to work too hard, setting unmeetable goals and becoming exhausted. I carried a lot of sadness. I was also, not surprisingly, given only positive reflections from Harbin.

Harbin remained consistent, in this regard, with the following four participants, who were described, consecutively, as (1) using smiles to hide sadness and keeping secrets; (2) dependent on others' praise for self-esteem and a little pessimistic and guarded; (3) closed, cold, unreachable, and full of pressure, like a soda can that has been shaken but not opened; and (4) lost without others' positive regard and deeply afraid of criticism.

When it was finally Harbin's turn, we were honest. Several participants, myself included, here commented first on his unwillingness to see anything negative in others. It seemed, said one group member, like he was unwilling to accept others for who they really were, including their shadow. This had something to do with his *own* lack of confidence and self-acceptance, another offered, suggesting that it was also a reflection of his deep, unacknowledged anger.

After we each cycled through once, we were directed to run through the exercise again, this time telling our group what we had felt upon receiving their feedback. We were to begin with whoever was in the hot spot at the time. In our group, Harbin admitted that he was not happy to hear our feedback. Many of us had been spot on, however, he said with a crestfallen look on his face. He did always feel like he could never measure up, and also harbored a great deal of anxiety and anger.

I spoke next, also telling my group that their reflections were accurate. I also shared, however, that it was a powerful experience to be seen in the space not as an anthropologist or foreigner, but as myself. Another group member noted that our observation of his fluctuating self-confidence helped him understand his persistent inability to find direction in life. The man who was told that he kept secrets in his heart confirmed that this was accurate. He did it in order to feel safe, he reflected. "If people knew my secrets," he said, "they would realize that I am not good."

Another group member simply confirmed that we had been right, further noting that nothing had been a surprise, while another began to cry, telling us that she really does feel unsafe, and that she *was* always hard on herself. She felt particularly guilty, she further noted, for always being annoyed with her parents. The participant who was told that she was afraid of criticism likewise noted, burying her face in her hands as she spoke, that it was true. It was because she was constantly criticized when she was little, she added. Others were more restrained in their responses. One group member said that she could only remember the words "cold," "serious," and "sad."

"When I heard these words," she told us, "I knew they were true. But didn't want to accept it. I'm willing to face my sadness, but don't remember where it is from."

Most of the participants in my group thus overwhelmingly expressed the sense that others had been accurate in their observations. There was only one group member who did not confirm or disconfirm our accuracy, telling us that she "forgot" what we said as well as her experience as we gave her feedback.

"It was like you were talking about someone else. This is my shadow," she said.

Demonstrating how intimate forms of psysociality developed at New Life emerged through interactions that involved a great deal of talk but were nevertheless deeply embodied in terms of affect, gaze, and positioning, this exercise underscores the ways in which novel "genres of listening" (Marsilli-Vargas 2014) were explicitly cultivated within this space, while others were eschewed. Listening genres, notes Xochitl Marsilli-Vargas, "create structures of relevance that provide *directionality*," attuning us to what to hear as well as how to make meaning of what we hear, who we hear it from, and the implications for us or others (2014, 42; emphasis mine). Asking participants to become vulnerable to the gaze of others in a way that vastly exceeded the norms of everyday interaction, such encounters also underscored the ways in which the *permeability* of participants' body-selves was foregrounded at New Life. Pointing to the ways in which emotions are "shared intersubjective states" (Haviland 2003; Wilce 2009; see also Ochs and Schieffelin 1989; Besnier 1990; Goodwin and Goodwin 2000; Wilce 2014; Pritzker 2020), such encounters also worked to enregister intimacy as a kind of vulnerable and provocative relationality within which we were invited and invited others to "see" and "hear" one another in novel ways.

ENACTING THE INNER OTHER

What I have been discussing as the expanded self at New Life also emerged in what I call, in this section, "enactments." Here, the inner experience or habitual tendencies of particular participants—their experiences, emotions, or even family members—were given outer expression as they were enacted by other participants and witnessed by yet others. Though often explained by instructors as a learning opportunity for *individuals*, exercises like these required focal participants as well as witnesses to stretch the boundaries of their normative body-selves in ways that often felt both unfamiliar and uncomfortable.

Lina's description of the exercise in which she was guided to approach a stranger as if she had embodied someone close to her is one example of a typical enactment at New Life. As described in detail in chapter 5, family constellation therapy or *jiapai* also hinges upon enactments in which others embody the living or deceased relatives of a focal participant. Enactments were also frequently more mundane, however, in the sense that they involved members of the group who embodied various aspects of the focal participant.

During the 2016 extended inner child workshop, for example, Teacher Jo invited participants to enact a troublesome tendency—specifically, the tendency to procrastinate—of one participant, a thirty-five-year-old man named Bin. One participant was thus called up to embody Bin's procrastination, while another enacted the "taskmaster." While "Procrastination" sat fumbling on their phone, then, "Taskmaster" spoke harshly, telling Procrastination that they should stop screwing around with the phone and be more productive. Another representative, meanwhile, was called up to embody Bin's feeling that he was never good enough, a feeling he had expressed in response to observing the scene thus far. Watching the enactment emerge from there, with each of the three aspects of himself struggling, as Bin later described to the group, was disconcerting. Once Bin's "True Self" was brought into the scene to engage compassionately with the others, however, it was deeply moving for Bin. Several witnesses also shed tears as they observed Bin's enactment.

In another example, an impromptu enactment took shape during a 2014 inner child salon at New Life. In this case, a participant named Ning was struggling with an ongoing dilemma related to her recent decision to leave her family for an entire year in order to study counseling in a European program. Teacher Du then called several attendees up to represent and enact Ning's fear, excitement, and anger. As they interacted with one another, quickly getting into a wordless struggle that led to them turning their backs to one another, Ning watched closely and intensely. The exercise eventually resolved once Du guided the participants enacting Ning's inner landscape to "walk together." As I have observed in a previous article (Pritzker 2016), such exercises might be seen, on one hand, as instantiating ideologies of individual self-management and expression that resemble the therapeutic process that E. Summerson Carr describes as "taking inventory." Taking inventory, Carr notes, involves "boring down through internal layers of denial, anger, and shame toward the innermost storehouse of the self" (2011, 94) such that it is the individual, rather than prevailing social conditions or forms of political/economic oppression, who constitutes the site of dysfunction. As I have also observed, however, such exercises worked to "distribute emotion across multiple bodies in such a way that inner/outer distinctions ... become blurred, and the experience of one individual emerges as a co-narrated interaction among many" (Pritzker 2016, 161). Evoking an intense reaction from Ning that, we later learned, had motivated her to rethink her basic orientation toward her culturally situated, gendered self, enactments thus often functioned, on the other hand, to reconfigure the boundaries of participants' body-selves in ways that both amplified and challenged traditional ethical-relational notions of the self (Chinese or otherwise), even if only for the length of a particular workshop or salon. Often exceeding norms of respectability and politeness, they invited participants, in other words, into an affective and relational experience of the kind of intercorporeal permeability that, in Leticia Sabsay's words, constitutes "a transindividual way of being in the world" (2016, 286) that, despite constituting a fundamentally dialogic human reality, can either be avowed or disavowed in ways that have relational and even political consequences.

TIME TRAVEL

In inner child exercises—whether conducted in groups, pairs, or individually—the past was often formulated as a space-time to which we were able to "travel" and within which we became able to interact not just with other participants in the immediate present: we were also able to enact an active dialogue with our past selves, our caretakers, our teachers, and our childhood environment, to name just a few. What I describe as "time travel" here specifically involved communicating *with* and *about* the past as well as travel *to* the past. Often enacted in individual exercises that involved "splitting" the self into different characters—for example, one's inner child and one's parent—time travel also took shape in dyadic and group exercises that involved both (inter)corporeal intimacy and discursive interaction. Framed as an individual endeavor within which the fixed nature of the past became malleable, it occurred in exercises that also enacted an increased permeability *with* the past.

Inner child work is often engaged as a problematically individualizing form of therapy that "reduce[s] pain into *solely* the matter of an internalized, familialized self" (Ivy 1993, 243) and evades consideration of the ways in which one's childhood suffering may have been caused by structural inequalities rather than individual experience. I discuss here, however, how the kinds of intercorporeal engagement and "feeling-with" that served to enregister intimacy at New Life also sometimes afforded a social, cultural, and historical interrogation that brought to light shared histories as well as shared forms of suffering in the present. Indeed, John Bradshaw, author of Homecoming: Relcaiming and Championing Your Inner Child, himself very clearly notes how one of the keys to successful inner child therapy consists of its enactment in a group setting, where witnessing others going through the process emerges as an amelioration of one's own suffering and isolation (1990, 267).

Encountering one's inner child at New Life, though sometimes occurring as individual exercises such as instructor-led journeys through our childhood homes, often required working in pairs or small groups. They were, moreover, always conducted in groups within which participants sat alongside others doing the same exercise. Affect—whether verbally, aurally, or through movement or facial expression—often overflowed the boundaries of the particular body-selves situated in the space. Someone would often cry out or moan, for example, or begin wailing. At the conclusion of such "journeys," moreover, there would often be some kind of group movement or release.

Encounters with one's inner child, in these cases, often involved direct engagement with another participant who might, depending on the instructions given, be embodying some aspect of oneself or close others from one's past. An exercise that was common, for example, involved working in pairs with one partner embodying the other person's inner child. Usually enacted predominantly in silence—as with Lina's hug described at the outset of this chapter—it often included an extended period of time in which partners would hold one another's gaze. It also gave rise to various facial expressions, spontaneous movements, and intimate, nonsexual forms of touch that were frequently deeply moving for participants.

This was evident, for example, in the vivid recollection of doing this exercise for the first time told to me by Chao—an intern at New Life in his late twenties during the latter part of this fieldwork—during a one-on-one interview in 2016.

"The most moving experience I had when I first started attending these courses was in an inner child exercise—the one where a representative of your inner child stands in front of you. So you are facing them," Chao began.

Chao opened by centering the *I* as it occurred in the past (e.g., "the experience *I* had when *I* first started"). He switches quickly, however, going on to describe the exercise as "the one where a representative of *your* inner child is standing in front of *you*." In Chinese, the use of the second-person pronoun, as in English, is often used to index a generalized person (e.g., "one") (Kitagawa and Lehrer 1990). The "you" here arguably also worked as a form of recognition, an acknowledgment of our shared experience of this particular exercise in multiple workshops and thus our shared knowledge. He switched deictics here, however, shifting back to a first-person account as he moved back into a description of his particular experience with his partner during his first experience of the exercise.

"We stood there facing one another," he said, "and I just looked at him—he had this vacant and dazed (茫然 *mangran*) look, ah? And I felt like that, *that* was *exactly* like me when I was a child."

Seeking (and gaining) recognition from me here by using a common conversational marker ("ah?"), Chao here invoked another deictic term ("that") to describe how he had experienced the dazed look on his partner's face as "exactly like" himself when he was young. Chronotopically drawing both the distant and more recent past into the present such that his own lived experience had suddenly become visible in the body-self of another, Chao then suddenly shifted back to using the second-person pronoun to describe the *feeling* that this encounter inspired.

"And then all of a sudden," he said, taking a breath, "in that moment when you suddenly see the way you were when you were young—the impact is so huge."

Chao's use of the second-person pronouns here extends his previous framing, proposing as common knowledge the fact that the exercise impacts the way one feels upon encountering the past. Chao thus frames this moment as evoking a *universal* experience, or at least one that might be general enough for me to relate to. Chao thus situated the exercise as a shared relational experience enacted through bodies and, importantly, *vision*. Indeed, the kind of vision that Chao highlighted here points to the role of "third-person self-witnessing"—as I discuss in detail in chapter 5—that often emerges as a therapeutic intervention of sorts and (at the very least) offers a new perspective on the self (Libby and Eibach 2002; Sutin and Robbins 2008; Pritzker and Duncan 2019). Chao switched back to a first-person narration here, however, offering a personalized description of what he had framed as a common experience.

"And I just walked over and embraced him. That was so moving (触动 *chongdong*) to me," he recalled, "and in a moment I *knew*—the inner child, in that moment, went from being an idea to a real presence."

Like Lina, Chao foregrounded the ways in which his sudden move to approach and embrace his partner was not only unexpected but also "deeply moving." Referring here in the past tense to describe *that* moment as one within which *that* child shifted from being an idea to a "real presence," Chao formulated the immediate and relatively profound embodied impact that he had experienced with his partner as a shift in his fundamental way of knowing *the* inner child. By linking his experience to the ways in which "the" inner child became real here, in other words, he scaled fluidly between the personal and general, moving on to describe how this past experience constituted the foundation for the kind of guidance he provided to *others* in workshops one he became an instructor. Chao thus noted how his own embodied experience of seeing the dazed look on his inner child's face informed the ways in which he had trained himself to attend constantly to participants'—especially *male* participants—subtle embodied expressions.

As I discuss in further detail in chapter 7, Chao here offered a range of insights about the ways in which gender differences are often productively and intentionally upended at New Life. He offered numerous descriptions of his new sense of the embodied, relational, and affective *hardening* effects of masculinity in China, as well as setting forth a nuanced theory of gender, embodiment, and political ideology that observed how political ideas have become entrenched within the body-selves of the adult men and women who come to New Life. This scaling or expansion of Chao's experience thus speaks to the ways in which the extension of the individual body-self in various configurations at New Life took shape as an embodied experience that indexed shared histories and common experiences in the present as well as desires for the future. Events, practices, and policies of the past, present (or both) mapped as occurring "outside" of the body-self as well as in the past, were experienced here as existing not only "inside" of particular individuals but also inside of the space itself.

Chao's observations here likewise suggest how experiences of embodying the past or communicating *with* or *about* the past sometimes moved participants toward shared understandings *of* the past and at least tentative ideas about the possible future. In this sense, it was often the *social* experience of embodying the extended self in time travel that afforded participants' insight into the ways in which their own intimate relationship with the past was often brought to life as a shared experience of an often similar past that had also affected others in the room.

In one exercise at a large workshop in 2016, for example, over fifty of us were seated in two concentric circles. Participants seated in the outer circle were to embody the mothers of those in the inner circle. The children were guided to all speak at once. I was, in this case, the "mother" of a roughly forty-year-old participant who began by asking me why I had left the country when she was young, only coming back occasionally for mere days or even hours.

"I was heartbroken—I never felt good enough," she said, suddenly becoming more animated. The volume in the whole room, in fact, seemed to become louder all at once.

"I'm angry now," my partner said after a deep breath, "that I had to take care of *everything*." Joining in the collective fervor that seemed to be taking over the room as some begin to yell, she switched to an accusatory stance.

"You should just face it, you have a better life than many," she yelled. "Why can't you be happy and just accept me?" Her voice was loud and sharp, but after posing the question, she began to soften. A sound like a squeak began to emit from her throat.

"I took care of everything when Baba needed the operation," she continued, beginning to cry softly. "When things went wrong, I blamed myself and all of you blamed me. But how come my older brother wasn't handling any of it?"

Unlike in other exercises, in this case we were given no time to "process." Instead, Teacher Jo rang a bell and those in the inner circle were told to move one seat to the right while those in the outer circle remained in place. We then repeated the exercise, again and again, for about half an hour. Time and space seemingly began to blur as those of us in the outer circle repeatedly occupied the role of so many different participants' mothers. As we did, we stepped into multiple different time-zones, for example, depending on the age of our partner and the period of their childhood that they brought up. The outer circle here also included both male- and female-identifying participants, who were thus situated repeatedly in a position where they were occupying a different *gender*.

When those of us on the outside switched to occupy the inner circle, additionally, we were able to occupy the body-selves of our inner children with each new interaction that we had with outer-circle participants. As a co-operative and emergent experience, however, it seemed—once I was in the inner circle—that both the emotions I experienced and the words that came tumbling out of my mouth upon encountering each new partner were not necessarily conscious or "intentional." Nor were they linear. Between "mothers" (some of whom were men), for example, I moved from being a six year old in one moment to a ten year old in the next, a teenager in the next, and a toddler in the next. It felt, honestly, like a frenzy of emotion in which the rapid movement between embodiments in time, space, and gender (or apprehension of gender, as the case was for me) seemed to strip away *any* sense of coherent selfhood.

To conclude this section, then, I want to linger in the sheer *complexity* of the shared spatiotemporal, visceral, and affective atmosphere of exercises in which we communicated with the past and, indeed, embodied the past. Time travel, here, was often wound tightly within hour after hour of different exercises. Some of these involved individual meditative movements that occurred within time and space; others included splitting our body-selves into pieces across time-spaces in which we and others have lived; and yet others invited us to engage with the past in explicit dialogues. As such, I suggest, such exercises were not simply sites for processing our own personal traumas or memories. They also became a site for witnessing others' complex histories in ways that blurred the normative boundaries that would have existed between the individuals if they had encountered each other in another public setting.

THE MADHOUSE

On the afternoon of the first day of the 2015 inner child retreat, Teacher Jo told us that we were going to be doing our first movement exercise.

"So in this exercise, we are trying to purify, to do house-cleaning," he said. He went on to tell us that we would use music to accomplish this "cleansing." Here, he explained, sweeping his hands down the length of his body, that "music has the power to touch these contents." He would therefore be playing a range of music that, he explained, would evoke a range of different emotions.

"Some music will be joyful, some will make you a little scared. Some may be sad. Some music is playful. Some are a little bit violent. Listen, but not only with the head—remember, everything is a vibration."

It was critical, he went on to caution us, that we listened with our whole bodies. He therefore advised us to keep our eyes closed, as much as possible, throughout the exercise. This way, he said, we would not be comparing ourselves to others. It would also facilitate our ability to *interact* with the music, rather than simply "receiving" it.

"And then we just move," he said. "It's very important that we move. Because if we are just receptive, if we just listen to the music, it is incomplete. It will not develop anything in us, or strengthen the I." He then paused, going on to contextualize our forthcoming activity in chronotopic terms. "In traditional societies, you didn't go to a concert and sit elegantly listening to the music," he said. "No—in traditional societies, there are drums and music and people moving! Dancing! Maybe instead of a concert, we could think of it as a *dis-concert*," he suggested, laughing and pausing to look around the room.

Teacher Jo's invitation for us to *upset* the kinds of control and self-restraint expected in the outside world seemed to generate a fair amount of anxiety in the room. There was, in fact, a feeling of mounting anticipation and tension in the space. As described in chapter 1, for example, my roommate, Hua Hua, later commented to me that she had been terrified upon first hearing about the exercise.

As if anticipating Hua Hua's concerns, Teacher Jo went on to explain how important it was to avoid "dancing" in any kind of organized fashion: "This is a very important principle. What you express, develops. What you live actively, strengthens, becomes more and more real in you. If you feel love, but you don't express love, it will not strengthen you. But imagine you work from love, then this love will be more and more a reality in your life, it will grow. So in this exercise we move. *The movement is spontaneous*," he emphasized. "It is *not* dancing—in dancing, we try to be rhythmic, harmonious—we are trying to look good, or at least look okay. But in this exercise it is not about how we look—no one will be looking except the assistant teachers. It is a spontaneous movement—ugly or beautiful, but it is free movement, like children. Small children. You play music and they will just be moving spontaneously. It is not dancing. Can you see the difference?"

There was nervous laughter. Several people giggled loudly and looking around them. Others nodded solemnly, still managing to look hesitant and doubtful. "This is not *China's Got Talent*," he said, "this is like a *madhouse*."

When the translator conveyed to the room that it will be like a "madhouse" (疯子院 *fengzi yuan*), the room exploded in nervous, boisterous laughter. When it finally began to settle a bit, Teacher Jo added a caveat.

"But we are mad *consciously*," he said. "I'm going to consciously let my impulses free. But when the teacher says stop, I can stop." Teacher Jo noted here that, in addition to allowing our full range of emotions to express, we were also to make sure to attend consciously to the ethical-relational commitment not to knock other participants down or harm them in any way. He explained then that, as children begin to attend to the project of not looking stupid in front of others, they lose the capacity for spontaneity.

"Life becomes quite serious," he said. "But psychologists—we find that adults have as many feelings and impulses as children. It's not that we don't have them—actually, you think you don't, because you are a mature responsible adult and good citizen who pays your mortgage, and is reliable, dependable, predictable. But we also have many other impulses. And those impulses need to have a space, an expression. If they don't, then they come out against us. Then I shout at my child, or feel anxious. Or all these things we've been talking about. Are you with me? You understand?"

Several participants nodded. Reminding us that the exercise would give us the opportunity to express the full range of our feelings, Teacher Jo here concluded with a warning that our efforts might be foiled by the kinds of critical voices that might interrupt our experience of immersion. Here, then, Jo invoked the internal voice of the Freudian superego, who will often "reprimand us for our disobedience and encourage us in the pursuit of impossible tasks" (Freud [1925] 1995, as cited in Marsilli-Vargas 2022, 41).

"We might hear this voice saying things to us such as 'you aren't doing it right'; 'you are not spontaneous'; 'you are a numb person'; or 'Why is the teacher looking at me? I must be stupid,'" he said. "All of this is normal, but my advice is that when you are lost in thinking, just come back to the music. Don't keep thinking."

The air was tense and full of anticipation as we started shuffling around the room, moving teacups and pillows so that the space was clear. The lights were dimmed. Music then began to play, blasting from four large speakers positioned in each corner of the room. It was, as Jo had promised, an eclectic range: from syrupy Chinese pop ballads to circus music to angry tracks from bands such as Rage Against the Machine. It went on for at least an hour, perhaps more. Time was difficult to track. At times I felt as if the boundaries of my own body were dissolving, as if we were somehow moving as one shared body. In those moments, I experienced the atmosphere of the "madhouse" as a form of emergent and collaborative process of embodied affect that was pushed forth by the music but also by the sounds emitting from the bodies surrounding me: loud grunts, wails, angry yells, crying, soft moans, indistinct mumbling, as well as jubilant cries of joy and even laughter. I also felt the *heat* of other bodies around me, further contributing to the sense that the boundaries of my body had begun to dissipate.

At other times, I felt the boundaries of my individual body-self intensely. Though I was *in* the experience as a total body-self, I was also acutely aware of my positionality as a participant-observer. It was if I could *feel* the thin line between participation and observation, which often seemed even thinner and more fraught than usual at New Life, appear and disappear within me. Although I did my best to keep my eyes closed, as Teacher Jo had directed, I peeked out from time to time in order to see as well as feel what was going on around me. Some people, I observed, seemed quite comfortable in the space, moving enthusiastically, flailing their limbs and leaping around the room, miraculously not bumping into anyone else despite the fact that their eyes remained closed. Still others had picked up pillows, carrying them in their arms while they wandered aimlessly around the room. At various points, a few people began shaking seemingly uncontrollably, emitting groaning sounds as they convulsed in place or fell to the floor. Some participants, I also observed, were obviously uncomfortable. A few kept their eyes open, looking at the scene in the room with curiosity and sometimes horror. Others kept their eyes tightly closed, standing in one place the entire time, barely moving or swaying ever-so-slightly side to side. I noticed that this was the case for my roommate, Hua Hua, whose brow was furrowed as she stood motionless in the middle of the room, her eyes tightly closed. It seemed clear, however, that Jo's direction to let it become a "madhouse" had opened up the opportunity for *something* in everyone present. Even those who stood motionless, it seemed, were affected by the experience.

When Teacher Jo told us to stop, however, everyone settled down. He then guided us to find a pillow to sit on. With the lights still dimmed, he led us in a meditation where we were guided to repeatedly speak the phrase "I AM" (我是 *wo shi*), or what Virginia Satir orients to, within the popular Satir method,[4] as the eternal self that lies underneath (or behind) the fluctuating emotional patterns that are seen as generating a sense of isolation as well as inhibiting everyday interaction (Akça-Koca 2017). "I am not the emotions," Teacher Jo thus said as we chanted, "I am the peace behind them, I am the strength behind them. I am, I am, I am."

Dis-concert

In considering the "madhouse" exercise, it is important to begin with a close look at Teacher Jo's introduction. It began, we recall, with Jo's invocation of a spatial understanding of the body-self, specifically a *house* that was going to be "cleaned" or "purified" by movement. As described above, Jo's framing here reflected a simultaneously psychoanalytic and embodied casting that chronotopically mapped the unconscious, as well as the body, as a space in which past experiences, both positive and negative, had accumulated. He thus often encouraged us to attend to our bodies, as he did here. Earlier that day, in fact, he had lectured to us about *implicit memory*. Such memories were often difficult to access, he had noted. In the context of China, Jo also knew, implicit, embodied memories were often even more difficult to *speak*. Participants were invited here, I suggest, to examine what prominent Chinese dancer Wen Hui, in the documentary *Long Way Home*, calls the "inheritance stored in [the] body" (Schaedler 2018). Describing it as an "ammunition warehouse" (弹药仓库 *danyao canku*), Wen Hui thus notes that many people are unaware of this simultaneously personal and collective inheritance in China. Emerging in and through intergenerational experiences that reverberate as movement rather than story, she argues that movement serves as a point of connection for young people to approach the personal traces of marks "left by society" that are necessary to confront before even considering the future. In this sense, Jo's introduction thus offered participants a kind of *permission* that might also be seen as an affordance or "trigger point" for the expression of complex feelings that often *could not be spoken* (R. Roberts 2013).

Here, we recall, Jo emphasized the importance of keeping our eyes closed. Noting first that closing our eyes would help us not compare ourselves to others, Jo's guidance here also seemed to align with the notion that therapeutic practices often hinge upon turning *inward*, and hence turning *away from* the world outside of the self (Teo 2018). As opposed to the kind of gaze that focuses "outward"—toward the kinds of structural inequalities and sociopolitical configurations that often lie at the root of individual suffering—the inward gaze encouraged in therapeutic settings is often interpreted as drawing people away from their entanglement in or their complicity with unjust sociopolitical configurations. An appreciation of the complexity of public secrecy as embodied memory in China, however, suggests a slightly different perspective. Specifically, rather than interpreting it "literally" as invoking or inculcating the "individualized self" we might consider the ways in which the guidance to keep our eyes closed actually invited people to move *toward* numerous unspoken aspects of both present and past Chinese society. Such a perspective requires extending our analysis beyond the "literal" or semantic meanings of "inside" and "outside," however, in order to understand the complex ways in which language in interaction emerges not just through its semantic content but through its *indexical* functions. Though always deeply constrained by a range of social, cultural, and historical processes, an indexical or pragmatic interpretation of co-operative (inter)action (C. Goodwin 2018) affords a reframing of Jo's introduction as offering a kind of possibility or invitation for participants to engage in an embodied, collective form of scalar inquiry with regard to their shared vulnerability to and implication within the kinds of pasts (and presents) that are usually kept well hidden.

Keeping our eyes closed, Jo had further noted, facilitated our ability to listen to and engage with the music, which he had advised was important to do. Teacher Jo had thus underscored that—although it did involve some amount of passive receptivity—the exercise also required our active participation, participation that could only be heightened by what he framed as "getting out of our heads." Again suggesting the cultivation of a distinct "listening genre" (Marsilli-Vargas 2014) or way of being-with one's own body, the music, and others in the space, Teacher Jo's introduction here also seemed to (re)formulate agency as *distributed* across the body of the practitioner and the music itself. Much like the ways in which *play* often serves to enact agency within the context of spontaneous "adjustment . . . to the conditions of a world-in-formation" (Ingold and Hallam, 2007, 3, as cited in Goodwin and Cekaite 2018, 195), Teacher Jo here invited participants to engage in a spontaneous kind of agency that he situated as emerging at the intersection of receptivity and activity.

Continuing to draw upon a kind of mind/body distinction that situated authentic emotion and authentic movement in the body rather than the "head," Jo had gone on to portray our upcoming exercise as wild, uninhibited, and participatory. Likening such movement to that which naturally occurred in "traditional" societies, he had contrasted this to the space-time of "modern" society, where *control* and self-management, he suggested, were required. Here, then, he had directed participants to think of the exercise as a *dis-concert* rather than a concert. As many readers will perhaps note, Jo's chronotopic formulation of *tradition* and *modernity* here seemed to correspond with an ideology that Heelas suggests is common within the New Age community and imagines cultural "socialization" as a kind of pollution or "contaminated mode of being" that contrasts with people's "authentic nature" (1996, 2). A generalized, universal, and perennial past is thus often idealized in terms of authenticity, agency, and embodied/emotional expression. For example, Gabrielle Roth—originator of the 5Rhythms method[5] of ecstatic dance—writes that dance might be understood as a therapeutic technology that repairs a breach exerted by "the patriarchs" who severely constrained earlier forms of dance that were "ecstatic and personal and tribal" (1997, 6). For Roth, spontaneous movement in and alongside of a range of different rhythms acts as an "antidote" to the "inertia" that she sees as caused by unacknowledged suffering (1997, 5).

This overall framing of "progress as pollution" thus arguably reified a simplistic historical narrative based in a romanticized framing of Western history in which people moved more freely in the past. This framing also works in a Chinese context, however. Bossler (2020), for example, suggests that Confucian patriarchs in the Han dynasty (136 B.C.E.–202 C.E.) enacted a similar breach when women's dancing came under scrutiny as particularly "threatening to [men's] morality" (2020, 27). Music and dance henceforth became "critical to proper governance" in China, a reality that persisted for thousands of years (2020, 26). Beginning as early as the Qin dynasty (221–206 BCE), Chinese philosophers thus emphasized the capacity of music to generate and maintain *order* in the individual as well as the social body. Classical Confucian scholars, moreover, elaborated on the notion that both music and movement enact a *moral* force with the capacity to regulate embodied/relational imbalances, including excesses of emotion or other forms of *qi*. Though enforced in different ways throughout history (Jiang 2020; Yeh 2020), dance in present-day Chinese society is likewise often a highly controlled and collaborative performative experience occurring in schools, state-supported corporations, and public parks (see C. Huang 2016)—or, as Teacher Jo noted here, on the TV show *China's Got Talent*.

Rather than engaging with Teacher Jo's formulation of tradition and modernity here in terms of its "accuracy," I suggest instead engaging with it pragmatically, a form of co-operative action (C. Goodwin 2018). From this perspective, his framing here arguably indexed what, in people's experience, has emerged as an enduring linkage between dance and governance in Chinese society. The contrast between traditional and modern thus served as a foundation for his chronotopization of the exercise as a "disconcert" rather than a concert. Teacher Jo's framing of tradition and modernity in these terms here arguably functioned, alongside the aesthetics and interactions examined in the previous chapters, to craft the New Life *atmosphere* as one that was radically different from the spaces of the outside workaday world. Recast here in terms of *inauthenticity*, Teacher Jo's formulation of the space as a dis-concert further centered the ways in which visions of a "harmonious society" as promoted by the Chinese state are often considered—though not necessarily explicitly or even publicly—empty and filled with "fakery" (Wielander 2018b). As both Kevin Carrico's research with participants in the Han clothing movement (2017) and Haiyan Lee's recent investigation of justice in China (2023) suggest, Chinese citizens are, importantly, often well aware of the gaps that exist between reality and fantasy. Teacher Jo thus implicitly seemed to acknowledge the way this was experienced as an omnipresent tension in participants' everyday lives. His invitation of *disorder* into the space thus might even be seen as effectively pulling *present*, in addition to *past*, Chinese society inside for scrutinization. In this sense, his introduction might be seen as offering participants an opportunity to simultaneously *move both toward and away from* "the social"—to disentangle as well as to entangle differently with past and present structures of governance.

Here, moreover, Teacher Jo seemed to suggest that we were going to *regress* in a simultaneously personal and cultural sense. In doing so, Jo also explicitly engaged the kinds of "seriousness" and rule-governed norms of responsibility often associated with harmony and order in both past and present Chinese society. Invoking the voice of authority here by drawing upon the pronoun "we" to situate "psychologists" as a group that included himself, he suggested that the kinds of impulses that exist alongside of and in relation to the kind of maturity that includes being a responsible adult (e.g., paying a mortgage, being a good citizen, and being reliable, dependent, and predictable) required a space for expression. Numerous times throughout his introduction he thus gave us permission to spontaneously express the full range of our emotions. He nevertheless anticipated that we might hear a "critical voice" trying to undermine our expression of emotion and free movement. Situating it as a spontaneously emergent, *internal* voice, his framing here also notably drew upon a psychotherapeutic register to refer to "the inner critic" as an internalization of parental and societal pressures. Placed in the context of his ongoing conversation with Chinese participants, however, it also pointed to the ways in which Chinese citizens often develop an overly "self-condemning" orientation that is amplified, over time, by the judgments and "requirements" issued by parental and institutional authorities (Yang and Lou 2013, 23). In this sense, it pointed to Jo's acute awareness of the competitive, comparative orientation often explicitly encouraged in Chinese institutions (J. Xu 2017; Wong 2020; Xie 2021). He thus positioned the inner critic as a voice that emerged from the *head* that would inevitably seek to derail the process we were trying to embody. In so doing, however, he also reinforced the notion that participants might enact a participatory form of agency by "coming back to the music" whenever they became aware of such intrusions.

The ideal of spontaneous expression of the full range of all emotions—including anger—here seemed to contradict the refusal of negative emotions often identified in "New Age" or other psychospiritual context (Simchai and Shoshana 2018). Notably, however, Teacher Jo also emphasized that the free expression of our impulses here needed to be filtered through the lens of *consciousness*. As a moral orientation or framework for interacting, the notion of "conscious madness" (有意识的疯 *you yishi de feng*) that Jo put forth here thus situated participants' desires not necessarily just to be "good citizens" but also to be the kinds of people who do not shout at their children. This underscored the ways in which the ethical, emotional, and relational atmosphere, or *qing*, of New Life emerged as one in which participants might experiment with new forms of spontaneous expression while simultaneously cultivating new forms of awareness about how such expression might help or *hurt* others. In Jo's introduction, then, the "self" was situated as a way of being that could be less performance-based and less orderly than usual, but which importantly was still not an "individualized" entity.

The self here was oriented, rather, toward relationality as *love*. As such, Jo was explicitly orienting to the possibility of group movement exercise as a simultaneously individual and collective process that has the potential to emerge, writes Gabrielle Roth, as a "love story between you and yourself, between you and everybody else, between you and the divine" (1997, 6). Pointing to the kind of "affective, expressive relationality" that Heelas discusses as central to the notion of love in similar European groups (2008, 26), "love" at New Life was, in this sense, often explicitly curated and cultivated. Such moments felt consequential in some way as a form of *communitas* or "the sense felt by a group of people when their life together takes on full meaning" (E. Turner 2012, 1). Calling into question the boundaries of the embodied self in ways that challenged available, normative cultural binaries distinguishing the "individual" from the "collective," the madhouse exercise can further be approached as a form of simultaneously individualizing and collectivizing experience that brings to light prevailing notions of the difference between self and other, freedom and control, and so on (C. Huang 2016).

Centering embodied, relational group practices of movement as an access point to encourage this kind of affective, embodied sense of connectedness or communitas has also, of course, been discussed extensively within anthropology for over a century. Group movement has been seen as inspiring a kind of "collective effervescence" (Durkheim [1912] 1995), for example. More recent research focused on the moving body has likewise highlighted how group movement affords participants the opportunity to enact a "dialogic relationship with other bodies" (Kazan 2005, 38, cited in R. Roberts 2013, 9) as well as a strategy for overcoming difference. In "integrated dance," for example—where dancers with disabilities are included in performances with nondisabled dancers—Gili Hammer suggests that collaborative movement affords the development of new kinds of "intersubjective bodily awareness" (Hammer 2020, 2021) that *bridge* or *translate* across difference. Often inspiring personal as well as cultural, historical, and even political forms of self-reflexivity (Hammer 2021), the capacity of collective movement here underscores the political potential of encounters within which entrenched ways of being in the world are "decentered" and disrupted.

Such encounters might thus be seen as the kinds of *agonistic* encounters discussed by Zeynep Gambetti as emerging in opposition to *antagonistic* or confrontational encounters within which some are "the predominant actors/doers" while others "are relegated to the place of endurers/sufferers" (2016, 36). Agonistic encounters, Gambetti observes, distribute vulnerability equally across interactants, thus generating new relational opportunities (36). Moments and social spaces within which customary boundaries are dissipated thus become spaces in which a direct engagement with differences—framed here as "differentials"—becomes "'generative' in such a way as to create something new" (2016, 35). Given the primarily Han, middle-class, and heteronormative constituency at New Life, I am hesitant to read the madhouse exercise as *inherently* agonistic or even one that afforded the kind of dialogue across difference that both Hammer and Gambetti emphasize as socially and politically productive. This kind of agonistic encounter thus arguably contributed to the framing of New Life as a space of collective development through which individuals frequently came to recognize themselves in those they would have previously considered different. Underscoring participants' shared vulnerability to ideological and institutional expectations about what the "Chinese self" is and what it is supposed to be, however, the exercise might still be considered culturally or even politically potent in terms of the way it afforded the unusual recognition of *sameness*, both in terms of past events and institutional experience as well as shared encounters with the effects of such institutions within families.

Such recognition, it is important to acknowledge here, was largely if not entirely implicit. Taking shape through an embodied register that hinged upon sound, movement, and intercorporeality, the "madhouse" here emerged as a complex intercorporeal synchrony of sound, heat, and movement within which, at least from my own perspective, the normative boundaries of the body-self were challenged, even if they did not completely fall away. There were also, notably, a number of people in the room who remained on the sidelines. Many of them, one might imagine, may have been having the kind of distant, disconnected, and ambivalent feeling that Ken described as "numbness" in chapter 1. Even for those who appeared not to have experienced the kind of dissolution of embodied boundaries (as I did) in the moment, however, witnessing others engaging in the process at New Life was often, as discussed above, a mysteriously collective experience. During a conversation we had a few days after the madhouse, for example, Hua Hua described to me how, throughout the exercise, she had been intensely self-conscious and could not let go. After witnessing others engage, however, Hua Hua had had the experience of being able to at least glimpse and possibly express her "inner self." She had experienced the madhouse as a witness, in other words, but nevertheless it had also become an embodied, relational experience that began to evaporate her sense of isolation. This demonstrates how, even for those who "just" observed, the exercise offered at least an affordance for all participants to reconsider their normative ways of being-in-relation with others and the world.

Hua Hua's explanation of her experience as opening up her "inner self," moreover, underscores the ways in which "love" at New Life—and even "strengthening the I," as Jo put it here—denoted a kind of *spiritual* freedom. Indeed, in Gabrielle Roth's terms such a process constitutes a kind of *soul retrieval* (1997, 6), reflecting, perhaps, the ways in which Teacher Jo linked the exercise to the cultivated ability to access what he framed as the "True Self" as well as the "I AM." Hua Hua's comments, finally, center the ways in which "freedom" and "opening," at New Life, were formulated as simultaneously individual and collective. As an embodied, chronotopic orientation within the space, New Life is thus notably distinct from the kinds of rigid order prevailing in other collective movements during the similar time frame in China. Within the Han clothing movement as described by Kevin Carrico, for example, there prevails "a standardized macrolevel mapping of relationship roles structured around preestablished microlevel etiquette that provides a clear social role for any and all people and flawlessly structured interpersonal relations" (2017, 75). Offering participants an atmosphere within which they were able to practice dissolving long-standing patterns of relationality and selfhood within intercorporeal exercises like the madhouse, I thus suggest in conclusion, exercises at New Life served also to institute—at least temporarily—an embodied experience of a different kind of *dawo*.

CONCLUDING REFLECTIONS

Throughout this chapter, I have discussed the ways in which, at New Life, participants experienced the expansion or recontouring of the boundaries of their body-selves within exercises that involved collaborative movement and the distribution of the feeling-self across bodies. These embodied shifts, I demonstrated, often worked to *unsettle* participants' normative embodied boundaries as well as dominant discourses of Chinese selfhood. Often uncomfortable and challenging, these experiences paradoxically also worked to *settle* participants, moving them out of isolation and toward the kinds of "collective development" (共同成长 *gongtong chengzhang*) mentioned both here and in the previous chapter. Multichanneled, embodied encounters thus frequently required participants to stretch beyond their comfort zones. Here, I suggested, the expanded *dawo* emerged or at least had the potential to emerge as a simultaneously cultural experience of the moving "we" as well as a deeply personal experience of the individual self.

This experience, I further suggested, implicitly invited but certainly did not require an interrogation of unspoken aspects of both the Chinese present and the Chinese past. I thus also showed how participants sometimes experienced inner child work, in a group context, in scalar terms that invited a (re)examination of specific ideologies of selfhood as well as gender. In this sense, it becomes possible to engage with New Life exercises not just as "technologies of the self" (Foucault 1988) but also as "technologies of the social" with the potential to "reconfigure participants' experiences of themselves as intersubjective beings in the flow of social, cultural, and historical space and time" (Pritzker and Duncan 2019, 470). I thus examined how somatic, relational activities such as Chao's encounter with his inner child sometimes "opened" participants to experiencing the ways in which, in the words of Rae Johnson (2018) " how we embody oppressive social conditions through nonverbal interactions, and how oppression affects our relationship with our own body" (Johnson 2018, 6). From this perspective, the notion that spaces like New Life are inherently "apolitical" misses the subtle and indexical ways in which exercises involving collaborative movement, mirroring, and the distribution of the self or emotions across other bodies often functioned to usher in rather than exclude other more public or political spaces. Demonstrating how various exercises took shape through discursive, affective, and intercorporeal co-operative action (C. Goodwin 2018), I have thus suggested that the kinds of therapeutic interventions enacted at New Life—often purportedly entirely focused on the individual—had at least the capacity to move participants toward considering or *scaling* their experience vis-à-vis broader inequalities and problematic histories.

Embodied encounters of the extended self at New Life, I argued, similarly afforded a rapid scaling process through which the personal was interrogated, or at least encountered, as broadly shared cultural experience. Here, however, it is important to return to a discussion of the ways in which such scaling, as I highlighted throughout the chapter, often emerged *haphazardly* and *implicitly* in the context of New Life. They were not, in other words, scaffolded by teachers or staff, and only rarely were invoked in textual materials. Alongside the ways in which New Life emerged as what I've dubbed a kind of "Hantopia" in which sameness (rather than difference) was central, this raises a set of serious questions about the potential consequences of such encounters for enacting more broad-scale shifts within Chinese society. In the following chapter, however, I present several examples of how conversations and narrative co-tellings at New Life *did* often explicitly interrogate broader, shared historical, cultural, and social ideologies and conditions. Such conversations, like the ones I have examined here, were often indirect and, generally speaking, were not supported by the kinds of explicit "political education" (Haines 2019) or "political mentalization" (Gaztambide 2019) that many within the fields of embodied social justice and liberation psychology suggest are necessary to support the kind of collectively scaled anticipatory modes that have the potential to affect society beyond the individual. In calling attention to the nuanced ways in which they moved participants to engage in simultaneous personal/intimate and public/collective forms of scalar inquiry, however, I nevertheless approach such conversations as constituting a critical step in the development of participants' *political subjectivity*.

4

Considering Culture

China becomes "China" in the world... only in the globally entwined material and ideological conditions created for the re-narration of the past in light of new demands on the present and new hopes for the future.
—REBECCA KARL

We are all amateur historians with various degrees of awareness about our production. We also learn history from similar amateurs.
—MICHELLE-ROLPH TROUILLOT

We were circled up for introductions one evening in 2014. A newcomer, who introduced herself as "Old Hong," began her introduction by noting that she was probably the oldest person in the room.

"I just turned fifty-five this year," she said proudly. We all laughed at the way she addressed us. A confident matriarch who spoke in a thick and animated northern accent, Hong then began to relate to us the circumstances that motivated her to attend the workshop that evening. Formulating her struggles in opposition to the previous participant—who had shared about her ongoing difficulties in her relationship with her mother—Hong proclaimed, "Actually, it's *us* who have a problem with *you*!"

The room erupted in laughter. Hong's alignment of herself as a "we," which placed her in a relationship with the previous speaker's non-co-present mother, as well as her deployment of the plural form of "you" (你们 *nimen*) to address the generation of children that the previous speaker was now situated as representing, centered both the temporality and historicity of the moment. Implicating us all in a shared cultural experience as well as an ongoing conversation, Hong went on to tell us about her ongoing tension with her adult daughter, issuing a series of complaints regarding the ways in which her daughter continually resisted what she framed as her *care*.

"For example, when she has issues at work," Hong said, "I am always wanting to educate her (教育她 *jiaoyu ta*)—it should be like this, it should be like that, it should be like this—but whenever I do this, she has a bad reaction. Me? I feel like I have to say these things, so you don't make a mistake. But she won't accept it, and she becomes furious with me. And I also become furious." Switching frequently between addressing her daughter as "you" and "she," Hong thus explained why she felt justified in offering this kind of guidance to her daughter.

"I'm doing it for your own good," she explained, again addressing her non-co-present daughter directly, carrying forth the "you" and addressing us as if we were her daughter. "I'm not wrong—how can you refuse to listen?"

The story Hong proceeded to tell us was peppered with local expressions and terminologies, and her narrative was framed as a simultaneously tragic and comedic clash of generational ideological perspectives. Throughout her story, moreover, she continually engaged with the group as a set of primarily younger people who she framed as *needing* to understand how this whole mess feels from her vantage point. She nevertheless made it clear to us that her struggle was also deeply personal, that the tension with her daughter was very much a daily struggle that disrupted her life. Earlier that day, in fact, Hong explained that her daughter—who she referred to repeatedly, using a common Chinese parlance, as "the child" (孩子 *haizi*)—had encountered some problems in her love life. They battled it out, as usual, but afterwards Hong had felt a great deal of regret. She had begun thinking more, she then told us in a more serious tone, about how her daughter had, on numerous occasions, tried to instruct her how to have more respect and sensitivity, to listen or "follow" (顺着她 *shunzhe ta*) rather than always trying to control the situation.

"So I'm in the midst of a struggle (矛盾 *maodun*)," she concluded, continuing here to offer a comparative perspective. "Actually—my relationship with my husband is good," she said, "my relationship with my mother-in-law—these are all quite good! It's just with the child that there are problems. So now I'm reacting (反应上 *fanying shang*). And I'm also anxious—like what can I say? I'm always worrying about her. I'm always concerned that she'll have problems. Because my daughter, she doesn't listen well (听力不好 *tingli buhao*). She's just gotten a new job, and I feel like I should appreciate that. But at the same time, I'm anxious. I'm always afraid that she'll run into problems at work, and I'm always thinking about how we can plan for these problems in advance—I just sometimes feel like—*aiya*—how can I have said so much, haven't I told you this? I told you this before! So that's the type of problem that often arises—and now I'm in a state of utter confusion (迷茫 *mimang*)."

Teacher Du, who was the instructor that evening, responded compassionately, initially addressing Old Hong with the informal "you" (你 *ni*) but quickly switching to the respectful form (您 *nin*). He began his remarks by complimenting her positive attitude and willingness to "at least try" to develop the kind of sensitivity requested by her daughter.

"I'm willing to try, sure," Hong said quickly in response, "but I often just can't make it happen."

This generated more laughter in the room. As it died down, however, another newcomer, Lan, interjected with an emotional plea:

"I'm just going to insert a brief comment here," she said. "I don't know if this is related to Chinese-style parental education methods (中国式父母的教育方式 *Zhongguo shi fumu jiaoyu fangshi*) or what—but I'm a daughter, and I actually really quite understand her daughter's feelings. We seemingly all have always been wanting to communicate with our parents, but actually it should be an *equal* dialogue (平等对话 *pingdeng duihua*). They should respect us, our individuality (个体 *geti*). So now, with regards to my own daughter's education—because I feel I'm lacking in this area, too—I've also always—it's like I don't want to—I *can't*—reproduce (复制 *fuzhi*) my original family's way of raising me and educating me. But it is so difficult."

Teacher Du was silent for a moment before responding by thanking Lan and then pausing for another moment before offering his own commentary.

"We definitely know," he said, ratifying Lan's experience. "Actually, our parents, that generation—the history that they've experienced—we have never endured that. That kind of pain they suffered—we have no way of understanding it. We have no way of even imagining it. So they have their own ways. They can teach us, and we—from here—we can begin to change. From here we can now be responsible for our own children and take responsibility for our own situation. We can create a good environment for them as they are growing up. So I'm so glad that we have so many classmates here sharing."

CHINESE EDUCATION METHODS ... OR WHAT?

In the epigraph above, Rebecca Karl notes how "China" has been made and remade, at different points in history, in the stories people tell about the past, always "in light of new demands on the present and new hopes for the future" (2020, 4). In navigating what Zhang (2020) refers to as "the inner revolution," I suggest in this chapter, participants at the center, along with instructors, were similarly engaged in a collaborative mapping of history, memory, and Chineseness itself in multiple ways. As they did so, they often simultaneously worked to preserve that which they value about the past at the same time as considering the possibility of a different, more just future, at least on an interpersonal level. Conversations variably drawing upon personal and shared experiences, desires, and fears here thus often constituted an active, embodied, and relational engagement with the core question "Who are we, and what makes us Chinese?," a question that Mayfair Yang identifies as often lying at the center of contemporary discourse in China (2020, 21).

In such conversations, I show, attendees frequently participated in what Stafford (2013) describes as a "more or less endless, spontaneous ethical commentary" focused on the *distance* or gap "between how things should be and how they really are" (15). Like many Chinese citizens in early twenty-first-century China, New Lifers here interrogated the endless "divide between the expectations of the nation and the realities of experience" (Carrico 2017, 33). Throughout the chapter, I thus adopt an ethnographic perspective that embraces such everyday dialogue as a key form of *theory-building* (Rosa 2019) through which participants, as "amateur historians with various degrees of awareness about [their] production," in Trouillot's terms (1995, 20), interrogated history both in interaction and narrative.

In the short interaction described above, for example, there was a great deal of emotional engagement with temporality, historicity, and imaginations of Chineseness in generational, gendered, and familial terms. From the outset of her introduction, for example, the pronouns that Hong used in her formulation of a collective "we" (the mothers) pitted in a struggle with the aggregate "you" (the daughters) brought shared generational differences to bear on a deeply personal and troubling pattern of interaction that she was experiencing with her daughter. This positioning, which was taken up by both Lan and Du in their responses, drew immediate attention to the ways in which recent Chinese history has influenced the ways in which parents "educate" (教育 *jiaoyu*) their children.

As Andrew Kipnis suggests, discourse on "educational methods" can be considered a form of *cultural intimacy* in China (Herzfeld 2016), within which "education is both a metaphor for governing and a tool of governing" (Kipnis 2011, 7). As discussed in chapter 1, "education" here refers not just to school-based instruction directed at youth but also to modes of relating that endure *across the life span*. Indeed, from Hong's perspective, the kind of guidance that she desired to give to her adult daughter represented *care*. Her daughter, who continually resisted such guidance, was thus represented as having poor skills in "listening" (听力 *tingli*), a term that often notably indexes both youth and obedience in China (D. Wu 1994). At one point, Hong further situated her relationship with daughter as an aberration in comparison to her good relationships with her husband and mother-in-law. Engaging here with the normative "mother-in-law script" in which tension with one's mother-in-law is expected in China (Mason 2020), Hong's description of her good relationship with her mother-in-law thus constituted a kind of evidence of her overall moral and relational character. It further functioned, I suggest, to recruit her interlocutors into the adoption of her perspective that it was her daughter who was ultimately culpable for their struggles, rather than herself.

Later in her narrative, however, Hong conveyed her daughter's efforts to try to teach her how to "follow" rather than constantly enacting a leadership role. In this portion of her narrative, the normative relational hierarchy between parent and child in China was, notably, inverted. Indeed, it was precisely this inversion that Teacher Du centered in his initial response to Old Hong when he seemingly endorsed her daughter's requests by complimenting her for being present and "at least trying." In so doing, I argue, Du gently refused to collaborate with Hong to document or ratify the intimate injustice that she had become subject to in her relationship with her daughter. Nor did he shame her for being "wrong," however. With his rapid self-correction in which he switched from the informal to the formal second-person pronoun that instantiated Hong's status as a respected elder, in fact, he discursively worked to reestablish the relational hierarchy that had been disrupted in her relationship with her daughter. In response to Du, Hong notably reiterated her willingness to try, a willingness that was nevertheless mediated by her overall doubtfulness about her ability to "make it happen."

At this precise moment, however, Lan interjected, notably breaking the usual participation framework of the opening circle, in which a single speaker addresses a group of listeners in an ordered fashion. As mentioned in chapter 1, this framework affords both spoken responses from the instructors as well as *unspoken* relational moves enacted by participants. In my three years at the center, it was only rarely diverted in the way it was here. Perhaps afforded by the jovial and informal mood that had come over the space during Hong's introduction, Lan began by enacting a stance of epistemic uncertainty with regard to whether her comment was related to "Chinese-style parental methods of education (中国式父母的教育方式 *Zhongguo shi fumu jiaoyu fangshi*) or what." With this positioning, Lan tentatively scaled the issue at hand as *cultural* and thus pertinent to the emergent conversation, which involved multiple cohorts of Chinese women, taking place at the time. Thus adopting a subjunctive stance, Lan admitted here that she identified with Hong's daughter.

Switching to a "we" voice that ratified the previously established orientation to the mother-daughter issue as a shared experience affecting co-present others, Lan went on to formulate a shared experience of *desire* among those in the generational cohort of Hong's daughter. The younger generation, she said specifically, had experienced a long-standing yet unrequited desire to "communicate with our parents." She then proceeded to enact an aspirational moral stance regarding the ways in which such communication should be "equal" as well as based in respect, on the part of the mothers, for the "individuality" of their daughters.

Pointing to the ways in which patriarchy in China includes both gendered and generational inequalities (Santos and Harrell 2017; see also chapter 7), Lan's comments here underscore the ways in which learning to love at New Life was often focused not only on marital relationships but was also inclusive of women's relationships with older women, especially their mothers. Thus highlighting the growing importance of *intergenerational intimacy* (Yan 2009; Evans 2012), both Hong's and Lan's comments here further show how the *striving* for intimacy, in Yunxiang Yan's own terminology, arises in the form of specific "ethical dilemmas and struggles" in the relational lives of Chinese citizens across generations (Yan 2013, 278). I therefore suggest that rather than reading Lan's articulated desire for "equality" as an attempt to insert so-called Western ideologies of personhood or intimacy into an imagined Chinese future, we might rather attend to the combination of real suffering and real desire that she, as well as Hong, was attempting to express.

Indeed, we then learned about how Lan's desire was rooted in her own challenge to enact this kind of intimacy with her own daughter. Here, she aligned with Hong, admitting that she, too, was "lacking in this area." Lan's admission here arguably points to an ongoing national conversation centered around efforts to produce higher "quality" (素质 *suzhi*) people through shifts in practices at home, within schools, and in society more broadly. Quality, very briefly, here points to "the innate and nurtured physical, psychological, intellectual, moral, and ideological qualities of human bodies and their conduct" (Jacka 2009, 524, as cited in Xie 2021, 52). As Xie (2021) thus notes, "quality" in China "has become a common description of individually embodied human qualities, with a sacred overtone." Liberal education or "education for quality," which primarily falls upon mothers to enact alongside school teachers, also constitutes a state-driven *nation-building effort* (Kuan 2015). It is important to note, however, that Lan went on here to emphatically articulate her desire not to reproduce such "methods" with her daughter. Indeed, she upgraded this desire, midsentence, to a *refusal*, saying that "I don't want to—I *can't*—reproduce (复制 *fuzhi*) my original family's way of raising me and educating me." Lan's chronotopic formulations of "Chineseness," from this perspective, can be seen as an ethical-relational and affective project of scalar inquiry in which she was attempting to make sense of the gap between how things had been, how they should or could have been, and how they *might become*.

Underscoring her experience of feeling (and having felt) pain within the structure of "Chinese education methods," the desperation of Lan's plea, I suggest, further highlights what Aileen, the director of New Life, once explained to me about the motivations of participants, both women and men, who came to the center because, in her words, "they don't want to repeat their pasts with their kids." Pointing also to what Santos (2016) calls "technologies of ethical imagination" within which "shared imaginary codes of conduct are systematized, objectified and made visible" (196), Lan's refusal here might be approached not (or not *only*) as an example of how mothers' self-development efforts in China constitute a form of interpellation or subjectification. Teresa Kuan, in fact, takes issue with this fundamentally "antihumanist" stance, emphasizing how efforts might rather be considered as constituting a form of *moral agency*. Detailing the ways in which one mother's grappling with a similar incident in which she assessed her expression of anger to her child as disproportionate to the circumstances, for example, Kuan describes the kind of ethical subjectivity that emerges as "a perception of an incongruity between emotion and situation" (2015, 103). Lan's comment—as well as Hong's story—thus brings attention to such incongruity as a phenomenological experience that emerges in everyday relational contexts or "situations." Her comment thereby reflects one of the central forms of suffering as well as one of the most intense forms of desire expressed by young mothers in contemporary China, who are often desperate to avoid reproducing what Katherine Mason calls the "ghosts in the nursery" (2020, 14). Like Lan and others at New Life, they did not, in other words, want to reproduce or witness their parents reproducing the kinds of shaming and violence that they had themselves experienced.

In invoking the past, I further suggest, Lan's comment served as an index of the kinds of sociopolitical suffering that people who were Hong's age in 2014 may have endured during the Great Leap Forward (1958–62) or the Cultural Revolution (1966–76). Highlighting his attunement to the complex ways in which "transgenerational memories are made both in the past and in the present" and are always "mediated through interpersonal communications between sentient bodies" (J. Li 2020, 6), Du's response to Lan likewise demonstrates how chronotopic formulations of culture, education, and family often served the *implicit* purpose of orienting interlocutors in the emergent interaction as well as vis-à-vis their emotional, embodied experiences of suffering in the past. Quickly situating Hong's generation within a history that "we have no way of even imagining," Du thus directed participants to try to appreciate "what they went through" without necessarily needing to know—or even imagine—all of the gory details.

Du's comments here highlighted the ways in which *the past* in China is not only a foreign country, so to speak (see Kuan 2015), but is also—for most people born beyond the late 1960s and 1970s—an *unknown* territory. In this landscape of secrecy, Jie Li notes, "What renders past reality 'inaccessible' to present consciousness is not only the immenseness of the trauma but also the inaccessibility of historical archives" (2020, 15). Articulations of shared pasts, however, often have pragmatic *relational* effects in the present. They also simultaneously work to "relationally configure" the past itself (French 2012, 345). As a collaborative form of cultural remembering in the context of so many unspoken secrets, Du's response here also arguably constituted an attempt to map shared experiences of suffering and desire in space as well as time while also maintaining respect for Old Hong. Initially inferring that the kinds of suffering that Hong's generation endured had generated a bad environment for children—and thus endorsing and even upgrading Lan's assessment—he also worked to preserve the state-supported narrative of the Cultural Revolution as a time of chaos within which everyone was a victim (Rofel 2007; Hillenbrand 2020). He thus absolved Hong from having to answer to her own attitudes and actions during that time, shifting discursive ground, in his conclusion, toward a more agentive framing that centered the immediate present. In shifting discursive ground, he also notably shifted responsibility from Hong's cohort to his own, suggesting that "we can take responsibility" for learning how to create a better environment for our children.

This interaction, I suggest, demonstrates how discussions about education at New Life frequently engaged with the intersection of care and governance (D. Wu 1994; Bregnbæk 2016; J. Xu 2017, 2020; Pritzker and Liang 2018). These conversations spoke continually, as I show in this chapter, to the notion of "politics and education as one" (*zhengjiao heyi* 政教合一) or "the way that politics and education aiming at transforming human beings mix together as a holistic whole" in both past and present Chinese society (Lin 2017, 24). "Education," within these encounters, functioned as an index for both past and current as well as *future* forms of governance. The interaction described above also shows how New Life participants, including older clients, were constantly wrangling with the ways in which culturally situated, parentally enacted "methods of education" (or what) landed in bodies as intimate, embodied ways of relating in the present. Often scaled fluidly and ambiguously between family, school, and state, such structures were engaged with, in other words, as individual and relational ways of thinking, feeling, and, indeed, *being* that had been influenced by past experience, continued to exist in the present, and constituted the basis for imagining different futures. Showing further how, as Yunxang Yan notes, "the predicament of *value entanglement* persists over time and cuts across generational lines" (Yan 2013, 278, italics mine) in China, the interaction further demonstrates how tentative statements and ambiguous references to relationships between the past and present constituted an intimate form of scalar inquiry through which people crafted ideas about their place within a situated spatiotemporal trajectory that continued from the past and stretched into the future. Especially in a context where public secrecy prevails through histories "that are broadly known but seldom said aloud" (Hillenbrand 2020, 21), such instances can further be interrogated as a kind of intimate *search* for ways of speaking about the past that simultaneously acknowledged both joy and suffering as well as it provided pathways for moving forward without being *bound* by suffering.

My emphasis in the following discussion, accordingly, revolves around a close study of how talk in the New Life space provided an opportunity for participants to wrangle with the project of (re)scaling their relationship to simultaneously personal and shared pasts, presents, and possible futures. Emphasizing the ways in which such conversations emerged as a kind of *dreaming* (Loizidou 2016) or "anticipatory mode" (Sumartojo and Pink

2019), I show how interlocutors drew variably upon both historically available ideologies as well as specific components of previous talk in order to interrogate "Chinese culture" in intimate ways that link shared histories to personal experiences in the present with deeply felt desires for the future. Throughout this chapter, I thus focus on the ways in which conversations at New Life often emerge as tentative (re)*chronotopizations* that (re)scaled interlocutors' ways of thinking about and relating with Chineseness within the emergent context of the present interaction and the present setting. Specifically, I examine how scalar inquiry took shape within conversations that involved participants' variably scaling themselves in relation to various forms of governance, secrecy, and trauma that had and *continued to* maintain a hold over their lives. Such scaling, I suggest, also often involved a collaborative envisioning of the possible ways in which they might enact governance differently within their own, albeit limited, milieu. This chapter thus further interrogates how both time-talk and place-talk sometimes serve to "reproduce, disrupt, and reconfigure" entrenched ideologies and structures (Rosa 2019, 4) while, at same time, contributing to the formulation of an ethnoracial identity of "Chineseness," that, like "the production of every ethnoracial identity . . . required the joint creation and erasure of difference" (2019, 107). Underscoring how cultural identity and political are both co-constructed in collaborative considerations of the ways in which the lived past permeated the present and the imagined future, this chapter thus emphasizes how such rechronotopizations simultaneously emerged as critiques and perpetuated a form of cultural identification that itself is deeply problematic.

WESTERN METHODS

I have suggested that attempts to locate "Chineseness" in simultaneously personal and shared pasts constituted an emergent, intimate, and collaborative form of scalar inquiry through which people discursively engaged in the project of situating their embodied and emotional experience in space and time vis-à-vis real and imagined narratives of "culture." Within this project, chronotopic formulations of Chineseness and "Westernness"—as well as "naturalness," "maturity," and "development"—at New Life underscored the ways in which scalar inquiry often works through tentative discursive projects that hinge upon and variably reimagine shifting sets of contrasts between past and present, self and other, and so on (Pritzker and Perrino

2020). Rather than endorsing rigid ideas or ideologies of culture, I suggest in this section, Chineseness was often examined *provisionally* at New Life. Both Chineseness and Westernness (or Otherness), in this sense, were often engaged with not as "actual things" in the world but as conceptual markers that worked indexically and chronotopically in interactions within which people attempted to spatiotemporally situate themselves in relation to others, the society around them, and the possible (or probable) future.

When I spoke with Du shortly after the event described in the opening vignette, for example, he shared his perspective on the ways in which "Western methods" are particularly well suited to the dilemma facing Chinese people who are seeking to better understand and express their emotions in early twenty-first-century China.

"In our traditional culture," he said, "there was a lot of emphasis on order (秩序 *zhixu*) within family relationships. But the feelings of particular individuals get overlooked (忽略了 *hulüe le*). So we can become pretty rigid (僵化 *jianghua*), and we can say we are filial to our parents—'Everything baba or mama says or does is right, period.' But we can't tell them anything that we aren't OK (不满 *buman*) with [what they've said or done], or express any anger (愤怒 *fennu*). Ever. And this creates emotional constraint (情感的压抑 *qinggan de yayi*). The communication is not smooth (畅 *chang*). Actually, as a result it accumulates, and we suppress even more problems. And we become even more alienated from one another (疏远 *shuyuan*)."

Du went on here to explain that what he finds appealing about "Western methods" is that they allow people to "return to the center of the self" (回到自己的中心 *huidao ziji de zhongxin*). They invite us, he suggests, to experience our emotions, to *acknowledge* these feelings. "And then we can begin to express them, release them," he said.

In constructing a chronotopic contrast between so-called "traditional" modes of relating and "Western methods" of awareness, Du began by chronotopically mapping an East/West dichotomy onto the landscape of Chinese individual and relational experience. Beginning with a general statement about "traditional culture" that ambiguously referred to both past and present, Du's perspective on "emotional constraint" here thus evinced a scathing critique of the ways in which an emphasis on *order* within the family—imagined here as demanding blind filial devotion—often required both silence and compliance from (adult) children. Within this structure, communication about disagreements and negative emotions is suppressed, which over time causes *rigidity*, *emotional constraint*, and *alienation*.

His explanation, notably, drew heavily upon a Chinese medical logic. Perhaps the most famous classic Chinese medical text, *The Yellow Emperor's Classic* (黄帝内经 *Huangdi Neijing*), for example, describes emotion as one of the major causes of illness. Excessive or constrained emotion, specifically, may cause emotional "counterflow" expressing as "anger, irritation, and an unsettled spirit" (Chace and Zhang 1997, 12). Excessive anger in particular "carries the *qi* upwards in the body, it makes you lose control of yourself" (Larre and Rochat de la Vallée 1996, 87). As in Du's explanation, the inner landscape of the person is thus imagined as a container for emotions that, when suppressed over time, become like "fuses," causing us to "explode" at often trivial matters, which over time affects the heart. Du thus deployed metaphors common to Chinese medicine, including rigidity, suppression, constraint, and the inhibited flow of emotion, as an entry point to discuss the effects of lack of emotional awareness or expression in traditional Chinese homes. Unlike Chinese medicine, however, where treatment of the individual body through "adjustment" or "harmonization" (调 *tiao*) of embodied imbalances is emphasized, Du here envisioned familial relationships as well as the family more broadly as if they constitute a single body through which *qi* must flow smoothly in order to avoid such rigidity. Here, one might suggest, Du was engaged in a kind of *bentuhua* (L. Zhang 2014, 2020) or "living translation" (Pritzker 2014) within which his roughly five years of participation in workshops at New Life and daily work with individual clients had specifically led him to the conclusion that "Western methods" such as inner child and family constellation therapy were critical for the transformation of negative relational patterns within the Chinese family as he imagined it.

After Du issued his statement about the utility of "Western methods," I became curious to hear his perspective on the ways in which (some) anthropologists have characterized Chinese citizens—at least in the 1980s and 1990s—as often expressing "psychological" suffering in "somatic" terms (e.g., Kleinman 1986). Intending to probe his chronotopic castings of Chineseness and Westernness, I thus asked him if he agreed with this observation. His "translation" here took on distinct *temporal* as well as spatial contours.

"Like us, in this generation," he said, including me in the cohort of people who were, like Du, in their thirties at the time, "even our parents, that generation, most of them don't look kindly upon the expression of emotion.... In their generation, it was all about prioritizing the benefit of the country, prioritizing the benefit of the collective. So you need to neglect or overlook individual experience/feeling in order to answer the call of the nation. And they used the same methods to teach us—so basically, we are like this, too. We want to study well and work hard and find a way to contribute. But our education, basically, lacked any focus on emotional experience."

Du here situated the problem both historically and politically. Issuing a historical critique that explicitly implicated the modern Chinese nation-state in the relational problems that he had previously identified as culture, Du zeroed in on a particular disruptive time period in recent history. Here, however, the conversation took a sharp turn in terms of Du's chronotopic framing of the socio-moral Chinese past. Extending his analysis even further back in time, Du thus began talking about the *ancient* (as opposed to more recent) Chinese past:

"In ancient China, people embraced the principle of the oneness of heaven and humanity (天人合一 *tianren heyi*), they paid a lot of attention to the ways in which the whole person could live in a natural, spontaneous, and harmonious state," he said, switching here from a description that referred to "people" to recasting the imagined ancient Chinese holism in exclusive "we" terms. "Whenever we would talk about self-cultivation (修身 *xiushen*) and nurturing life (养性 *yangsheng*), we paid a lot of attention to the entire body, including the relationship between body and emotions—like in Chinese medicine."

"But in recent times," he then said, zooming back in time to the relative present, "we've had an entire generation completely deny Chinese traditional culture. It actually started in the beginning of the twentieth century, and then in the second half of the twentieth century, our education—it started to change such that we were taught we should deny the self and emphasize the nation. When I think about the last hundred years," he finally added, "the reason is pretty obvious." Du paused here, seemingly checking to make sure I was "with him." He then moved into a chronotopic analysis of the latter portion of the twentieth century, within which the great Chinese "we" was transformed into something other than ideal.

"So by the time you get to the 1970s and 1980s," he continued, "people weren't willing to talk about their feelings. And besides, there was nowhere you could go to talk about them—in every work unit, every housing unit, every organization—there were people who did thought work (思想工作 *siwei gongzuo*). If you had worries, they would talk sense to you (给你讲一些道理 *gei ni jiang daoli*), in order to turn your thoughts around (转化 *zhuanhua*)."

At the outset of this segment of his interview, Du cast a simplistic chronotopic formulation of an ancient utopia within which harmony had presumably prevailed. Mirroring contemporary discourses that revolve around the imaginary notion of a continuous and harmonious legacy of "Chinese tradition," he arguably invoked the kind of "nostalgia for the imaginary past" (Lin 2017, 26) that has been observed to function as a form of affective governance in China since the early twenty-first century (Carrico 2017; Wielander 2018a). He thus proceeded to craft a chronotopic formulation of the past century as a *deviation* from some "ancient," "pure," and fundamental Chineseness that involved a core commitment to self-cultivation (修身*xiushen*) and nurturing life (养性 *yangsheng*). Du's presentation of the harmonious ancient past here thus notably seemed to systematically erase the complex diversity of gendered, class-based, and ethnic experience over thousands of years.

It is further important to recognize, however, how the spatiotemporal perspective that Du set forth here was arguably strategic, emerging as a subtle and strategic sociopolitical critique directed toward both past and even *present* structures of governance. In this sense, Du's comments here demonstrate how scalar, spatiotemporal configurations of ancient "harmony" not only serve as reifications of an idealized ancient China but afford narrators the ability to critique specific aspects of the recent political past that are ongoing in the present. Demonstrating the nuanced ways in which critique operates within the constraints of "knowing how to say without directly referring" in China, one might also engage with Du's chronotopic formulations as his entry point for discussing highly controversial and even unspeakable matters.

These kinds of "chronotopic calibrations," Wirtz suggests, point to the changing ways in which people co-construct their "experience and subjective feel for history" (2016, 344). It was also likely the case that Du was working dialogically to co-construct the conversation within the bounds of safety and appropriateness. Here, it is safe to assume that Du was himself highly aware that he was constantly walking a political tightrope in publicly discussing the traumas of the recent past in a group context (or in conversation with an American anthropologist). In the opening vignette, for example, he very clearly but indirectly suggested that Hong's excessive control over her daughter related to historical experiences that younger generations "cannot even imagine." He very swiftly moved on to set Hong at ease, however, with his suggestion that knowing any details is not required in order to shift the kinds of relational patterns that emerged in the past. In that case, Du insinuated his understanding of both past and present mandates to maintain public secrecy as a form of respect, politeness, or care.

Du exhibited a distinct form of chronotopic dexterity, however, within which he also refused to turn away from the particular kinds of suffering that existed in the past and persisted in the present. After framing his explanation vis-à-vis the chronotopic contrast between the (imagined) ancient past and the more widely understood but rarely discussed recent past, for instance, Du completely dropped all further references to the kinds of ancient harmony he had previously suggested were critical to his analysis. Du spoke explicitly, here, to the kind of "thought work" (思想工作 *siwei gongzuo*) that existed within every work unit in the past, and to which people were subjected as an official form of mental health "treatment" during the Mao years. In both his pitch and prosody as well as his gaze, he likewise indicated the ways in which such thought work remains prevalent today in various forms (Cheek 2019; L. Zhang 2020). Insinuating that this kind of control relates to or has invariably influenced the kinds of "emotional constraint" in the Chinese family, Du thus drew, here, upon relatively formulaic castings of "East" and "West" to articulate a critique that was expertly scaled to relate history, politics, society, gender, intimacy, and health while remaining appropriately ambiguous.

Throughout his narrative, in fact, reified notions of culture here arguably served as resources (rather than realities) for Du, who drew upon them to engage in a kind of on-the-ground sense-making process in which he investigated the ways in which so-called Chineseness had developed, in particular in comparison to the West, over time. His chronotopes were flexible, in other words, such that he became able to speak about more sensitive, complex realities without saying anything (much) about them. At the same time, Du's narrative undoubtedly engaged in a range of troubling pragmatics. His formulations from Chinese history arguably erased the systemic exclusion of non-cis-gendered elite, Han men (e.g., himself), from the idealized narrative of "nurturing life" in "traditional Chinese culture," for example. It also arguably flattened Chineseness into a singular spatial temporal trajectory within which "the Chinese family" and "the Chinese body" were the primary victims of global political processes in the first half of the twentieth century. While nuanced and strategic in some ways, then, it also problematically reproduced and reified Chineseness in a simultaneously spatial as well as temporal recursion that, in casting binary oppositions between past and present as well as East and West, at least discursively erased persons, places, and times that did not correspond to the broad categories of either Han-ness or whiteness (Irvine and Gal 2000; Rosa 2019).

PROGRESS PLUS SOCIAL DAODE

At one of New Life's longer inner child retreats with Teacher Jo, I met Lao Fei, a fifty-something-year-old life coach, and his colleagues, all life coaches as well. Hailing from a large city in the south, the group worked primarily with business executives who wanted to achieve financial and social "success." One evening, we sat together in their hotel room, snacking while we conducted a group interview. At one point in our conversation, Lao Fei began sharing his perspective on what he glossed as "the real problem" in Chinese society.

"In China, closeness within the family is very rare, especially with our parents. This has a big influence. And so we use these exercises to—because you don't have a lot of intimacy in your life. In the more traditional cultural places, the poorer places, there is actually very little expressing of emotion, so people suppress (压 ya) it in their hearts. I love you a lot, but I can't go across and hug you—I feel that that isn't OK, it isn't polite. Or I can't directly tell you that I really, really love you, I really really like you. People will feel that is impolite, or it's too casual."

Opening with an assessment of prevalent expressive norms within "the Chinese family," Fei here noted that peoples' lack of emotional expression—framed here as "suppression"—has had a negative influence on the amount and quality of intimacy within Chinese relationships. Fei's formulation of "Chineseness" here cast a distinctly chronotopic perspective on the Chinese social landscape, within which the restraint of intimacy was (and is) more prevalent "in the more traditional cultural places" and "the poorer places." Like Du in the previous section, he also constructed a chronotopic mapping of the Chinese affective-relational body-self. In contrast to the feelings of anger, dissatisfaction, and pain that Du emphasized, however, Lao Fei here foregrounded the ways in which *positive* emotions, including love and appreciation, are also suppressed in the heart when one cannot physically or vocally express them. Whereas Du attributed the lack of emotional expression to a traditional emphasis on "order" within the Chinese family, however, Fei related it to a sense of propriety or etiquette wherein most people deemed it "impolite" to spontaneously express feelings of positive regard to others. Spontaneous expressions of emotion, Fei suggested, might seem "too casual" to many people.

Another coach, Wenling, weighed in here: "Chinese culture is like this, Chinese people are very embarrassed/shy (害羞 *haixiu*)."

Lao Fei continued, overlapping her speech, "Yeah, it is not very open (开放 *kaifang*)." Equating shyness with a lack of interpersonal *openness*—an interesting terminological framing that arguably indexes the "reform and opening" (改革开放 *gaige kaifang*) period initiated by Deng Xiaoping after the Cultural Revolution—Fei here built upon his earlier chronotopic casting of "the more traditional places" by invoking a temporal frame that situated such places—and the Chinese norm itself—as outdated and even backwards.

"But in our thinking, we are open," he further added, now casting himself as part of this broad "we."

Wenling agreed, "Yes, our thinking is open-minded. And in our hearts, it is there. We have love for our families, but our methods for expressing it are limited."

Lao Fei interjected again here, pointing out that since these kinds of classes have been offered in China, Chinese culture was becoming more open.

"We all know that we really need these exercises in emotions. But we *also* want to have social morality (道德 *daode*). We want to combine them together." Pausing here, he continued his formulation of a broad "we" that he went on to spatialize, broadly, as located "in China."

"Actually, in China, we also rely a lot on emotions. In the family, we have strong ethics (伦理 *lunli*). We all want to love and protect the others in our family."

Drawing upon the deictic form "we" to construct a shared epistemic stance within which Chinese people all presumably *know* that such training is necessary, Fei here suggested a shared form of awareness as well as shared form of *desire*. Chinese people, in his framing, were imagined as wanting to preserve the extant forms of "social morality" (道德 *daode*) that, in Fei's frame, were both loving and ethical, even if they extended only to the boundaries separating the (national?) family from "others." The grammatical structuring of Fei's statement—which began with a claim of (known) deficiency but was followed with an emphasized desire for "also" maintaining social morality—is key for understanding his subsequent chronotopic casting of "East" and "West" as contrastive moral domains that can be "combined." Fei thus highlighted the desire to preserve indigenous ethical modes of feeling and being while also learning new relational modes through which ethical Chineseness might be extended rather than replaced. Fei and his colleagues thus positioned themselves as active agents who were working to combine cultural approaches to the emotions in ways that preserved the dignity of "Chinese tradition" while also expanding its scope. Once he had established this ethical stance, however, Fei began discussing Chinese society, drawing upon a comparative perspective to call attention to what he positioned as problematic expectations issued by "the collective."

"In some places, you have to respect what people express. If I say no, you can't force me," he said, "but in China, if I say no—if you are part of the collective (集体 *jiti*)—then I have to go along with it. I have to say yes. But now a lot of people have started to respect themselves, and are learning how to say no."

In a broad chronotopic contrast between "other places" and China, Fei here issued a critique of Chinese "collectivism," framed as a perennial cultural truth rather than linking it to any specific periods of history. A tension thus seemed to emerge in Fei's narrative, within which social morality was itself impeded by forces that disrespected the individual's right to refuse. This latter framing further invoked the *agency* of individuals, who had "started to respect themselves" and were thus "learning" how to refuse the demands of the collective. The chronotopic formulation of "combining East and West" that Fei had previously articulated, here served as a framework for successfully resolving this tension. It did so by situating agency or resistance, or both, as a form of self-respect that, though it originated in places beyond China, was a teachable skill that could be productively combined with indigenous forms of moral relationality without undermining them.

I asked, here, for Fei's perspective on how his own and others' contributions toward teaching this kind of material in China might affect Chinese society.

"It will bring great benefits," he replied, "because, number one, I am certain that thousands of years of Chinese cultural development—it won't easily change. But if you allow each of us to study this stuff, and put it into our culture, I feel that we will be much stronger. Every person will be stronger."

In this statement, Fei effectively flattened "thousands of years of history" into a unified depiction of "Chinese cultural development" that was recalcitrant to change. In this frame, if people shaped by this history were "allowed" to gain knowledge of the "Western" material, they would "pull it into" the culture. This, notably, chronotopically mapped Chinese culture as a unified *container* into which forms of knowledge could be deposited through the individual efforts of people, each of whom would thus contribute to strengthening "it." Scaling rapidly between "the individual" and "cultural change," Fei here situated his and his colleagues' work as "spreading the message" that we were learning at New Life.

"Because if you spread it enough, you can create qualitative changes (质变 *zhibian*), and then the government will recognize that it has a good effect for people, and all the schools will start to include it. There is this intention, this is our goal. East and West are just representative of cultures," he added. "But people—every country wants its people to progress. I feel that it's the same everywhere, but it's just the cultural background that is different." Going on to point out how my very presence in the hotel room with them then demonstrated how foreigners gained from the study of China, he concluded by positively framing the ways in which "we are learning from each other, but we are the same."

In analyzing Fei's and his colleagues' comments, it is important, first, to foreground the dialogic situation and the background of the interaction. Here, then, it is relevant to recall that Lao Fei and his colleagues were salespeople who were attending Teacher Jo's workshop in order to accumulate technologies that they could then export to their hometown. It is also, however, important to consider the discursive challenge created by the situation, which involved me—a white, American woman—in a hotel room with several Chinese life coaches whom I had only recently become acquainted with. They had no idea, in fact, how much I knew or understood about Chinese history or Chinese society (a knowledge that I myself also frequently question). It is thus fair to assume that their positions were strategic and careful. They were also, it is fair to assume, pragmatically oriented toward the very forms of politeness and social morality that they described. Such norms likely guided Fei toward his relatively neat affiliative conclusion in which he and I were positioned as "opposite but the same."

Any of these considerations might lead one, perhaps not unreasonably, to discount Fei's narrative as a historically situated performance that, given his position as a life coach for business executives, was organized around the kind of "emotional capitalism" described by Illouz (2008, 60). His reflections might also lead to a consideration of the ways in which he positioned therapeutic ideologies that problematically imagine "individual agency" and "personal responsibility" as the solution to a form of systematic injustice that he formulated as occurring entirely within the bounds of Chineseness. While this view cannot be entirely discounted, it also elides a historical perspective that acknowledges Chinese citizens' "acute awareness" (Kuan 2015) of their own entanglement with systems of governance. Reading Fei's narrative as a form of scalar inquiry within which constantly shifting sets of contrastive chronotopes function as critical scaling devices affords insight into the ways in which seemingly simplistic ideologies of culture at New Life were often *provisional* discursive tools through which people developed emergent theories that afforded cultural critique in a setting where public secrecy—especially with regard to recent and present systems of governance—prevailed. As I detail in the next section, such social structures were often a critical part of the personal and collaborative "work" that functioned to co-constitute participants' political subjectivity as an intimate, ongoing experience that was continually up for retheorization.

FAKE FLOWERS

The process of flexibly drawing upon available geographical binaries in order to formulate distinct forms of political subjectivity, among New Life participants, did not always point outward (e.g., toward Westernness or whiteness). My conversation with Sylvia—a professional forty-eight-year-old woman who had been engaged with self-development for more than ten years—drew upon both temporal and spatial contrasts between urban and rural sites in China in order to scale her ongoing interrogation of Chineseness.

When we met in the conference room of her thirty-fifth-floor office to conduct our interview, Sylvia began by telling me about her history. She had first sought help, she told me, because she suffered from excessive anxiety, which she described as a persistent feeling of *terror* that had not necessarily related to any specific situation in her otherwise successful life. At first, she had seen an "image therapist," who—she succinctly explained—had supported her in coming to see how her "inner self," at the time, was "trapped" within and *under* a dark, pressurized force of some kind.

"Because I was born in the 1960s," she explained here, pausing as if to confirm with me that I understood the meaning behind her chronotopic shift. I offered a brief nod, suggesting that I was clear that she might be making a reference to the political environment and events leading up to the

Cultural Revolution, which officially began in 1966. Sylvia thus began to scale rapidly between her childhood and the political ideologies of the time.

"Our education at the time had to do with loving the country, loving the collective. Take your life and offer it as a tribute to humankind." She laughed sarcastically here. "You—you were to give your life as a tribute."

Indeed, writes Feuchtwang (2013) of the dominant culture that prevailed in the 1950s and 1960s, people often suffered from intense humiliation and shame when they were seen as unenthusiastic in the kinds of "self-sacrifice" and "revolutionary ardor" required of them not just by the state but by also by their own family members, colleagues, and neighbors (225–26). The ideology of "self-sacrifice" that Sylvia referred to thus pointed to systems of governance that instituted scalar intimacies linking the family to the state in specific ways. Within this environment, Sylvia suggested, she never had the opportunity to develop a sense of "self." Her selfhood, in this framing, had been *oppressed* under a murky force, a depiction that emerged from her initial encounters with her image therapist. Her experience of her self expanded with therapy, however, especially once she began participating in group sessions organized around the Satir method. These encounters, indeed, had felt like an almost immediate "revelation" for Sylvia.

"I realized [felt]—oh!—I am a person with *value*. I'm not so insignificant, not so—[in the past] even though I studied well, and worked well, deep in my heart I felt I was less than others, insignificant."

She no longer thought of herself as "less than others," she then told me, but she did still have moments when she felt unworthy and insignificant. In these moments, she admitted, she still experienced some anxiety. She interjected her own narrative here, however, to share a recent realization with me,

"Maybe through these classes," she said, "this is just my own embodied experience (体验 tiyan)—all these years, observing things outside, observing people. And there's also—I also frequently go to the park or whatever to see trees—every year, they blossom. They just naturally blossom. When it's time to blossom, they blossom.... They don't care about other people—they don't need others to need them to blossom. We—people are also a part of nature, we aren't different from that tree. But if there are people who make us blossom—you have to blossom! I need you to blossom! We can blossom, but they aren't real flowers. They are fake."

"Maybe, like in the countryside," she continued, "there aren't people *managing* children. Maybe compared to the city—sometimes I think, like the plants in a hothouse who are managed by a gardener—they have to blossom by May First—sometimes they have to, for National Day (国庆节 *guoqing jie*), they have to decorate the public square. They have to blossom at this time, so they will give the tree a hormone (激素 *jisu*) or whatever. So people, sometimes, are like this. In school, I feel like sometimes they give you this kind of thing," she laughs, "you have to—they force you to blossom, but they are not pressuring something original to one's nature (原性 *yuanxing*)."

This segment of her interview constituted a "tangent" that Sylvia had initiated while discussing her own experience with recognizing and developing her "self." As such, I engage with her remarks here as the kind of incomplete, constantly shifting ethical theory-building that I have discussed throughout this chapter. As a form of scalar inquiry, such theory-making efforts were deeply entangled with the intimate, embodied, relational, and affective selves of participants at New Life.

Indeed, Sylvia launched, here, into the formulation of a comparative framework linking people to trees, describing how the "natural blossoming" of trees occurs without concern for what people "need." People's own growth was similarly natural, she then suggested, noting here that the primary difference was that, unlike trees, we become subject to the desires and demands of others, who insist that we "blossom." Voicing their desire here ("you have to blossom! I need you to blossom!"), she then quickly switched back to an inclusive "we" voice to share her recent realization that the flowers blooming as a result of such demands were "fake."

Indexing the kind of "fakery" that Wielander (2018b, 37) suggests inheres in several state narratives in contemporary China, Sylvia went on here to develop a tentative chronotopic contrast that might be used to support the theory she had clearly been recently developing. Invoking a geospatial distinction between "city" and "countryside," she proposed that "maybe" there were not people constantly *managing* children in the countryside. Though she had not directly invoked children before, in this portion of her narrative it became clear that she was considering the nature analogue in developmental terms that (perhaps) related to the struggles she had faced as a result of the ways in which ideologies of self-sacrifice had permeated her own childhood. Sylvia spoke here, however, of a ruthless urban environment that was familiar to her. In the city, she observed, children were like plants in a "hothouse," continually managed by a range of entities that Sylvia linked to the space-time of "school." As I have discussed throughout this chapter, however, "school" here arguably indexed much more than simply K-12 educational environments. Indeed, in a swift and deft set of scalar shifts, Sylvia linked the kinds of manipulation enacted by the *state* upon plants—for example, gardeners who give "hormones" to trees and flowers at the behest of authorities who need them to be ready for the festivities of national holidays—to the pressures existing within the (urban) education system.

Sylvia's theory took a chronotopic turn here that seemed to hinge on a naïve idealization equating naturalness with "the countryside." Having come to know her deeply over the course of a weeklong inner child workshop, I couldn't help but challenge her on this. I thus asked if she really felt that life in the countryside offered children the kind of "room to grow," so to speak, that she had been describing.

"It's not like that—the countryside also has a lot of problems—rural parents, they all come to the city and leave their children at home," she admitted, "But there's also some people who stay, right? And some places that are more prosperous." She paused before continuing.

"I don't know—I just think that if their parents are there—even if they aren't very prosperous, the kids don't have so much pressure to study. They don't necessarily give them so much programming—'you have to become a doctor, or a lawyer, or whatever high-level person.' But maybe in terms of their *spirit* (心灵 xinling), compared to these kids who are *forced* (强化 qianghua), they are more free. Because I feel I'm just—from the time I was young, I studied well . . . but later I felt that my spirit wasn't that free. So I want people to be able to take the initiative, to choose—I couldn't see clearly what I wanted, what I could do."

In Sylvia's response to my question, there was—notably—a great deal of hedging. Apparent in the way she repeatedly interjected her own flow of speech as well as in her posing of questions and admission of epistemic uncertainty (e.g., "I don't know"), it also inhered in her subjunctive framing. Hedges, as Goffman contends, "introduce some distance between the figure and its avowal" (1981, 148). Sylvia can be seen as distancing herself, at least initially, from an identification with the chronotopic ideology of absolute difference between urban and rural societies. Given the very real sociohistorical conditions that often necessitate the separation of rural families in China, she acknowledged, it couldn't possibly be as straightforward as her nascent theory had suggested. She went on, however, to formulate a set of conditionals that (might) corroborate her theory. Turning to me to confirm or at least entertain the notion that *some* parents do stay with their children, she also addressed the constraints that poverty placed on the actualization of her theory by pointing to the fact that there were some places that were "more prosperous." *If* the parents are there, even in the case of poverty, she then suggested, children in the countryside could be seen as receiving "less pressure to study" (notably from their *parents*) than their urban peers are systematically subjected to.

"Conditionals can be examined," write Don Kulick and Bambi Schieffelin, "for the categories of concern that they express" (2004, 363). Underscoring how they often index the pragmatic as well as moral values that a speaker holds—or is experimenting with upholding with their utterance—this perspective on conditionals points my analysis toward the sociopolitical and moral implications of Sylvia's mapping. Her development of a theory here had, at this point, moved fluidly between the family, the state, and the educational system. In doing so, she invoked the intimate ways in which they became merged into a single hegemonic force exerted upon the imagined (urban) child.

Sylvia also developed a nuanced temporal perspective here, further linking her own childhood experience of pressure to sacrifice herself for the nation to contemporary pressures set upon urban children. Neither form of pressure supported the kind of *freedom* that she went on to imagine was possible. It was here that Sylvia distinguished the ways in which her theory centered around the notion of "spirit." Specifically, she formulated freedom here as a spiritual freedom that contrasted, ultimately, with her own experience growing up. She seemed to argue, however, that it also aptly applied in present-day society. Describing her desire for "people to be able to take initiative, to choose"—unlike she had been—Sylvia's theory here emerged in an "anticipatory mode" (Sumartojo and Pink 2019) within which freedom was imagined. Rather than invoking an idealized or absolute freedom or the kinds of "freedom of choice" often associated with consumer society, however, Sylvia theorized freedom as a relationally grounded form of agency. Demonstrating how scalar inquiry emerges as the kind of *dreaming* that Loizidou (2016) argues constitutes a form of political subjectivity, Sylvia's theory—rooted in her own everyday experience of observing plants and her reflections on her past *as image*—here notably built up to a vision that extended, ultimately, to *all* people.

Sylvia thus seemed to be formulating a scalar vision of the possibilities for "individuality within collectivity" (C. Huang 2016) in China. Her vision, indeed, also resonates with Vivek Murthy's (2020) formulation of a possible "third-bowl society" that balances the intense relationality and strict demands of "traditional" or "first-bowl societies" and the isolation and loneliness of "modern/urban" second-bowl societies. Sylvia's chronotopic framing here must therefore not be read as an indication of her "literal" understanding of the Chinese national landscape. Her comments, rather, point to the ways in which such mappings worked pragmatically as a form of scalar inquiry in which speakers made an effort to understand the past as well as the present in order to imagine alternative cultural possibilities. In the end, however, Sylvia drew back from the activity of theory-building to reflect upon the ways in which her vision was not, ultimately, realistic.

"But it's not that easy," she added, laughing ironically.

Underscoring the realistic picture that participants in the current study had regarding the *actual* possibility that their visions for the future might take hold in Chinese society, Sylvia's ironic stance here points to the ways in which New Life participants faced a set of very real constraints that, in comparison to a U.S. context, for example, extended far beyond their own self-obsessions or refusals to participate in collective forms of political action. Raising the question of the ultimate implications of such dreaming, as I further discuss below, it also underscores the ways in which widespread cultural transformation rarely constituted an explicit focus at New Life.

CONCLUDING REFLECTIONS

I began this chapter with two epigraphs. In the first, Rebecca Karl suggests that Chinese citizens' discursive engagements with the past variably offer them the opportunity to reenvision the future in specific ways. In the second, Michele-Rolph Trouillot observes how all people are "amateur historians." I have drawn upon both insights here to investigate the way New Life participants collaboratively and continually narrated and renarrated their relationship to the very notion of Chineseness. As ethical agents confronting and thinking about ways to approach and adjust their relationship to the structures comprising Chinese society, people thus drew upon multiple, flexible chronotopic frameworks to position imagined and tentative forms of "Chineseness," often set in binary relation to "Westernness," in order to build emergent theories.

Here, however, I demonstrated the ways in which participants often understood, related to, and struggled with these systems not only as external structures, but rather as intimate and embodied aspects of themselves.

As they scaled fluidly and ambiguously between family and state, past and present, I thus emphasized how much was at stake for participants within conversations about the kinds of scalar intimacies that are, in normative everyday interactions, often maintained and upheld. Conversations within this context, I thus argued, emerged as a kind of collaborative "theory-building" (Rosa 2019) within which binaries such as East/West, urban/rural, past/present, or governance/freedom are interrogated and reformulated in ways that undermine their absolute distinction as cultural "facts" but rather reveal the ways in which they provided "benchmarks" upon which to build further theories (Hollan 1992).

Formulations of East and West at New Life, for example, often made use of simplistic dichotomies that hinged upon the construction of East and West as distinct but constantly moving moral spheres. China or the "East" was thus sometimes framed through a lens corresponding to state-supported narratives of an "enduring, timeless Chinese culture" (Karl 2020, 190) within which traditional "Confucian" ideals of relational, holistic personhood are emphasized as morally superior to the crude individualism and corrupt capitalism of Western ideologies. At other times, the East was imagined as a site of extreme repression, governance, and constraint whereas the West was positioned as a space-time of freedom and agency. The spatiotemporal and moral territory attributed to each thus shifted constantly in various "fractal recursions" that involved the "projection of an opposition"—in this case East/West—onto other kinds of relationships, for example, between freedom and oppression (Irvine and Gal 2000, 38; see also Gal 2002, 2016). As such, East and West emerged as fractally iterated contrastive chronotopes that were constantly made and remade in ways that oriented the intimate, relational experience of interlocutors. The shifting nature of such recursions, I argue, relates to the ways in which particular speakers or groups of speakers engaged in conversations as simultaneously personal, cultural, and historical scaling projects that sought to evaluate, critique, and even transform their relationship to various structures of governance, enact such transformations in their everyday lives, or both.

Suggesting an investigation of the gap between the ways in which cultural, geographic, or even temporal binaries were imagined and the ways in which they were experienced, these conversations further often confronted the very real gap that existed between what was known and what was only vaguely known about the real Chinese past. Throughout the chapter, I have thus shown how conversations at New Life frequently engaged, though often implicitly, with histories "that are broadly known but seldom said aloud" (Hillenbrand 2020, 21). Here, then, I suggested how the various forms of public secrecy that exist in the Chinese "cryptocracy" (Hillenbrand 2020) were actively engaged as providing a (if not *the*) key to reimagining the past and present as well as anticipating the future. Rather than a one-sided orientation toward the past that sees it all as "constraint" (Rofel 2007), collaborative scalar inquiry here offered the opportunity for participants to (re)imagine alternative possible futures that simultaneously preserved that which they valued (e.g., the "social morality" mentioned by Fei) at the same time as addressing what they understood, often provisionally, to have caused or to be causing suffering. Such (re)imaginings here pointed, I suggested, to a simultaneous process of self-development and intimate cultural reflexivity within which participants' political subjectivity was (de)constructed, examined, and interrogated collaboratively in moment-to-moment conversations as well as over time in interaction with surrounding environments. As an anticipatory activity of *dreaming* (Loizidou 2016), learning to love for participants like Lan, Du, Lao Fei, and Sylvia thus included envisioning a future Chinese society within which individuality and collectivity might officially coexist (C. Huang 2016; Murthy 2020). As a simultaneously personal and collective process of self-development, participants at New Life enacted, in other words, a form of moral agency or "ethics of trying" (Kuan 2015, 18) or "microintervention" (R. Johnson 2023) that was often centered around the self but also extended, at least in theory, far beyond the self.

To the extent that it either implicitly or explicitly extended only or primarily to the kinds of elite, middle-class, Han constituency represented by center participants, however, it is also important to consider the ways in which such conversations, which were often intentionally ambiguous, also served to reproduce and reinforce a Hancentric version of Chinese history (Carrico 2017; Friend and Thayer 2017; Cheng 2019). In this sense, iterative (re)chronotopizations of East/West like those described in this chapter simultaneously worked to perpetuate problematic ideologies of Chineseness and Westernness at the same time as their very uptake emerged as a strategy for enacting scalar inquiry and the development of nuanced forms of political subjectivity. It is further important to note that as much as participants might be seen as engaging with *public* secrets within such conversations, engagement with what might be considered "actual" secrets was, not surprisingly, entirely absent in the space. Although I am, of course, not privy to all of the actual secrets held in place by the intricate machinery of governance in China, the ways in which oppression is being enacted through forced labor, imprisonment, and "negative eugenics" in Xinjiang Province (Byler 2018, 2021a-b, 2022) comes to mind as something that was sorely missing from the public ethical-relational consciousness at New Life. Though arguably absent for good reason, the sources and resources that New Life participants had to "think with," so to speak, as they formulated their visions of the future, constituted a serious constraint upon the possibility that their engagement in scalar inquiry and development of political subjectivity might contribute to the kinds of social transformations that impact society beyond elite, Han, middle-class institutions. Even if they were to have access to such information, moreover, it is also important to consider the ways in which entrenched ideologies regarding racial and ethnic hierarchies might have, "unintentionally" or not, circumvented the extension of the love ethic to people and places understood and experienced as "different." As central as these caveats are to my analysis, the kinds of scalar inquiry that emerged at New Life, I argue, still do not warrant dismissal as inherently "apolitical." As I discuss in the following chapter, the kinds of "conversations with ghosts" that emerged within family constellations, in particular, often served as a basis or affordance for at least partial acknowledgment of what Peggy McIntosh refers to as the "colossal unseen dimensions" that must be recognized before any type of social transformation can be realized (1989, 12).

5

Wrangling with Ghosts

Only the imagination and promise of an alternative future allow historical and present suffering to emerge and speak. Only this can give meaning to past and present movements.... And only a nonteleological future vision can free history and time from the custody of power and violence.

—DAI JINHUA

The time of the "learning to live," a time without tutelary present, would amount to this . . . : to learn to live *with* ghosts, in the upkeep, the conversation, the company, or the companionship, in the commerce without commerce of ghosts. To live otherwise, and better. No, not better, but more justly. But *with* them.... And this being-with specters would also be, not only but also, a *politics* of memory, of inheritance, and of generations.

—JACQUES DERRIDA

One afternoon in 2015, we were sitting on the floor of the large banquet room of the hotel. The blinds were drawn closed across the wall of glass doors that looked out upon the perfectly constructed lakeside, where a wedding party had just drawn to a close. For most of the past few hours, we had been working together in groups doing family constellations. There were eight people in my group. In one constellation set up by Ding, a woman around sixty, I was chosen to play a representative. As usual in family constellation therapy, however, I did not know who I was. She simply placed me, at the outset of the constellation, standing up alongside a woman and a man. Two other women in our group were then guided to lay down on the floor. We were silent for a moment and then, for no reason that I can explain, I moved to lay down next to the other two women. It was then quiet in our constellation. No more movement ensued.

Teacher Jo rang a tiny bell, and we transitioned. We became ourselves again and huddled up to debrief. Ding was very worried, she told us, because

I had been playing her little sister, with whom she was quite close and who, we also learned, was currently suffering from some kind of serious illness. We learned, too, that the two women on the floor had been her mother and another little sister, one who had died when she was young.

"When she died," Ding explained, "my mother's heart seemed to go with her—even though my mother is still alive." Ding was thus worried that my behavior in the constellation meant that her sister was going to die. I told her, quite honestly, that during the constellation I had not *felt* like I was dying. I had gone to lay down with the other women only because I had wanted to feel safe, and it had felt comfortable there. This only superficially comforted Ding.

The bell rang again. The next constellation in our group was for a man of roughly seventy, who I will call Lao Hua, who placed me in the center of a group of four others. The moment we started, they turned their backs to each other. I tried to reach out to them, to turn them back to face one another. I felt like the embodiment of sticky glue, and I became increasingly anxious as my efforts were ignored. When we debriefed, Lao Hua told us that I had been playing a sister of his who acted just like I did. She had always tried desperately to keep everyone together, Lao Hua commented. We all found this remarkable, even after I disclosed that my experiences in my own family could very well have influenced my behavior in the constellation.

As we were discussing it, with a feeling of closeness and camaraderie among us, the group next to us was still in the midst of a constellation. They were huddled together, gazing intensely at one another without saying a word. Farther back in the room, we could hear another group in the midst of a constellation.

"Why are you looking at me?," a middle-aged man yelled. "I hate you. Go away!"

His voice seemed to hang over the whole room, as if time was standing still. At some point, however, someone opened the blinds and pulled the glass doors open slightly. Light poured in, highlighting the dust hovering over the tissues, pillows, water bottles, teacups, and journals scattered throughout the room. There was a lull in the room, and many of us just sat and gazed curiously outside to see a family walking by the lake. The man was wearing a suit, walking several steps ahead of his wife and son, gazing forward. Hips jutting forward, arms wrapped comfortably behind his back, he seemed immensely confident in his masculinity, despite (or perhaps especially) the way his wife's designer pink handbag dangled from his hands. He glanced back from time to time at his wife, who was wearing a fresh white linen dress. She walked slightly bent over, taking small, awkward steps as she tried to grab ahold of a little boy's arm. He kept escaping, I noted, and running—or teetering, rather—back and forth between his parents and the lake.

CONVERSATIONS WITH GHOSTS

According to the founder of family constellation therapy, Bert Hellinger (1925–2019), phantoms of our ancestors' grief, guilt, and cruelty—their burdens and secrets, their uncertainties, but also their curiosities, their connections, their solutions for making sense of the world—live on inside us, informing the way we move, the way we connect with others, and our everyday desires. These phantoms also include past and even ongoing events in the lives of our living relatives, both those that resonate with what Hellinger (1998) calls "love's hidden symmetry" and those that do not. These ghosts, in other words, constitute the intimate, embodied lens through which we see, hear, and otherwise engage with the world. In order to begin to heal any pain that these residues continue to cause in our daily lives, we must therefore bring these ancestral energies to life in a "constellation." American family constellation practitioner Mark Wolynn thus cites psychiatrist Norman Doidge when he frames the method as a psychotherapeutic process of turning "ghosts" into "ancestors" (2016, 49). Often described as a *mysterious* experience in China as well as globally, family constellation therapy—translated into Chinese as 家庭系统排列 (*jiating xitong pailie*) or simply "*jiapai*" (家排) as I refer to it throughout this book—involves focal participants choosing representatives to enact their family members, both living and dead. The participant, as described above, then watches or *witnesses* the primarily silent but intensely embodied and emotional interactions.

As Whitney Duncan and I have noted, constellation work asks participants to embrace a novel understanding of the self as one that "extends backwards in time and space through an unimaginably dense network of events and relationships that are, at the time of the conversation, obstructed from view" (2019, 473). The self as enacted, embodied, and experienced in *jiapai* was thus frequently framed in *spiritual-relational* terms that involved past temporalities and non-co-present and sometimes nonliving or even nonhuman entities in the immediate embodied experience of participants.

Although this self was understood to be inclusive of the individual families of *particular* participants, moreover, in practice the boundaries of the body-self were distributed across the bodies of others who are co-present during constellations and workshops (see chapter 3). Consisting of verbal expression, physical contact, and coordinated movement, Duncan and I thus discuss *jiapai* sociality as involving a type of "entrainment" in which "self and other . . . are closer, more similar, more intertwined" (Davis 2004, 33). In an intensive process that involves "third-person self-witnessing" in which participants had the opportunity to see "themselves" from different angles (Libby and Eibach 2002; Sutin and Robbins 2008; Pritzker and Duncan 2019), this intimate form of sociality or "register of intimacy" also notably affected the bodies of participants who simply observed and those participating as representatives.

Pointing to the kinds of intersubjective, intercorporeal "melting" or permeability that informed mirroring, enactment, and "time travel" exercises, as described in chapter 3, the expanded self in *jiapai* thus significantly recast normative Chinese notions of the familial *dawo* or "big self." In classical terms, of course, such a self is rightly understood as capable of "trafficking" between the worlds inhabited by the living and those inhabited by the dead (M. Yang 2020). The interface between humans and ghosts is not, however, customarily framed as a continuous *location*, nor is it situated within the bodies and minds of descendants. Though bearing some resemblance to the ways in which, in classical Chinese cosmologies, the relational process of "influence and response" (感格 *gange*) is understood as an ongoing communicative channel between living and dead relations (Gardner 1996), the kinds of resonance (感应 *ganying*) understood to prevail in *jiapai* are novel in China. Hellinger's understanding of the ways in which bodies are *occupied* by and continually enact the experiences of their relatives, for example, is very different from the kind of practical relationality imagined as obtaining between the living and dead in classical Chinese formulations. Ghosts, in this traditional frame, as Song dynasty philosopher Zhu Xi (1130–1200 C.E.) succinctly explained, constitute a form of *qi* that is dispersed rather than condensed (Gardner 1996). Appeasing them through various ritual practices, moreover, might be crudely summarized as "preventative" in that keeping one's ancestors and other ghosts happy helps them avoid becoming "hungry ghosts" (饿鬼 *e gui*) who wreak havoc in the lives of the living (Gardner 1996). In *jiapai*, however—as I have joked—"the ghosts need therapy, too" (Pritzker 2019). At New Life, constellations thus emerged as a way of helping both deceased *and* living "ghosts" resolve their complex interpersonal and psychodynamic entanglements.

Despite this strangeness, *jiapai* has become incredibly popular over the past decade in China. The reason for its popularity, expounds prominent Chinese therapist Zheng Lifeng—who leads *jiapai* workshops throughout China—is because of the method's ability to generate "harmony" 和谐 (*hexie*) in the home/family, which serves as the basis for harmony in other areas of life, including career, finances, and citizenship more broadly. Zheng's framing of *jiapai*, alongside Confucianized renderings of the method (J. Yang 2020), thus notably aligns with state discourses of "harmonious society" (Wielander and Hird 2018; J. Yang 2018a-b, 2020; L. Zhang 2020). The intensive interest that Chinese citizens have taken in the method cannot therefore be separated from such discourses. The immense *drive* that many of the people I met had to engage in hours upon hours of constellation work—even sometimes continuing on their own after the conclusion of a workshop—suggested to me, however, that there had to be something *more* that compelled such an obsession.

In this chapter, I thus propose that—in addition to or perhaps *because* of the ways in which it overlaps with hegemonic state discourses—*jiapai* is also immensely successful in China because it offers participants an opportunity to "wrangle with ghosts" in an intimate, embodied, relational as well as anticipatory register that requires very little explicit communication. Indeed, the director of the center, Aileen, once explained to me that *jiapai* is particularly appealing to clients because it constitutes "a straightforward method" for seeing "what places are blocked" within the complex terrain of an often only partially understood family past.

This strange intervention, which required participants to expand their fundamental spatiotemporal orientation to the body-self, afforded what Duncan and I suggest might be considered as a *technology of the social* at New Life. Technologies of the social, specifically, refer to the ways in which group psychotherapy, in particular, has the capacity to "[reconfigure] participants' experiences of themselves as intersubjective social beings in the flow of social, cultural, and historical space and time, even if only for the length of a workshop" (Pritzker and Duncan 2019, 470). As a technology of the *social* self, *jiapai* served to draw participants' attention toward culturally and historically shaped, habitual ways of being-in-the-world. Constellations at New Life also, however, offered a unique opportunity for participants to access or witness the enduring effects of the past not just as a personal project but as an intimate and collaborative as well as a collective or social anticipatory mode.

As I suggest throughout this chapter, *jiapai* here afforded participants the agency, within an intensive relational and embodied context, to face events and emotions of the past, or ghosts, that had long been and were largely destined to remain buried. The central, foundational goal of *jiapai* was thus often framed at New Life as the possibility of accessing what Hellinger called the "underlying love and life power" that exists at the level of the broad family system. Drawing on Hellinger's spatialized notion of "symmetry," the love of the "clan" was thus often envisioned as a location that is temporally enduring within the extended familial body-self and which could be accessed only through the identification of hidden family dynamics, traumas, and secrets. Cast as a process of *movement* that "[allowed] historical and present suffering to emerge and speak," as Dai Jinhua frames it, *jiapai* was thus often chronotopically formulated as an embodied, sociospatial, and temporal process through which we might "free history and time from the custody of power and violence" (2018, 21). *Jiapai*, in other words, invited participants to practice "being-with specters," in Derrida's terms, and offered a pathway toward learning to live—and learning to *love*—both "better" and "more justly" (1994, xvii–xviii). As Teacher Du framed it once during a highly charged group discussion about the interpersonal, affective, and embodied effects of forced abortion, for example, we were engaging in *jiapai* in order to create a more "just" (更大公平 *gengda gongping*) environment for future generations.

Constellations and conversations about constellations, I thus discuss in this chapter, often implicitly, and sometimes explicitly, invoked the kinds of more-or-less public *secrets* that I have discussed, throughout this book, as related not only to the risk or fear involved when speech is censored or otherwise coercively suppressed. Public secrecy, rather, underscores how speech is often *impossible* because there is so much that is unknown, or at least not *explicitly* known. Communicated within the kinds of mundane everyday interactions that suggest but do not directly refer to the events, emotions, or experiences of the past (Feuchtwang 2013), public secrecy here becomes "like the ghost . . . a thing that hovers between the visible and the occluded, the known and the unsayable" (Hillenbrand 2020, 37). In this chapter, I thus suggest that constellations promised (and sometimes afforded) participants the opportunity to address secrecy in embodied interactions that did not require explicit dialogue. Indeed, in Hellinger's terminology, the focal participant benefits from adopting what he calls a "phenomenological posture," a highly intense state in which they become able to grasp "the vastness and complexity of the greater whole" (Hellinger [2001] 2007, 2). As opposed to the kind of "processing" that occurs through explicit inquiry, Hellinger explains, the phenomenological posture moves us toward a state of openness in which "we pause in our efforts to grasp the unknown" ([2001] 2007, 2). American practitioner Mark Wolynn thus contrasts the kind of "intellectual understanding" often considered crucial for healing to occur with the centrality of "visceral experience" that prevails in *jiapai* (2017, 22).

Because the details of the past in China often quite literally *could not be spoken*, the "wrangling" that I am referring to must be understood not as a direct engagement but, rather, as a kind of sidelong glance. Such a process, as I discuss throughout this chapter, often functioned through the kinds of "indexical traces" that, Jie Li writes, "make metonymic inferences from fractured records, while also acknowledging the gaps and limits of our knowledge" (2020, 10). As apparent in the opening vignette, however, constellations at New Life also invoked a collaborative process that was no less real than that which occurs in any other conversation. Rather than being primarily referential, this dialogue took shape as a pragmatic and deeply indexical form of collaborative *questioning*. Though such questions were often ambiguous or poorly articulated, they nonetheless constituted *embodied* questions that aligned with the definition of a question as "an utterance that 'craves' a verbal or other semiotic response" (Bolinger 1957, 4). Whether the questions were spoken aloud or not, constellations here thus offered an opportunity to grant *epistemic authority* to the various ghosts and ancestors who then replied to us through other participants' bodies.

The notion of epistemic authority here points to a kind of relational gradient within which one party has information or *knows* something (K+) that the other does not (K-) (Heritage 2013). Within the discursive processes that emerged in *jiapai*, the ghosts (who had the knowledge we lacked) thus occupied the K+ side of what Heritage (2013) refers to as "the epistemic gradient." Like mediums in spiritualist séances, moreover, *agency* here was "distributed" across the spirit-minds of living and dead interlocutors (Manning 2018). The bodies of representatives, from this perspective, worked like mediums who served as the vehicle for *permeability* between human and nonhuman (or posthuman) entities in late nineteenth- and early twentieth-century spiritualism (Puglionesi 2020). Unlike spiritualism, however, in *jiapai* the conversation is rarely framed as direct contact with "actual dead people" but is rather conceived of as the continuation of a range of people's energies as ghosts that continued to reside within the self. We might therefore perhaps understand jiapai to be a kind of lived biosemiotics of ghost/human communication or "genre of listening" (Marsilli-Vargas 2014) in which participants learned to "hear" ghosts—our own and those of others. Shaped by the emergent context of participants' desires to get a glimpse into the past, wrangling here thus emerged as participants engaged with their personal ghosts—the illness of Ding's sister, for example, or the dynamics in Lao Hua's childhood home—as well as more public or *shared* ghosts that were not only collective but are also, as Andrew Hoskins suggests, "connective" (Hoskins 2011, as cited in J. Li 2020, 18).

The answers we received from the ghosts in jiapai, admittedly, were incredibly ambiguous, requiring more conversations to decipher tenuous associations and possible meanings. Like the rapid "debriefings" between constellations in the opening vignette, these dialogues were often at least somewhat less obtuse and significantly more casual as participants worked together to make sense of the constellation as if it was a puzzle we could, at least tentatively, collaboratively solve.

As part of this quest, such conversations frequently involved a shared mode of inquiry or collective subjunctivity in which we engaged curiously with what Jie Li calls a "memory ecology" or an "environment in which . . . a dynamic constellation of political, economic, cultural, and technological forces affects the survival and perishing, reproduction, and dissemination of memories" (2020, 9). Throughout this chapter, I thus draw upon Margaret Hillenbrand's notion of "revelation," which she describes as "conjoin[ing] the notion of uncovering what was hitherto hidden with startlement or shock ('the big reveal'), with a sense of fear and wonder . . . and with a whisper of the numinous" (2020, 143). Even without such explicit invocations, however, Hillenbrand emphasizes that both individual and collective experiences of revelation in what she calls "the cryptocracy" of contemporary China "do more than merely rip back the veil" (2020, 143). "Revelation *does* things to the secret," she writes, "not simply turning a laser light on it, but sculpting unexpected angles of illumination: it performs a more processual and *responsive kind of labor*" (2020, 143, italics mine). Similar to the ways in which the collaborative enactment that other group exercises motivated (but did not necessarily require), jiapai invited participants to rescale their intimate relationship to concepts about selfhood, relationality, gender, education, and governance in China. Constellations, in other words, requested a similar type of "time travel" labor from participants in which they might wrangle with rescaling their intimate relationship with Chinese histories that endured in their own as well as in *other* participant's bodies. Striking at the heart of participants' deeply felt desire to reorient themselves within a distinct personal or biographical space-time, the indexical function of obscure images in *jiapai* here initiates participants into a more broadly shared *cultural* time that endured in their physical, emotional, and relational body-selves.

Inasmuch as this process often took shape through implicit references or indexes that could have pointed to multiple possible "secrets," it is difficult to describe it in a "scientific" manner that stands on the sturdy grounds of either "evidence" or "outcomes." My observations here, however, derived from watching countless constellations as well as listening to hundreds of conversations about the modality and conducting interviews with longtime participants who—as I discuss in chapters 6 and 7—experienced *jiapai* as an entry point into an embodied interrogation of intergenerational trauma. As I discuss below, moreover, founders and leaders in *jiapai* very explicitly engage with the ways in which the extended space-time of the familial body-self is inclusive of a range of broader cultural and historical experiences. My observations, in this sense, were both empirically grounded and situated in a conversation that is not entirely novel, broadly speaking. In examining the "how" of the processes through which this emerged at New Life, however, my goal is to engage specifically with the reason(s), beyond state-driven pressure to establish harmony within the family, that people at this center—and perhaps China more broadly—find *jiapai* so unceasingly compelling.

THE AGENCY OF IMAGES

I was never allowed to photograph or video-record any of the constellations I witnessed over three years of fieldwork. Constellations nevertheless often seemed—as I have previously noted—like old family photographs coming to life (Pritzker 2019). They were distinct, however, in that—when observing or participating in constellations—it seemed as if one was suddenly able to witness, or at least ponder, all the unseen dynamics operating *beyond* the frame. Lilly, for example—a twenty-four-year-old student from a large urban center—framed her relief when she first encountered *jiapai* several years ago.

"I've always felt that relationships between people are not as simple as they seem on the surface," she explained. *Jiapai* had helped Lilly to begin to see, however, the unspoken complexity that she had always felt related to what she called her "family karma" (家族业力 *jiazu yeli*), further offering her insight into what she called her own, hidden "dark side."

"Photography disrupts conventional notions of experience," writes Robert Desjarlais, "as photographs so often involve complex foldings of past, present, and future, self and other, the actual and the imagined. Photographs upend set ideas of selfhood, temporal clarity, and steady, continuous streams of experience" (2019, 20). Constellations seemed to hit all of these marks. They were particularly brilliant at disrupting the conventional experience of temporality as well as embodied selfhood. Even conversations *about* constellations, as described above, often upended normative ideas of time, space, and the possibility of accessing the past, not to mention the normative boundaries of the body-self. Indeed, it sometimes felt like the dynamic, nonlinear, space-time gave rise to a sense of being entirely "out of time." By "out of time," I should clarify, I do not mean to suggest that time in such exercises, as Derrida—or Hamlet—might say, fell, somehow, "out of joint" (Derrida 1994, 20). Here, however, it often felt like the liminal time-space of the constellation caused everyday time to fall somehow more *into* joint,

Similar to the ways in which, as the sense of *communitas* co-created and collaboratively maintained in the context of transformational festivals in the West gives rise to liminal "moments in and out of time," constellation-time here seemed to fall into alignment with the temporality that Derrida associates with "learning to live" as a "being-with specters" (1994, xviii). It felt, in other words, like we were confronting the "ghosts"—the secrets, the unspoken alliances and feuds, the kinds of agreements made long in the past and never articulated but always felt. As suggested above, the social and historical implications of this process were key. Before moving into a discussion that centers the ways in which "being-with specters" constituted what Derrida also identified as "a *politics* of memory, of inheritance, and of generations" (1994, xviii; italics in original), however, this section engages with the agency that constellations—as images—enacted in the personal and interpersonal worlds of participants.

"What does an image want?," Desjarlais asks. He answers immediately: "An image wants to be noticed" (2019, 137). Images, in other words, maintain a kind of evocative *agency* that requests, if not demands, recognition

(Gell 1998). Indeed, throughout this fieldwork, I frequently heard about the ways in which particular participants had responded to the images gleaned from or shortly after their own or others' constellations. In one opening circle for a *jiapai* seminar in 2016, for example, an attendee shared how the method had helped her see that she had needed to resolve her strained relationship with her father in order to feel genuine intimacy with her husband. Julie—one of the head administrators at the center—likewise reflected upon the ways in which witnessing her first constellation had worked to alleviate the tension she had previously always felt with her mother-in-law. What I suggest here might be considered in terms of the "agency" of images that emerged in constellations at New Life, however, was rarely as explicit or straightforward as these condensed reports suggest.

I introduced Lina's impressions of the "mysteriousness" of the atmosphere at New Life in the opening vignette of chapter 3, for example. There, I detailed a short exercise that she described engaging in during her first visit. In our longer conversation, however, Lina described how the experience of witnessing her first constellation also contributed to her sense that New Life (and *jiapai* specifically) offered her a sense of "productive confusion" that was both disarming and compelling.

"This thing captures—the stuff it presents—it made me feel—it gave me a lot of feelings," she said, "and a lot of very confusing problems. They all come out from this kind of process—I can say I am relieved to some extent. And then—but afterwards I also felt even more confused."

Lina then briefly described her first constellation, which I had unfortunately not been present to witness. First, she detailed her initial encounter with the facilitator, a process that involves a publicly initiated back-and-forth dialogue in which the participant poses a central question or series of questions that they want to focus on in their constellation. Lina had told the facilitator that she wanted to focus on her relationship with her estranged husband, who was living overseas with their son at the time. More specifically, she had wanted to figure out if she should initiate a divorce.

Despite this specific focus, Lina explained, the constellation had unexpectedly taken shape as an encounter primarily between Lina's representative and the representative embodying her mother. Lina was put off by this at first. She was frustrated that the "answer" she was receiving seemed irrelevant in terms of offering anything specifically about her marriage. As she observed the interaction between "herself" (as embodied by another participant in the workshop) and "her mother" (again, another participant), however, she had begun to feel curious about the intensity of emotion that flowed between the two women.

"That's why it's very interesting—the reaction, the connection between me and my mom," she said, speaking in English. "Because, you know, I would never hold my mom and cry, that kind of thing. We are kind of, like, not very *close*—because I never—we're never, like, *physical* . . . and I can never say—I don't say 'I love you' to my mom, my parents. Ever. They can't do it either."

Explaining how her mother had "lost her trust" long ago, Lina went on to describe a particular moment, during the constellation, that "hit hard." It happened when the participant representing her mother told the participant representing Lina that she thought that she (Lina) was a better mother than her (the mother). Hearing her "mom" acknowledge this resonated deeply, despite the fact that it was a stranger playing a role.

"I kind of like—because I would never hear that from my parents. So I kind of feel, like, *relieved*," she said. It had only occurred a month prior to our interview, however, and Lina remained both confused and skeptical. She nevertheless went on to describe a strange shift that had seemed to occur in their relationship since the constellation. It began when her mother had called to warn her to return a piece of ("cheap") Ikea furniture due to a recall, evoking what Lina cast as her "typical response" to her mother: resistance and irritation.

"But when I hung up, for a while I even thought maybe I should just, like, return it—because even with all the hassles, if returning the thing makes her happy," she said, interjecting her sentence to comment on how "I would never—I would never think that way before."

She laughed heartily here as she described how she began to rethink the intimate meaning of returning the Ikea product in the context of her relationship with her mother. The effect had been subtle, but interestingly, and again to Lina's surprise, it persisted in the interactions that she had with her mother during her weekly obligatory (and dreaded) visit with her parents a few days later. Her mother, at one point, had suggested that the two of them go for a walk.

"Normally, I would've been nervous to be with my mom alone," she explained, noting that her mother always seemed to find a way to put her down within the first five minutes of their conversations. This time, however, she went. "And we didn't say anything particularly, but kind of, I kind of feel happy, almost—I don't know, for a long time. Like, you know, it doesn't have—I had the kind of feeling like I don't mind being with her."

Describing how the shift must have had something to do with her involvement at New Life, Lina adopted a chronotopic framework to contrast her past way of being with her mother with this new orientation. In doing so, she notably framed a kind of *hope* that she had begun to feel in relation to *other* relationships, including her marriage. Speaking to the mysterious "efficacy" of *jiapai*, Lina's story underscores how *witnessing* constellations also often evoked emotional and physical shifts for participants. Ping, who I introduced in chapter 1, thus described witnessing a constellation for the first time at New Life as evoking a powerful "mood" or "atmosphere" (气氛 *qifen*), even though she was only watching from the sidelines.

Importantly, people who had only served as representatives or witnesses *also* frequently noted the therapeutic benefits of their participation. During a closing circle, a participant named Bunny thus once poetically described how, in serving as the representative for another woman in the group, it felt like she had become "a conduit" (管道 *guandao*) through which the pain as well as the love of the other "flowed into her" such that she felt "more complete." This experience, Bunny further noted, felt like a form of *healing* that somehow relieved the pressure she always seemed to feel to do things responsibly and correctly. She felt, she concluded, like she could finally *breathe* and move naturally. As the participant quoted in chapter 3 noted once during a closing circle, moreover, even just "sitting outside and watching" others' constellations had been "a deep experience."

To be clear, constellations did not, by any means, always guide participants toward the kinds of closeness or intimacy that Lina and others here described. The confusion they generated was, furthermore, not necessarily always "generative" in a positive sense. In one constellation I witnessed, for example, the focal participant, Lucy, had opened with her desire to address her persistent stomach pain, the cause of which multiple diagnostic tests had been unable to reveal. During her consult with the facilitator, however, she did admit that there had been, for several years now, a great deal of tension in her marriage. Lucy's constellation thus initially included just two representatives, one for her and one for her husband. Lucy placed them far apart from one another, facing in the same direction. As the constellation took shape, her "husband" repeatedly tried to bridge the distance separating them. Each time he crossed the room to stand next to her, however, her representative would shift slightly away from him. When this continued without any further resolution, the facilitator asked Lucy about her relationships prior to marrying, and Lucy reported that she had been in a serious relationship with her boyfriend in college. A representative was then called up to represent Lucy's previous boyfriend. Immediately upon his entrance into the constellation, her representative began to move slightly closer to him, ending up by his side with her back to the representative of her husband. Here, the facilitator halted the constellation and asked Lucy if she could "see" the situation.

"She doesn't even care if the old lover is paying attention to her, she is just happy to be close to him," the facilitator observed. Lucy responded with immediate distress.

"I don't know what to do with this—I wanted resolution with my husband. I just wanted to have a happy home with my husband and child," she said, tears forming in her eyes.

The facilitator asked her, here, if she was able to say out loud, in front of the entire group, that she wanted to be with her husband. Lucy folded her face into her hands, repeating that she just wanted to have "a happy home" (幸福的家 *xingfu de jia*). The representatives became listless in response, and the facilitator walked over to Lucy and extended her hand. She then led her, still in tears and still mumbling that she just wanted a happy home, toward the representative who had been enacting her. When they reached the inner circle, the facilitator then guided her to utter the phrase "I want you to be happy" over and over until something began to shift. As this unfolded, her representative observed that she felt resentful.

The representative for Lucy's husband then spoke, "If you really love him and want to be with him, I can accept it."

The constellation took shape, from here, as a conversation in which Lucy expressed considerable distress at the "reality" that the scene seemed to indicate. Clearly unwilling to embrace the notion that she was no longer—or perhaps never had been—in love with her husband and, indeed, was yearning for her previous partner, Lucy continued to express hesitance (if not resistance). When we moved on to the next constellation, moreover, she was still clearly stirred up. Indeed, as she observed the following constellation, Lucy began to burp loudly. She also ran outside to the balcony, at one point, to issue a guttural wail. Speaking to the embodied and affective resonance that often prevailed during constellation work, Lucy's closing comments also underscored the ways in which the experience did not always translate directly into clear answers.

"It is ultimately up to me," Lucy, who had regained composure, said during the closing circle. "But it was helpful for me to say that I wanted to have a happy home with my husband."

Lucy's closing comments point to the fact that, despite the agency of images in *jiapai*, participants still retained a great deal of their own agency in responding to them. Indeed, as one participant named Tee remarked once during a private conversation—after an unusually conclusive *jiapai* session in which we had observed her representative become frustrated and walk away from her partner—"I never make decisions based on this." Facilitators and participants alike thus often noted the importance of *discernment* when making sense of constellations. Even Tee's refusal, I suggest, constituted the kind of response to the agency or even insistence that *jiapai* images enacted. Perhaps it was related to the ways in which such images seemed to move us into a different relationship with temporality. Or perhaps there was more to the story. Perhaps, I suggest below, the images in constellations worked like the aesthetic images that Hillenbrand (2020) refers to as *photo-forms*.

In Hillenbrand's definition, photo-forms are images that "take 'a secret about a secret,' and encrypt it further still" (2020, 210). Though often highly occluded, photo-forms are "adept at shadowboxing with those things that people find difficult to say aloud," she explains, "because they are visual objects that 'speak' the language of secrecy" (2020, 5). Underscoring the ways in which constellations often invoked obscure references to past social traumas or "social ghosts" (R. Roberts 2013), the consideration of *jiapai* images in terms of photo-forms highlights how "aesthetic encounters," as Marianne Hirsch writes, "elect a sense of vulnerability that can move us toward an ethics and a politics of open-mindedness and mobility, attuning us to the needs of the present, to the potentialities for change, and to the future" (2016, 82). Both in terms of what they revealed—or at least seemed to reveal—and the ways they embodied or *indexed* that which was *excluded* from a photograph, the following section thus engages with the ways in which the intimate geography of New Life continuously emerged, during constellation work, as a social, even political anticipatory mode that chronotopically situated reckoning with the past as a mode of imagining and even creating a better future.

THE INDEXICALITY OF GHOSTS

Drawing upon the notion that "numen-seeking . . . is often a communal experience," Hillenbrand highlights the ways in which photo-forms and other "works that use encryption to take on public secrecy" work to "enjoin new ways of looking" (Hillenbrand 2020, 21). Photo-forms, Hillenbrand

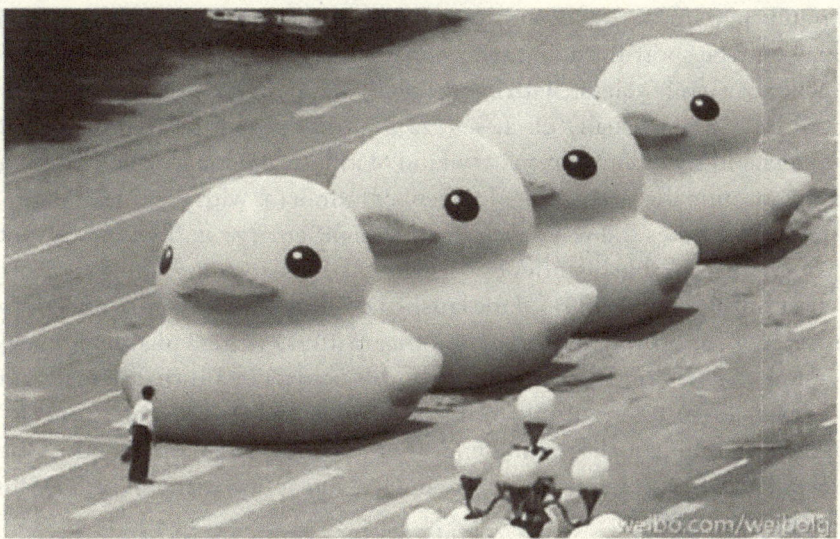

Figure 5.1. Photo-form of Tank Man with tanks replaced with giant rubber duckies.

writes, have a kind of *revelatory power* that betrays "the brittle character of public secrecy" (216). She details, for example, how photo-forms that variably obscure the man, the tank, or the street from the famous Tank Man photograph taken during the massacre at Tiananmen in 1989 (commonly referred to as "six four" or June Fourth) have the capacity to reveal, to at least some viewers, "the cracks in the carapace," so to speak (179). In her discussion of the widely circulated photo-form in which the tanks are replaced by giant rubber duckies, for example, Hillenbrand underscores the image's apparent "anti-spectrality" (see fig. 5.1).

"Indeed," she writes, "if ghost had an antonym, it might well be rubber duck" (Hillenbrand 2020, 190). Especially when they are witnessed collectively, Hillenbrand observes, photo-forms thus afford "an encounter whose phenomenology is akin to the experience of the shared secret" (210). Creating "conduits of solidarity" among viewers, Hillenbrand thus suggests that photo-forms have the capacity to "forge coalitions of shadowboxers, made up of artists and audiences who are willing to experiment together with being more candid about those things that are broadly known but seldom said aloud" (21). Foregrounding the experience as a *communal* experience that variably extends across space as well as time, she thus observes how those who collectively experience such revelation might even be seen as "minor publics," or groups "whose coalitions naturally ebb and flow and may only be short-lived, but who nonetheless cohere as blocs that experiment, for a while at least, with being honest about the things that they know well but do not usually discuss" (222). Further proposing that we might understand such photo-forms as a kind of indexical flood barrier that often pivots around the strategic deployment of humor (as with the rubber duck), she further notes the ways such images might emerge as "metonyms" not just for unspeakable histories but also to "all the many other things that are unsayable in China" (188). "If the crushed protests of 1989 were to enter into sayability, so, too, might these many other matters," writes Hillenbrand, suggesting that the indexicality of photo-forms points not only to the secrets of the past but also to multiple forms of ongoing and "only partially visible" injustice and inequality in the *present*, including (as per Hillenbrand) the marginalization of migrant workers and the corruption that prevails in state institutions (188).

The group context is thus critical to my analysis of what I frame here as the *indexicality of images* in *jiapai*. Though workshops inevitably included participants from multiple generations who had experienced different aspects of Chinese society based on gender, class, and political background, the collaborative engagement with ambiguous yet indexical images, I suggest here, might be understood as at least affording (if not necessarily guaranteeing) a similar dynamic. Pointing to the ways in which the acknowledgment of various forms of *shared vulnerability* afford a unique space for enacting a kind of intercorporeal, collaborative scalar inquiry, the notion of constellations as images that are often more like photo-forms than family photographs further draws our attention to the ways in which *indexicality* works, within particular constellations, to invoke public secrecy by pointing to pain existing in the shared personal pasts of participants, as well as shared (political, social) suffering in the present.

The presumed sharedness of such histories, I argue, afforded a broad form of cultural affinity within which implicit messages could be intuitively "translated" across bodies at New Life. As I discuss further below, it also arguably functioned to erase or simply further occlude the historical and present forms of either interpersonal or political injustice that were *not* imagined to be either shared or public. In examining the indexicality of images, however, it is critical to attend to the ways in which such images pointed to a range of both real and imagined shared social histories as lived by the ancestors of the predominantly Han-identifying group.

One constellation described in detail in Pritzker and Duncan (2019), for example, involved an enactment that included a long line of maternal ancestors and the metonymic representation of the "baggage" of inherited trauma with attendees' backpacks, yoga mats, and purses. Representatives for these ancestors, notably, had been added by the facilitator in response to what appeared to be a stand-off between the representative of Mei, the focal participant, and the representative enacting her mother. When the facilitator had observed that the inclusion of additional representatives in the position of the mother's ancestors did not elicit much movement between "Mei" and "her mother," she had asked the rest of the group (including myself) to bring our bags and whatever else we had brought with us and place them upon and at the feet of Mei's representative. As we proceeded to drape backpacks, yoga mats, and purses upon her, the participant enacting Mei began to droop, eventually falling to the floor under the weight of the "baggage." This moved Mei's "mother," who said that she was becoming able to look at her "daughter."

"She is pitiful to me," said Mei's representative in response, speaking from beneath the pile of backpacks and purses in her arms.

While Mei herself looked on with intense fascination, the facilitator then asked us to continue piling anything we could find—flyers, books, magazines, scarves—on top of Mei's representative. When there was nothing left to add, a heavy silence fell upon the room and the representative began shedding tears. After a few moments of silence, the facilitator then took Mei's representative's hand and calmly moved her—slowly, since she was carrying so much stuff—toward her "mother" in order to remove the bags, one by one, and lay them at her feet.

"I didn't know," said Mei's representative, without prompting, also beginning to shed tears. As she spoke, several women in the room began to cry as well. Though they did not weep, several men in the room sat up rigidly, jaws tight and fists clenched.[1] The representatives of Mei and her mother then moved, slowly but spontaneously, toward one another. They embraced.

"I love you," said Mei's representative, again without prompting.

"I love you, too, and I just want you to be happy," said the representative of Mei's mother.

The two women remained holding each other in a full body embrace for several minutes, both of them weeping along with others in the room. Even when the facilitator reached in to separate them, they held on. When they were finally wrenched apart, the facilitator brought the real Mei into the circle to stand next to her representative, facing the representative of her mother. She was then told her to repeat the words "Mama, thank you for giving me life" several times. After she did so, the representative playing Mei's mother was told to repeat after the facilitator: "I've decided now to release your life—I want your happiness." After she spoke these words, all of them—including Mei, her representative, and her mother's representative—were guided to bow deeply to one another. Feelings of joy and relief seemed to flood the room. People were still crying, but I also noted that there were several deep, audible sighs.

As noted in Pritzker and Duncan (2019), Mei's constellation demonstrates how constellations were often or even *always* enacted as intensely relational encounters. Showing how the "self," in *jiapai*, was reframed in intersubjective, intercorporeal terms that pointed backwards and forwards in time and space (e.g., vis-à-vis the family line), Mei's constellation also suggests the ways in which the process often emerged, not unlike photographs or photo-forms, as a set of obscured, encrypted, and incomplete images that required *labor* on the part of representatives, facilitators, focal participants, and witnesses to decipher. Pointing to the kinds of "responsive labor" that Hillenbrand suggests is evoked by photo-forms, the affect in the room was apparent from the outset of the constellation. Lucy—introduced above—had begun to burp suddenly and continuously during Mei's constellation, for example. This began the moment the baggage was set down at Mei's "mother's" feet, and constituted a *physical* response that might also be framed as an embodied-affective "release" that emerged in "resonance" (感应 ganying) with Mei's constellation. The intimacy that emerged between Mei and her mother, moreover, points to the kinds of relational shifts that occur within constellations and were sometimes carried forth in real relationships (e.g., between Lina and her mother). Such shifts—quite literally in this case—were often *weight shifts* wherein imbalances were corrected and new possibilities emerged for mental, emotional, and relational "balance" (平衡 pingheng) to form.

The resolution, in this case, seemed to suggest that the mother, for whatever reason, had been unable to carry the weight and had thus transmitted it unknowingly to her daughter. The question of *what*, exactly, was contained in the "baggage" Mei returns to her mother was never explicitly addressed. Recall, however, that the kind of "phenomenological posture" (Hellinger

2007) required for healing to occur in *jiapai* rarely requires such discussion. The kinds of "secrets" that came to light in constellations thus often remained shrouded in precisely the kind of ambiguity that, as Hillenbrand (2020) notes, preserves public secrecy in China. As indexes whose meaning may not have been articulable, however, the "burden" borne by Mei's mother and then by Mei could point to a range of events, encounters, and ideologies. As discussed in the following section, however, the "baggage" might have indexed particular gendered burdens that prevailed in Chinese history and continue in the present. It could also have served, however, as an index of any of the particularly troublesome periods in recent Chinese history, which Mei's mother undoubtedly endured. Without knowing *what* it ultimately referred to, however, the baggage here might have worked, at least for some, like photo-forms, to "encourage viewers to gaze anew at the social world precisely within its settled groove and thus allow the elephant in the room, the nudity of the empire, to crystallize into an apparition worthy of notice, thought, even action" (Hillenbrand 2020, xix–xx). It is, in the end, impossible to say with any confidence how particular participants might have variably engaged with the indexicality of the baggage in Mei's constellation, and how.

It is important, here, to note that the notion that constellations offer a pathway to engage with the lasting embodied impacts of cultural experience is not entirely novel. Indeed, as I discuss in the following section, the method very explicitly confronts the ways in which the extended space-time of the familial body-self is inclusive of a broader "cultural time." Indeed, it is widely known that Bert Hellinger, the developer of *jiapai*, was inspired by Zulu practices of ongoing relationality between deceased and living family members that he observed while working as a missionary and priest in South Africa. Upon quitting the priesthood and becoming a psychotherapist in his native Germany (in the 1990s), he was thus eager to incorporate a form of this relationality with the kinds of phenomenological interventions he considered most effective.[2] He was also, importantly, interested in developing an intervention that could address a particular kind of suffering affecting many Germans who were—and *are*—wrangling with the inherited consequences of their parents' and grandparents' experiences during the Nazi regime (Cohen 2006; Hellinger 2007). Though thoroughly organized around balancing an individual's family lineage, *jiapai* is thus also intentionally crafted to afford engagement with broader sociocultural histories.

CULTURAL TIME IN JIAPAI

As described above, the founder of *jiapai*, Bert Hellinger, specifically considered how constellations, beyond addressing personal traumas, offer participants a unique opportunity to interrogate the ways in which violence experienced or enacted by one's ancestors persists within one's own everyday lived experience. The notion of "trauma," in this intergenerational framing, importantly, also points to the way both the experience and perpetration of violence endure as inherited suffering well into the future. In Germany, for example, intergenerational suffering often emerges within constellations within which "the consequences of the Third Reich come to life before our eyes" (Ulsamer 2005, 33). In one constellation that Bertold Ulsamer describes, for example, there seemed to be an immense amount of guilt being enacted by the representative playing the role of the focal participant's grandfather. The grandfather had, indeed, been a Nazi, and it seemed like there was an immense amount of pain and suffering caused by the persistent feelings of guilt related to the deaths he condoned, caused, or both. Just as aborted children must be placed back within a system, Ulsamer explains here, anyone whose death was caused by a family member must be reckoned with as an *enduring presence* within the system. All parties in the system must therefore come to terms with the way this violence and suffering persists, not just as an abstract spectral presence but as an entity that resides in the bodies of descendants.

In the English translation of his book, Ulsamer—who has traveled around the world with Hellinger offering *jiapai* workshops—likewise comments generally upon the way constellations in the United States often underscore how "dispossession, murder and slavery form the basis of American history" (2005, 96). Underscoring the ways in which psychospiritual and somatic healing milieus in the United States are often "white utopias" within which whiteness is not only ubiquitous but often unquestioned (Lucia 2020; see also williams et al. 2016; R. Johnson 2018; Haines 2019), Ulsamer nevertheless comments that the few Black participants he has had the opportunity to work with have amply demonstrated the ways in which the "pain, hatred and shame" of white supremacy as enacted in the past persists in the present (92). "It seems evident from the little work that I have done in this area," he writes, "that enslaving a population surpasses murder in its deleterious effects on the dignity of the victim" (92). He notes, moreover, that the white Americans he has worked with often demonstrate a lamentable lack of awareness about how the violence perpetrated by their ancestors, particularly against indigenous Indian populations and enslaved people from Africa, persists as a form of embodied suffering (210).

Indeed, Ulsamer's observations here point to the perspective offered by somatic therapist Resmaa Menakem. In his widely acclaimed book *My Grandmother's Hands*, specifically, Menakem engages with the ways in which history resides as a form of *visceral* trauma that affects both Black and white Americans[3] (2017, xvii). Speaking from the perspective of a Black American, Menakem thus writes about how "white-body supremacy" exists as "the equivalent of a toxic chemical we ingest on a daily basis" (xx). But "white-body supremacy also harms people who do not have dark skin," Menakem also emphasizes, describing how this "legacy of trauma" also underlies a persistent form of suffering in the bodies of white Americans (11). Acknowledging here that the trauma persisting in Black bodies is "often (and understandably) more severe" (18), Menakem nevertheless underscores the ways in which white Americans can contribute to "greater freedom and serenity for all of us" (11), specifically by coming to terms with this enduring trauma in their (our) own bodies.

Ulsamer likewise minces no words in imploring readers to attend to what he frames as a refusal on the part of white Americans to confront the burden and consequences of imperialism, capitalism, and white supremacy as *personal* issues. Both Ulsamer and Menakem thus highlight how constellations emerge as a multimodal form of scalar inquiry wherein present forms of personal suffering are rapidly and instantaneously scalable to past *social* atrocities. For both practitioners, moreover, individuals must reckon with the deeply personal, embodied ways in which "cultural time" and "biographical time" interweave in ways that have urgent consequences in the present. Though neither suggests such a reckoning replaces other forms of social or political action, their perspectives frame the kind of wrangling involved in *jiapai*—especially when conducted in groups—as an intimate form of scalar inquiry that not only interrogates the personal past but also engages with it as a historically and culturally shaped register of embodiment.

Ulsamer, who has accompanied Hellinger in leading a number of large workshops in both mainland China and Hong Kong, notably also writes about how he has witnessed this kind of scaled intergenerational suffering in China. In the Chinese version of his introductory text, for example, Ulsamer discusses his observations regarding the ways in which the Chinese past persists in the present. He details, for example, how he has witnessed the effect of "past" forms of patriarchy upon both men and women in contemporary Chinese society. "Traditional Chinese feudalistic ideas regarding the value of boys and girls has been very clear in the constellations," he writes (2009, 81).[4] Noting the ways in which this affects women in his workshops, Ulsamer here points to two prominent effects that he has observed. First, Ulsamer suggests here that many women seem to have accepted this ideology and "believe they are actually lower [than men]." At the same time, he posits, the ideology has generated feelings of "humiliation" and "rage" in the same women (82–83). Ulsamer observes, finally, that Chinese patriarchy has also deeply affected men as well, giving rise to a persistent and troublesome feeling of "inferiority" (自卑 zibei) that lies beneath a surface sense of superiority (82–83).

Ulsamer also addresses the ubiquity of abortion in China as a deeply gendered, embodied rupture that creates ripples throughout the entire family (2009, 79). Abortions, he explains in the English version of the book, "are often perceived as a trespass against someone or an injustice" (2005, 79). The commonness of abortion in China, he concludes, has left a legacy of pain among individuals as well as within families, disproportionately affecting women in ways that travel into the future through living offspring. Though arguably attempting to address the issue of *forced* abortion, Ulsamer here reinforces *jiapai's* naturalization of women's unique role in childbearing as well as their embodied role in epigenetically transmitting traumatic burdens to their children and serving as the nurturer for the family once a child is born (Wolynn 2016; see also Duncan 2018; Pritzker and Duncan 2019). As Whitney Duncan and I have noted, however, there is often a somewhat ironic twist in the ways in which family constellation workshops can simultaneously be seen as perpetuating problematic gender roles while also making room for participants to engage in both direct and indirect interrogations of such roles (Pritzker and Duncan 2019).

In a *very* brief section of the Chinese version of his book, finally, Ulsamer suggests that constellations afford witnesses the opportunity to observe the effects of both political events and policies in the recent or (relatively) more distant past in China. He thus very generally notes the multiple ways in which the tremendous unrest and upheaval over the last century in China emerges as disharmony in the family system. Specifically, he mentions how constellations demonstrate the lingering effects of the Second Sino-Japanese War (1937–45), for example, as well as the Great Leap Forward (1958–61) and the Cultural Revolution (1966–76). For perhaps obvious, strategic reasons, he does not discuss more recent traumas, such as the crackdown on student protesters in Tiananmen Square in 1989. Nor does he engage in the nuanced kind of ethnoracial analysis evidenced by Menakem, wherein also the embodied legacy of both Han and non-Han participants has been shaped by historical violence enacted upon bodies scaled as "barbarian" in contrast to the "civilized" Han (Carrico 2017; Cheng 2019).

Ulsamer nevertheless seems to understand the ways in which public secrecy functions in China, noting how rare it is for any of these events to arise for explicit discussion in workshops, especially on the first day. Occasionally, he writes, related cases will come to the fore on the second or third day, once "a deep feeling of mutuality" has developed between attendees and facilitators. When they do, Ulsamer notes, the specifics are invariably both obtuse and obscure. "This history won't immediately surface and express," he observes, "and will commonly express in a feeling of numbness or heaviness deep in the body" (2009, 84). Ulsamer gives an example, here, of what he refers to as one of the most "profound and deep" constellations he facilitated in China. It occurred during a workshop consisting of nearly one hundred people from both Hong Kong and mainland China. On the third day, he explains, a man wanted to do a constellation because he was angry with his family for reasons he did not understand. As the man spoke of his anger, Ulsamer writes, he kept holding and wringing his hands.

This embodied expression prompted Ulsamer to direct the participant to see if he could feel the emotion in his fingertips. "When he did this, the rage suddenly turned into terror," he writes (2009, 85). Ulsamer then asked him a number of questions about his childhood. The stories he shared, however, seemed not to offer any firm conclusions. Inserting a comment here about the ways in which trauma transmitted across generations is often amplified by "keeping secrets and avoiding topics," Ulsamer notes that this kind of silence "only causes trauma to become deeper" (85). Since the man in the constellation had no clear or specific information to offer about his family's past, however, Ulsamer chose an additional representative to act as an "unknown entity" within the constellation, which already included representatives for the man as well as his parents. The participant representing this unknown entity instantaneously felt fear upon entering the constellation. Eventually, Ulsamer was able to guide all the representatives to enact a ritual "release" by bowing deeply toward one another (as the facilitator did in Mei's constellation). This offered an experience of catharsis for the focal participant, he explains. "Genuine bows have a very mysterious healing effect," Ulsamer concludes, explaining that "[they] allow us to step back from our past entanglements" (86). With this, the section concludes.

Ulsamer's depiction here notably implies that the focal participant had been affected by traumatic historical events (we do not know what) that someone in his family (we do not know who) either enacted or endured (also unclear), but was able to find release from his terror through the process of constellating the (still) unknown. Whether or not this process was effective in the long term for the man or not, however, it is relevant to reflect upon the ways in which perceived efficacy occurs not *despite of* but precisely *because of* the kinds of ambiguity that often prevail during constellations. Such ambiguity, I suggest, afforded an indirect and implicit but nevertheless powerful and *collaborative* engagement with public secrecy at New Life. The resolution of the pain caused by secrecy, importantly, can be achieved without explicit discussions about specific events or actors. Suggesting how even indirect or "small acts of speech" sometimes offer a "vital relief" to the burden of silence in China (Hillenbrand 2020, 223), it further indicates how the complex intercorporeal dynamic of *jiapai* offers such a deeply compelling set of practices to Chinese participants, many of whom do not know exactly what happened within their own families in even the recent past (Rofel 2007; Feuchtwang 2013; Hillenbrand 2020; J. Li 2020). As I demonstrate in the following section, however, conversations *about* constellations were sometimes (and often just slightly) more straightforward about the ways in which the method provided a uniquely appropriate affordance for (Han) Chinese participants to engage with both past and present forms of public secrecy.

Big Data Cloud

It was the morning of a daylong *jiapai* salon at New Life in 2016. After our opening circle, Chao, one of the chief interns at the time, gave a brief lecture on family constellations. He began by telling us how we might understand Hellinger's notion of the common soul using computer terminology. Here, he posited that the common soul is something like a "big data cloud" (云端大数据 *yunduan da shuju*). He then rhetorically asked us what kinds of information might be stored in the big data cloud, going on to provide an answer for the twenty or so participants raptly attending to his every word.

"The information in this is how your father was and is; how your mother was and is; the way your mother and father started up together; whatever kinds of relationships your father had with previous girlfriends; how they separated; how your mother was when she entered their marriage; what happened to them during the Cultural Revolution—any injustices faced by you and your family, how your family was during the Cultural Revolution—did they hurt others? This is all recorded in here, the big data cloud." Going on to describe it as a "ledger" within which all of one's business is recorded, Chao underscored how death did not constitute the end of such a record. It continued, rather, into the future as it merged with the thorough records of other family members and those they had been in contact with.

In this case, Chao was relatively explicit in discussing the ways in which both gendered and political histories are recorded, in gory detail, in the all-encompassing "data cloud." Though never departing from the kind of heteronormative script that is central in *jiapai* (Pritzker and Duncan 2019), Chao's list nevertheless further emphasized the complexity of marital relationships, which here were chronotopically situated as inclusive of *previous* relationships, conditions, and events, including possible separations. Chao's introduction also, however, included a rapidly spoken and deeply embedded but unambiguous acknowledgment of the ways in which personal family histories, here in relation to the Cultural Revolution, included both injustices suffered or perpetrated by one's family.

Though his question (*"did they hurt others?"*) was arguably strategically placed *after* his reference to injustices suffered, his inclusion of this perspective stood out boldly against official state discourses that problematically frame *everyone* as having suffered during the Cultural Revolution (Rofel 2007; Hillenbrand 2020; Karl 2020). As several scholars both in China and abroad have noted, this dominant narrative, which strategically sweeps everything "under the rug" so to speak, affords the avoidance of what Hillenbrand describes as "the vexed questions of guilt and complicity that lie at the most sensitive core of Cultural Revolution experience" (Hillenbrand 2020, 94). As Lisa Rofel further argues, when embraced by descendants of people—many of whom had in fact both enacted and suffered violence during this part of Chinese history—this narrative can be seen as an affordance for the kinds of "apolitical" consumerism that came to dominate Chinese society in the early twenty-first century (2007, 61). In Rofel's study of daughters' understanding of their parents' experiences during the Cultural Revolution, for example, she notes that although they "are often unclear about the details," they commonly imagined this past as "nothing but a life of sacrifice and constraints" that they then sought to overcome with their own "cosmopolitanism" (118). Occluding the reality of their parents' possible participation in violent political campaigns in which "many of them denounced their [own] parents for having the wrong politics" (127), Rofel concludes that the generalized image of ubiquitous "constraint" generated precisely the kinds of ignorance that precluded the development of the daughters' political subjectivities and drew them away from concerted forms of political engagement.

In contrast to the kind of "historical forgetting" that Rofel (2007) found among young Chinese women in the early part of the century, however, Chao's suggestion of the possibility that one's family may have *hurt others* during the Cultural Revolution foregrounded the ways in which things that we "know but don't know" (e.g., public secrecy) were given at least some space during *jiapai* events. Public secrecy here, Hillenbrand argues, is "a felt but elusive force" (Hillenbrand 2020, 4). Pointing to the ways in which "public secrecy is . . . everywhere and inescapable, as are its off-shoots in the strategic silences that prevail in communities, in families, in our most intimate relationships" (Hillenbrand 2020, 206), the emotions of the past here—whether because of one's own or one's ancestors' positioning as either "victim" or "perpetrator" in particular encounters, remain *present* in everyday interactions that travel across generations in "verbal or non-verbal and everyday ways" (Feuchtwang 2013; see also Mason 2020). As a kind of *warning* as well as a promise, his comment pointed to the ways in which conversations about *jiapai* at New Life spoke simultaneously directly and indirectly about areas of private life that have been *felt* but which have remained unspoken. Chao's reference to the violence (possibly) enacted by one's family members during the Cultural Revolution also, however, arguably called upon co-present participants to interrogate everything they did not know or could not say, but, indeed, *needed to* know.

There was barely a pause, however, before a newcomer—a roughly forty-year-old man—intervened with a comment/question that centered around the fact that, no matter how much they might want to know the kinds of details Chao described, the reality was that *access* to such information was invariably restricted. Building upon Chao's data-cloud metaphor, he further asked Chao how *jiapai* approached the problem of "big data."

"So in *jiapai*, when we are processing data and trying to conduct an analysis," he said, "it is likely that there will be *a lot* of data. Maybe as much as 80 percent of it will be irrelevant—if it is all intercepted."

"Right," Chao responded quickly. "We will not intercept all the data.

We will intercept the relevant data just based on the issues of the person, and their goals." This was necessary, he further noted, because people in the midst of a particular situation or enduring family drama often suffer from "incoherent thinking." Their data, he reflected, will thus be similarly "chaotic" or "messy" (乱 *luan*). Chao thus suggested that *jiapai* facilitators serve the purpose of *filtering* information, helping focal participants discern which data to "pull out" (拿过来 *na guolai*). He went on to compare facilitators to a "firewall" that helps prevent irrelevant data from passing through into the constellation.

Chao's response here, in formulating the expertise of *jiapai* facilitators as a "firewall," invoked an understanding of firewalls as inherently *protective*. As I was taking rapid-fire notes on this interaction, it stood out to me as an index of the ways in which the state, in constructing China's "Great Firewall," often situates itself as enacting a kind of benevolent authority rather than a restrictive force (M. Roberts 2018). Alongside his previous comments, however, it also suggested that the notion that facilitators help "filter" information could also be interpreted as highlighting their nuanced skills in guiding participants *toward* rather than away from relevant data. We might then understand that Chao was positioning facilitators in the role of virtual private networks, which indeed often afford access to censored information in China, at least for those who can access them.

Chao shifted here, however, to offer a more inclusive perspective on the ways in which the agency to turn toward or away from particular data points was always distributed among the bodies of focal participants, representatives, *and* facilitators. Invoking Hellinger's phenomenological stance, he thus explained that, in order to make sense of any of it, the focal participant must work toward adopting a "panoramic view" (全观的视角 *quanguande shejiao*) that encompasses and yet transcends specific data points.

"It is all very mysterious once you say it, though," he finally admitted, pausing briefly before going on to present a complex lecture on linear versus multidimensional space-time, complete with diagrams that he drew rapidly on a whiteboard that had been rolled in from another room at some point. Participants, including myself, leaned forward as he lectured, many of us with furrowed brows and pens suspended above notebooks as we tried to follow Chao's rapid-fire explanations, which cohered around the notion that *jiapai* offered the possibility of remaking the future by understanding the past (at least as it existed in the present). This generated a conversation about three- versus four-dimensional temporalities that—had it unfolded in

English, my native language—I would have still found difficult to follow, let alone reproduce. The way his diagrams seemed to overturn normative and even logical notions of temporality, however, seemed to confirm my impression of constellations as feeling, often, "out of time."

When he concluded, there was a lull in the room. A middle-aged woman, speaking into the silence, commented on how Chao's lecture was a "big shock" for her. Her eyebrows raised, she further noted that a number of the specific examples as well as the metaphors (比喻 biyu) that he had used sounded "like truth" to her.

Frameworks of Thought

After Chao's lecture on the same day described above, Teacher Du, who was the usual chief instructor for the sessions and had been letting Chao lead thus far, made a comment on Chao's lecture, which had drawn us into an engagement with time, space, and materiality that had seemed to render even long-term participants speechless with its complexity and unorthodoxy as well as (at some points) apparent abandonment of all logic. Specifically, Du drew on a common Chinese trope mapping ideas, behaviors, and thoughts as either reasonable or "scientific" (科学 kexue) or unruly and "unscientific" (不科学 bukexue). Placing *jiapai* somewhere between these two poles, he observed that the method was "far from scientific," adding that, even among instructors of the method, "there is no completely accepted argument." He went on to recommend a book, however, in which a world-renowned facilitator offered insights into the ways in which researchers in many scientific disciplines had begun to explore similar issues regarding temporality, materiality, and intergenerational trauma. He concluded by drawing our attention toward the pragmatic "truth" of the method. Here, he noted, the value of *jiapai* was not necessarily situated in the kinds of *certainty* that it provided (in scientific terms) but rather in the *opportunity* that it offered participants to look at problems from multiple perspectives.

"It is really good, though," he continued. "It has pushed me to start to get in touch with a lot of things I didn't know before." Thus offering a personal endorsement of the method, Du went on to scale his individual experience in a chronotopization that was vastly more collective:

"In the past," he said, "we all lived under our parent's educational frameworks of thought (教育的思维框架 *jiaoyu de siwei kuangjia*), the educational frameworks of thought of the schools, and society's 'cognitive frameworks'

(社会认知的框架 *shehui renzhi de kuangjia*). But now we can increasingly open ourselves (打开自己 *dakai ziji*), and we are able to accept (接受 *jieshou*) all kinds of different possibilities (可能性 *keneng xing*). There are so many things we can come to understand—to maybe understand what actually happened [in the past]—but we have to become willing to open up. This in itself is a kind of inner psychological development."

Arguably invoking the *desire* to understand "what actually happened [in the past]," Du's remarks here, I suggest, demonstrate the ways in which investigations of relationships between the past and present often constituted a form of scalar inquiry through which speakers collaboratively crafted and refined theories about their place within an (imagined) spatiotemporal and cultural trajectory. Positioning himself as someone with, in David Divita's words, "an authoritative stance" in relation to knowledge about the past (2019, 64), Du specifically situated the entire room of participants (or all, perhaps, except me) vis-à-vis a trifecta of family, school, and society. As detailed in the previous chapter, conversations about such institutions, structures, and frameworks or methods—here presented as a *unified force* that acted upon the individual—can be seen as "technologies of ethical imagination" (Santos 2016) that "[link] intimate family life ... to the wider political economic landscape against which it plays out" (Stafford 2013, 17). Individuals, in Du's framing, were furthermore chronotopically situated, in the past, as having lived "under" or having been contained "within" such structures. His statement crafted a contrast with the present, however, in which "we" had the opportunity to "open ourselves." With this contrast, his remarks thus situated him, as a kind of ambassador of hope, a "conductor" (to use Heelas's metaphor) who was able to offer a specific kind of horizon or vision of the ways in which possible futures are embedded in the activity of *jiapai*.

With this statement, Du further articulated a well-known chronotopization of Chinese history within which the past was "closed" and the present is "open." His comments here notably seemed to draw upon a readily available chronotope of "progress" in China (Rofel 2007; Yan 2018; Karl 2020). As argued by Rofel (2007), the chronotope (or "trope") of progress in China is often undergirded by revisionist histories, strategically and selectively pieced together with scraps of state-mediated information. Generalized narratives of "constraint" during the Cultural Revolution, for example, here afford the framing of the present (as well as the future) as a total break from "the constraints of the past." Rofel thus highlights the ways in which popular notions that China had entered "a new era" were often engineered, often quite successfully, to direct people toward the private life of the self rather than engaging in more public or political configurations of personhood. Du's comments might thus be read as a fairly typical reproduction of such narratives, especially in the context of a discussion about a therapy that is seemingly entirely focused on the family and "the self." His phrasing, for example, which invoked "frameworks of thought" and "cognitive structures," arguably indexed the kinds of "thought reform" (思想改造 sixiang gaizao) that are well known for prevailing during Mao's regime as well as the ways in which such thought work remains prevalent today in various forms (Cheek 2019; L. Zhang 2020).

It is worth dwelling here, however, upon the ways in which his chronotopic mapping did not in any way suggest that the structures themselves—the frameworks of the family, school, and state—existed *only* in the past. His statement, for example, was rather (intentionally?) ambiguous about where and when "the past" began, or where it ended and the present began. When spoken in a room containing individuals ranging from age twenty-five to seventy, in other words, his statement left open the question of the existence and persistence of state-mandated structures of society while also seemingly referring to the past. Perhaps, like his carefully ambiguous response to Lan in the previous chapter, the comment might thus be interpreted as a strategic way of critically addressing present structures of governance while seemingly talking about the past.

Du's statement was nevertheless unambiguous about the ways in which he positioned the individual vis-à-vis such structures, past or present. Overall, then, his statement emphasized the ways in which a collectively formulated "we" can now engage differently *with* such structures. In his phrasing, Du notably formulated an agentive self who could (now) relate to and within Chinese "frameworks of thought" but could also engage with "all kinds of different possibilities." Suggestive of the ways in which New Life was systematically organized around introducing non-Chinese "difference" to participants, Du notably positioned himself and his interlocutors not as passive recipients of foreign knowledge, but as active, culturally situated participants whose access to such knowledge could help them transform suffering endured in the past. The term for "possibilities" that Du used (可能性 keneng xing) further importantly worked to formulate a kind of "maybeness" about the present that pointed to that which might become possible in the future through the embodied, collective experiences available at New

Life. In so doing, his comments further worked, I suggest, to "relationally configure" (French 2012, 345) the immediate context through the invocation of the *horizon* chronotope, which I discussed in chapter 2 as a collaborative anticipatory mode or atmosphere (Sumartojo and Pink 2019).

In situating participants as agents in this historical process of coming to understand the past, moreover, Du's comment thus joined with Chao's in productively complicating the kind of "historical forgetting" discussed by Rofel (2007). Rather than forgetting, in other words, Du here foregrounded the strategic importance of *remembering* the past—or trying to, at least—and *considering the present*, both of which were positioned as "a kind of inner psychological development." Suggesting an awareness of the ways in which the traumatic events of recent Chinese history were often felt but not spoken of (Hillenbrand 2020), the agentive effort to "break free" from the past here was framed by both facilitators as an efforted struggle to *understand* the past. If nothing else, it was situated as an attempt, at the very least, to gain a better sense of what, generally speaking, the "energetic" deal actually is (or was), even if such understanding was never going to be completely possible. Spoken in a group context, his comment finally suggests how collaborative theory-building *about the past* might also have served as a relational as well as an ethical affordance for participants to recalibrate their own intimate relationship *to the past* and thus, simultaneously, to one another in the present and the possible future.

The room was quiet for what felt like a long time after this. It seemed, to me, like people were still taking it all in, as if they were unsure what to say, or whether to say anything at all. After a few minutes, a relatively new participant began to speak tentatively, however.

"I think that maybe, in fact—actually this was all quite unexpected (挺意外的 *ting yiwaide*) today. I feel like Chao is talking about all of these abstract ideas—things that are incomprehensible," she said, trailing off and looking around before going on. "But okay, so during the *jiapai* process, we can maybe also use the images to move closer (贴近 *tiejin*) to some of the *current* people in our lives. Some of that data can certainly be interpreted—I do believe this kind of high level exists, but—well, first of all let's just be more concrete, because time is limited."

In offering a metadiscursive commentary upon the *unexpectedness* of the interaction thus far, this participant's comment highlighted the ways in which conversations at New Life, despite their often-implicit references, frequently diverged from topics and ways of relating that were "expected."

Going on to situate the complex notions of multidimensional space-time that Chao had introduced as "abstract" and "incomprehensible," however, she seemed to dismiss much of what had just been discussed in order to foreground the practical possibilities that *jiapai* had for enacting increased intimacy within the structure of relationships with "current" or living others. She then admitted that the more abstract "data points"—the kinds of things we do not know or understand—might sometimes be interpretable at a "high level" of practice that she had not (yet) experienced. Nor, her final remarks suggested, was she particularly interested in attempting to do so. In concluding that we should "just be more concrete, because time is limited," she thus issued a chronotopically framed directive that not only pointed to the urgency of participants' desires to reorient themselves within particular relationships (e.g., to heal the "distance" between intimates by moving "closer" to them) but also effectively directed the group's attention back toward a safer goal that aligned more with current state discourses of family harmony. As a whole, then, the interaction—especially its abrupt conclusion—points to the ways in which wrangling with ghosts at New Life often intentionally constituted more of a sidelong glance rather than an explicit or direct form of collaborative engagement with public domains that participants were well aware they had no business interrogating.

CONCLUDING REFLECTIONS

Throughout this chapter, I have shown how "wrangling with ghosts" occurs in both active and collaborative interactions within constellations as well as in the "witnessing" and "digestion" of particular constellations by participants over time. I also examined the ways in which constellations, like photo-forms, worked as an affordance for (re)directing participants' attention toward the kinds of public secrets that undermine at least *some* official narratives permeating Chinese society. Often pointing to both past and present forms of public secrecy, moreover, engagement with "ghosts" here, I suggest, "reveal[ed] the insufficiency of the present moment, as well as the disconsolations and erasures of the past, and a tentative hopefulness for future resolutions" (del Pilar Blanco and Pereen 2013, 16).

Pointing to the often-implicit ways in which participants developed a distinct form of political subjectivity at New Life, in this chapter I also offered a detailed example of how conversations about constellations were sometimes considerably less coded and ambiguous than the constellations themselves. Though still careful and frequently indirect, strategic, or implicit, such conversations foregrounded participants' shared vulnerability to and within the relational, embodied chronotope of the public secret in China. I thus argued that such conversations often functioned, like constellations themselves, as a "technology of the social" within which participants might be said to have become what Desjarlais (2019) frames as "anthropologists of the phantasmal," attending to the ways in which their own lives have emerged not just as a familial structure extending backwards and forwards in time, but as a product of shared histories and shared cultural *presents*. The question of how such histories and presents both were and are shaped by violence enacted in the name of Han "civilization," however, was never explicitly raised. Indeed, the systematic erasure of this embodied legacy arguably reduced it to a form of nonknowledge that cannot, therefore, be a "secret." In addition to a critical perspective that acknowledges such erasure, however, one question that arises is whether and how, under different conditions, such engagement might be incorporated into *jiapai* spaces in China and beyond.

The question of the generalizability of my argument here, however, is also relevant. As mentioned repeatedly throughout this book, I have knowingly and intentionally offered a study of the "perplexing particulars" (Mattingly 2019) rather than the dominant reality of *jiapai* in China. From a generalized perspective, then, the process that I have discussed here as "wrangling with ghosts" must be seen more as a potentiality than a determinable outcome. Though it seemed clear that particular instructors were often fairly explicitly encouraging such engagement, it is thus important to highlight how the ambiguity and dual indexicality of their commentary was also often deeply problematic in the way it at least explicitly worked to reify problematic state discourses, for example regarding gender. The ways in which it sometimes *also* functioned to bring more public "ghosts" to participants' attention, however, suggests how such encounters offered a revelatory experience of engaging with the so-called elephant in the room. Like photo-forms, the ghosts who spoke to participants and who were frequently spoken *about* here afforded co-present attendees the opportunity to see the affective portrayal of their own and others' histories and presents that perhaps were only vaguely known or poorly understood. Pointing to the fundamental indeterminacy of atmosphere (Sumartojo and Pink 2019), the open-ended nature and ambiguity of constellations at New Life thus calls into question the notion that psychotherapeutic group work, in China or elsewhere, is ipso facto "apolitical."

The ultimate question, however, points to what, if any, impact such conversations might have in terms of *addressing* injustice in ways that might travel beyond the realm of interpersonal or "low justice" (Lin 2017; Lee 2023). I return here, however, to Hillenbrand's analysis of the political possibilities that photo-forms afford. As noted above, Hillenbrand suggests that collective encounters with photo-forms generate "minor publics" or groups "whose coalitions naturally ebb and flow and may only be short-lived, but who nonetheless cohere as blocs that experiment, for a while at least, with being honest about the things that they know well but do not usually discuss" (2020, 222). Further suggesting that the indexicality of photo-forms points not only to the secrets of the past but also to multiple forms of ongoing injustice and inequality in the *present*, Hillenbrand emphasizes how such acknowledgment in and of itself constitutes a kind of action or "countermove" (153). Collective encounters with photo-forms that variably reveal public secrets, she suggests, "belong to a series of networks-in-incubation, awaiting the notes that will draw them into linkage" (100). Hillenbrand takes care, however, not to suggest that the collaborative viewing of photo-forms points to broad-scale political capacities for transformation. "It would be foolish to suggest that photo-forms might one day bring an end to public secrecy in China," she writes, acknowledging the ways in which "the impact of the photo-form must be limited because its audiences are typically small" (222). Emphasizing the *processual* nature of photo-forms as a "continuous event" in its own life as well as the lives of its beholders, however, Hillenbrand leaves room for the possibility that the impacts of the kinds of revelations that photo-forms afford—and the kinds of "minor publics" they generate—while not constituting social action or activism per se, are still significant and worthy of attention.

As Whitney Duncan and I note, theories of *ritual theater* as a communal experience of witnessing the social (e.g., Boal 1979; V. Turner 1969, 1985; Nussbaum 1994; Mattingly 2014) are helpful here. Analyses of the social effects (and efficacy) of ritual theater, specifically, invite us to think about "the potentiality of socially situated witnessing" in *jiapai* as affording an opportunity "for the workshop community to collaboratively, as [Victor] Turner might say, 'bend existentially back upon itself' in order to examine social, moral, and emotional alternatives that [might] heal the past and develop culture in specific desirable ways" (Turner 1985, 124, as cited in

Pritzker and Duncan 2019, 487). As with photo-forms, however, *jiapai* also warrants a considerable degree of skepticism regarding the ways in which such practices might ever bring an end to public secrecy, real secrecy, or injustice in China. As noted throughout this book, the ways in which Chinese social history was often framed as a shared past that attended specifically to the injustices that prevailed in the Han past can be said to have worked, here, to erase the ways in which both past and present injustices target ethnic or gender minorities and others chronotopically positioned as lower in "quality" (Carrico 2017; Cheng 2019; Grose 2019; Byler 2021a; Evans 2020). Often formulated as a predominantly personal, agentive endeavor, moreover—as in Du's comment about how engaging with *jiapai* made us capable of creating a more "just" future for descendants—discussions about constellation work (or any other kind of therapeutic endeavor) at New Life did not, at least in my experience, engage with the problem of how to create such justice without addressing or challenging the state-driven policies that gave rise to them in the past or which generate new forms of injustice in the present. As discussed with regard to Sylvia's dreams for the future of "spiritual freedom" in China (see chapter 4), this points to how participants' desires often involved (or evoked) the desire to change what, in essence, they did not have the power to change. To focus simply on that which one *could* change, in this sense, constituted a limited compromise that, as Zhang (2017) highlights, Chinese citizens engaged in therapeutic "transformation" are often quite well aware of. For many of the people I met over the course of this research, however, such engagement also points to an ongoing rescaling process through which participants come to understand their own embodied experience in relation to particular forms of injustice in Chinese history—forms blurring the lines between "high" and "low" justice—in ways that afforded nuanced forms of intimate rescaling. Though not always or even often as politically charged as many of the photo-forms that Hillenbrand discusses, the potential sociopolitical efficacy of *jiapai* might thus be considered in similar terms, with regards to the coalitions it builds among people "who are willing to experiment together with being more candid about those things that are broadly known but seldom said aloud" (2020, 21). If such conversations were expanded to include those things that are *not* broadly known and thus *never* or only rarely said aloud, moreover, the processual power of *jiapai* might just be similarly expanded.

6

These Burdens We Carry

If, as history, the past lies behind us, as memory it remains with us, not only in words but also in our neuromuscular patterning and kinesthetic memories—the way in which specific experiences and concepts of time/space are built into our bodily modus operandi.

—BRENDA FARNELL

One afternoon during my first inner child retreat at the hotel outside the city center, we returned from a short break. Instead of settling on our cushions, however, Teacher Jo instructed us to begin jumping around the room while loud, boisterous music played.

"Pretend you are an animal," he directed us, "a kangaroo, a dragon, a phoenix!"

We began to bounce around awkwardly, laughing hysterically as we each played with embodying different animals. Jo suddenly stopped the music, however, and told us to find a random group of three people. One of us would be the "baby," he explained, and the other two would be "Mama" and "Baba," regardless of gender. Baby was going to then crawl into the arms of his, her, or their loving parents.

We shuffled around quickly and began the exercise, still laughing as we embodied the imaginary, joyful trinity of a baby resting in the arms of loving and available parents. Not long after we had started, a middle-aged woman named Bao became very distressed. She began to wobble, and then fell suddenly to the floor, and remained laying on the ground, seemingly convulsing. Without a thought, I moved quickly to Bao's side. No longer a proud new "father," nor even an anthropologist, I moved in that moment as a clinician.[1] The rest of the room dropped away as I felt her pulse and listened to her breath. I scanned her face and body, and breathed a sigh of relief once I recognized that she was not having a stroke or a heart attack, nor had she gone completely unconscious. I noticed more about *her* now. She appeared to be in her mid-fifties and had short, permed hair. She was wearing polyester black pants, sensible black flats, and a standard sheer, loose, dark blouse. She had thick makeup on, but she was so pale that it seemed as if it was floating on top of her face. She is somebody's mother, I remember thinking.

Bao was still trembling mildly all over her body, her eyes opening and closing intermittently. Julie (a lead staff member at the time who was serving as an assistant teacher) was there with us, crouched down holding her right hand and looking at her intensely. I took her left hand and began to lightly massage certain points on her face, hands, and the bottom of her feet (Du 26 人中 *renzhong*, H7 神门 *shenmen*, and K1 涌泉 *yongquan*, for the clinical record). Julie remained calm, chatting with me and asking for my guidance on where to massage. She smiled and joked that I would need to come back to all of New Life's events to serve as their clinician. Apparently, this kind of thing happened enough that I would come in handy in that role. I shuddered at the thought.

When I finally looked up and noticed the room again, I spotted Aileen, the center's director, watching us intently from the other side of the room. She seemed calm but very focused on us. I noted this with curiosity. I also observed that Teacher Jo had kept the rest of the class focused on the exercise, though he was glancing at us from time to time. He was clearly concerned. Both, however, seemed quite comfortable to let Julie and I handle the emergency. Still, it felt strange to me that Aileen was just sitting there. It seemed, however, that—like Teacher Jo—she was quietly ensuring us that we were not alone and would come over to help if she was needed.

Bao was in and out for a while, though from my perspective it was hard to tell if it was five minutes or twenty. Eventually, she opened her eyes. She was dazed, but able to talk minimally. She moved to sit up, with our assistance. Julie then ran to get her some warm water to drink, and I suggested a few physicians of Chinese medicine who I knew were particularly attuned to the embodiment of psychoemotional distress. She took their names, which I quickly jotted down on a small paper, nodding politely while simultaneously disregarding my referrals by telling me she did not live anywhere near the city.

I never had the opportunity to track Bao further. A few weeks later, however, I learned that Aileen also had a strong memory of her collapse. We were seated in the comfort of the New Life headquarters. Though we had had many casual conversations by that point, we had finally been able to schedule an official, recorded interview. After talking for a short time about her background, the history of New Life from her perspective, and the reasons she had persisted in a field that—at least in the beginning—was not very lucrative, I asked her one of my standard questions.

"Do you think this kind of work is particularly important in China?"

Aileen paused for a moment, looking across the room, and bringing up Bao. After a few moments, she asked me if I remembered who she was talking about. I nodded, curious.

"I saw that woman," she said. "She has come four times already. I knew there were a lot of complex emotions she had to deal with." Aileen had watched the woman closely each time she had participated, she explained. Despite still not knowing *exactly* what the woman had experienced, she thus understood the type of intensity that was "opening up" within her as she had participated in this workshop.

"Being a Chinese woman," Aileen then said, "the things left to us by our ancestors—maybe it's all there—in our bodies." She explained, here, how she had come to understand the ways in which traumatic histories become, quite literally, entrenched in Chinese women's bodies and minds.

"We are carrying so many burdens (负担 *fudan*), from our ancestors. They endured so much heavy stuff. Maybe, in our subconscious, we also carry these burdens."

I said nothing, giving her an opportunity to say more. She quickly offered a qualification of her statement, telling me that, until recently, she had not been particularly aware of any troubling histories within herself or anyone else. In her first inner child workshop, in fact, she hadn't felt much of anything.

"I was closed up," she told me. "I would see other people crying, and I would ask myself why they were so upset. I was laughing at them, honestly." Her customary evaluative stance had suddenly shifted about a month later, however. It began one afternoon when she had suddenly begun to feel feverish. The fever was accompanied by what she describes as a persistent "emotional ache" that had continued to increase in intensity until it hit a peak. Suddenly, unexpected torrents of emotion had emerged, seemingly out of nowhere, from within her.

"I cried a lot. I was crying, crying, crying, crying—so much I felt like the police would come banging on my door, I was crying so intensely. It went on for almost a full twenty-four hours. And then the next day," she continued, "in the morning, I discovered that my fever had disappeared. It was like it was the first time these feelings ever came out. And then my body changed. It just changed. It was very mysterious, and I've never been the same."

Over the subsequent days, Aileen told me, she began to connect the dots, linking her emotional release to everything she had witnessed and experienced in the course.

"*Aiya*," she said, finally, "I just felt, wow, people are so hurt. We have so much hurt (悲伤 *beishang*)."

"WE HAVE SO MUCH HURT"

It struck me that, even though Aileen had remained physically distant when Bao had collapsed, the event had stood out to her as an example of why the kind of work they were doing at New Life was important in China. Even more striking was that, in her response, Aileen essentially collapsed the space between herself and the woman, both in terms of the distance that separated them in the room on the day of the workshop and the familial and spatiotemporal distance distinguishing them as separate body-selves. Beginning with a subjunctive frame in which she posited that the burdens "our ancestors" carried *maybe* continued to be "there, in our bodies," Aileen at least tentatively opened by scaling Bao's extreme physical reaction in relation to a vast collective of gendered individuals who shared a similar kind of inherited, embodied suffering.

Suggesting how the atmosphere at New Life often indexically invoked a shared history, Aileen's description here further foregrounds the ways in which memory, as Brenda Farnell writes in the epigraph to this chapter, remains with us "not only in words but also in our neuromuscular patterning and kinesthetic memories" (1999, 353). Her response here also suggested a kind of intimate *spatiotemporal intercorporeality* that prevailed across time in a shared form of embodied, gendered memory. Aileen's remarks further seemed to suggest the ways in which the workshop itself had afforded the normative boundaries of her own "Great Self" to extend not only across genetically unrelated bodies but, indeed, across time, at least within the confines of an imagined Chinese past. Aileen thus interpreted the woman's intense response that afternoon as an index not only to kinds of "burdens" that Aileen understood herself, as a Chinese woman (later scaled more broadly to "Chinese people"), to be carrying.

One could certainly argue here that Aileen was projecting her own experience onto the woman, who may have simply been dehydrated or physically undernourished. She could have been exhausted in some way that had nothing to do with the workshop or she could have had an underlying condition that we did not know about. To belabor this point, however, misses the ways in which Aileen's narrative emerged as an intimate scaling project in which she very fluidly moved between Bao, herself, and Chinese women—even Chinese *people*—more generally. While the ethnoracial formulation of Chineseness in Aileen's narrative further bears consideration in terms of the ways in which it erases the burdens carried by non-Han bodies (as well as the ways in which the "Chinese burden" itself relates to the violence enacted upon bodies situated as "other"), the ipso facto condemnation of such an erasure also ignores the ways in which "openings" such as Aileen's might be investigated as forms of embodied political subjectivity.

Here, then, I turn toward an analysis of how Aileen deployed the narrative framework of *metamorphosis* to illustrate the contrast between her previous and current orientation to and within the world. As Bakhtin notes, stories of metamorphosis, at least within novels, emphasize "how an individual becomes other than what [they were]," often in relation to various crises (1981, 115). Authors writing within different genres construct the contours of the more-or-less "private" individual, as Bakhtin observes, by situating characters' metamorphoses in relation to personal encounters, more broadly public events occurring on the "road" of life, or both (1981, 98). Like novelists, anthropologists have observed, speakers in the context of emergent, lived conversations also frequently draw upon the chronotope of metamorphosis to situate themselves along the pathway or "road" of their lives (Perrino 2007; Woolard 2013). In doing so, as Woolard (2013) notes, people often draw upon either "biographical" or "sociocultural" chronotopic frames to understand themselves in relation to their own personal or "psychological" development or in relation to more public (e.g., historical, political, and economic) processes. Aileen's story, however, seemed to depict a kind of scalar state change within which her metamorphosis *moved* her from a more biographical or individualized perspective to one that was significantly more sociocultural and historical, even if it was not entirely complete.

Aileen's "backstory" thus began with her initial experience of being an isolated individual observer who apprehended workshop participants' expressions of emotion with a judgmental, critical, and even mocking gaze. She went on, however, to offer a rich description of an embodied crisis involving a mysterious fever and tumultuous emotional upheaval that arose only *after* the workshop. In her illustration of the intensity of this experience, Aileen here drew upon images of *rupture* and destabilization. Noting that she had been crying so fiercely that she thought the *police* would come banging on her door, for example, Aileen invoked culturally salient chronotopes of "chaos" that arguably indexes the ways in which extreme emotional expression, especially among women but not necessarily limited by gender, often signals a disruption of the "harmonious" social order in China (see, e.g., Kuan 2015; Fu 2020).[2] Over time, however, Aileen suggested that she had come to understand her response not as an unraveling into chaos, but rather as an "opening" that instigated a fundamental shift in her embodied way of being-in-the-world. Specifically, Aileen positioned her embodied-affective unraveling as having afforded an increased empathic awareness of the ways in which shared histories of gendered experience persisted within the bodies of the living. Indeed, Aileen situated the "heavy stuff" that the ancestors experienced as a shared and embodied *weight* that bodies, especially women's bodies, continued to bear. The burden of this weight was real whether particular individuals were aware of it or not, Aileen then asserted. Underscoring her own previous lack of awareness, Aileen thus went on to describe how her fever and emotional unraveling had engendered a fundamental shift in orientation that attuned her to the enduring forms of pain that "people" continued to bear.

Aileen's experience corresponds to what I discuss throughout this chapter in terms of the concept of *embodied defrosting*. I take up this term, specifically, to refer to the kind of multistage embodied, affective, relational process of scalar inquiry and personal transformation described by multiple longer-term participants at New Life. Whether occurring over time or instantaneously, participants often described a kind of *melting* of that which had previously been or remained "frozen" in their bodies. Such experiences furthermore often afforded movement out of what was variably described as a physical and social frozenness, as aptly depicted by Aileen's shift from her tendency to judge and even mock others in her first workshop to her later experience of having fundamentally changed such that she had suddenly become more empathetic to the suffering of others.

As a key turning point in her process of learning to love, Aileen's "meltdown" was also an *opening* that offered her the experience of *entangling differently*, well beyond the space-time of a particular workshop, with both others and the world more broadly. Indeed, experiences of embodied defrosting were often described as having afforded a kind of *settling* or "warming" that was simultaneously physiological, affective, and social. By "social" here, I mean both the sociality of everyday interaction as well as the sociality invoked by Aileen in terms of the way her experience moved her to rescale her relationship to Chineseness. In this sense, embodied defrosting guided particular participants to become more aware or *attuned* to the fact that their suffering was indeed both their "own" in a personal sense and something more collective.

Like the kinds of "somatic openings" associated with the formal practice of Somatics (e.g., Strozzi Heckler 1993), embodied defrosting often propelled participants into what somatics practitioner and social activist Staci K. Haines describes as the "unbounded terrain" that exists "between known ways of interacting or coordinating" and a range of as-yet *unknown* possible alternatives (2019, 25). Further allowing them to "listen, somatically process, and transform" the "stories" held in our bodies (26), experiences of embodied defrosting described by New Lifers—like somatic openings—further invited both the experience and interrogation of the ways that multiple forms of oppression (as well as resilience) had become entrenched within the "shape" of participants' body-selves (20).

In the following discussion, I thus underscore the ways in which the kinds of embodied defrosting that afforded such investigation emerged, notably, without the kinds of "political education" advocated for by Haines as well as others in the emerging field of embodied social justice (see, e.g., williams et al. 2016; brown 2017; R. Johnson 2018, 2023; Magee 2019; Fikes 2021a-b; Ndefo 2021; King 2021). Although I align enthusiastically with the call to include more scaffolding for people to adopt an explicit sociohistorical and political perspective to make sense of their embodied experience, throughout this chapter I nevertheless emphasize the ways in which New Life participants described embodied defrosting as a more or less "spontaneous" or "mysterious" experience. The temporality here emerged much like the kinds of unpredictable "revelations" that occur in the case of psychoanalytic listening over time, in which something unexpectedly "gives directionality to a situation that [one] was previously unable to codify" (Marsilli-Vargas 2022, 65). Embodied defrosting, in other words, occurs in particular moments, often suddenly and surprisingly, and is only interpreted over time.

Here, then, embodied defrosting bears a resemblance to the kind of defrosting that Hannah Arendt associates with the willingness to interrogate or "unfreeze" culturally dominant ways of knowing (1971, 433–44). Defrosting, as described in the introduction, constitutes a fundamentally *ethical* process in which "evil"—as frozen thought-forms—is interrogated in ways that afford sometimes dramatic and sometimes subtle interventions. Despite the similarities, I nevertheless hesitate to ascribe an absolute moral meaning(s) to the kinds of embodied defrosting I discuss in this chapter. Indeed, as noted by Bloom and Moskalenko (2021), the "unfreezing" of dominant cultural discourses often gives rise to a deeply uncomfortable embodied, affective, and relational state that drives people to embrace bizarre and radicalized political conspiracy theories (see also Carrico 2017). Here, however, I emphasize how embodied defrosting was often situated as the "spark" or "opening" that afforded explicit, ongoing forms of moral interrogation or scalar inquiry. Often further leading to adjustments in the ways in which participants enacted scalar intimacy vis-à-vis a range of culturally salient ideologies, in other words, experiences of embodied defrosting served as "entry points" of sorts for an ongoing, deeply intimate, and at least somewhat intentional process through which participants experimented with distancing themselves from certain culturally salient ideas while embracing others. Though arguably evoked intentionally by various teachers within workshops at New Life and other sites, in other words, moments or processes of embodied defrosting here notably seemed to emerge organically from within the situated body-self, but also served as a kind of unscaffolded "pathway to the collective" that afforded a sustained vulnerability, at least for some participants some of the time. As I have made clear in previous chapters, I am not suggesting that there is a direct causal link between experiences of embodied "opening" and more broadly cultural forms of scalar inquiry that is, in any way, "generalizable." In my research, it was predominantly only long-time, experienced participants, such as Aileen, who made the connection (at least explicitly) between their embodied experience and various forms of real or imagined oppression in Chinese history. I therefore adopt a "long view" perspective in this chapter, emphasizing the ways in which particular or more diffuse experiences of embodied defrosting "landed" within the bodies of two women, Ting Ting and Sulin, over several years.

In this sense, this chapter embrace's Cheryl Mattingly's (2019) notion of the perplexing particular to investigate how experiences of embodied defrosting moved Ting Ting and Aileen to gradually rescale their relationship, often without any explicit political education, not just to other people but also toward the enactment of oppression both historically and in present-day society. The long view, I suggest, helps situate the narrative construction of "metamorphosis" in relation to numerous and shifting personal and social timescales, as well as "space-scales," if you will. Rather than the kind of one-time, all-encompassing or complete "transformation" that Aileen depicted in her brief story above, the linkage between embodied defrosting and scalar inquiry is demonstrated, here, as an often nonlinear, uneven, and emergent process of continual unsettling or uncovering.

In this sense, I further suggest, these longer narratives call into question the notion that the kinds of psychotherapeutic, embodied, and relational practices enacted at New Life and other similar sites are inherently "apolitical." Though undoubtedly lacking in explicit forms of guidance, their stories rather offer insight into the possible ways in which therapeutic engagement not only (at least sometimes) affords the kind of psysociality that Duncan (2018) defines as "grappling with the social" and that Kate Wright (2010, 220) suggests might ultimately work *against* the kinds of individualization and depoliticization commonly associated with psychological self-examination. This became true especially when—as suggested in the previous chapter—such conversations were expanded to include the kinds of past and present forms of injustice that are neither public nor secret but rather exist as forms of "nonknowledge" in contemporary China. I hesitate, here, to suggest that any of these women (or anyone in this book, for that matter) were especially "politicized" by their experiences at New Life or beyond. Indeed, most New Life participants, as well as instructors and staff, as I discuss in the conclusion to this chapter, would undoubtedly resist such an implication. I do emphasize, however, the ways in which experiences of embodied defrosting afforded the opportunity for Ting Ting and Sulin, as well as Aileen, to develop a kind of "critical consciousness" that continued to emerge over time and across sites. Rather than invoking the idea of "politicization," throughout this chapter I thus embrace the notion of *embodied political subjectivity* as an emergent, situated, and yet somewhat haphazard process that, as suggested above, often related to the felt experience of the melting or transformation of that which had previously been or remained "frozen" in their body-selves.

SPEAKING OF SHAME

Before diving into a detailed analysis of Ting Ting's and Sulin's narratives, I offer a brief section examining the ways in which *shame* was one of (if not *the*) most common things that people discussed as having become frozen within them. I found this particularly notable because of the ways in which shame—as many readers are undoubtedly aware—is often represented as a positive, even moral emotion or force in "Asian" cultures (Seok 2017; Lo and Fung 2012). Such ideologies are often grounded in the notion that the so-called "Asian self" is "relational, interactive, and interpersonal" (Seok 2017, 104). In contrast, the so-called "Western self" is imagined as "self-contained, autonomous, and atomic" (2017, 104). Philosopher Bongrae Seok, for example, suggests that shame elicits a "moral injury" for Westerners that does not affect Asians in the same deleterious way (2017, 104). Anthropologists Adrienne Lo and Heidi Fung similarly suggest that the notion that shame is inherently "maladaptive, counterproductive, antisocial, primitive, and even pathological" constitutes a Western cultural ideology that cannot be exported to East Asian settings without qualification (2012, 170). In nearly every kind of workshop I attended, however, New Life participants continually invoked shame—both being shamed and shaming others—as a complex embodied, relational, affective experience that variably inhibited participants' engagement in the vulnerable exercises often required in the space. Shame was also frequently discussed as that which "came up" within particular exercises.

The centrality of *shame* in discussions about embodiment, memory, and collective experience at New Life, moreover, often related to personal and cultural forms of violence that had been transmitted to them either directly or indirectly. Shame was frequently associated with the experience of physical violence at home or in society, for example, or the experience of parental or institutional "care," or both, as a form of governance and "control." Shame was thus often described as an enduring assemblage of broad historical events and more particular relationships that continued to affect participants' experiences of themselves as well as others. When participants spoke of shame, in other words, it became clear that such experience pointed not only to the past but also described the kinds of pain and low self-regard that had continued long beyond a particular incident or period of time.

Shame at New Life thus pointed to an anxious feeling or, as Sylvia put it, a persistent feeling that one's self did not have any kind of inherent worth or value. For Hua Hua, it was the sense that she was fundamentally different from others, that she was not as good as them. Others, like Aileen, emphasized the ways in which their socialization into shame had resulted in their adoption of a habitual shaming stance toward others.

Despite recognizing the importance of questioning anything imagined (by Western theorists) as a "universal" human experience, I resist interpreting such conversations as evidence of the fact that participants have been "inculcated" with Western ideologies of the self that have reoriented their understanding—indeed, their very memories. I do so not because I embrace a naïve perspective regarding what might be imagined as "cultural autonomy" among New Life participants, many of whom had been steeped in Western literature from a range of disciplines throughout their lives. There are multiple reasons influencing my choice to resist the designation of conversations about shame as a form of Westernization. First, following the broader theory on the culturally situated self offered by Hollan (1992), I argue that the reified and entrenched search for culturally enduring definitions of "shame" overtly erases the ways in which *both* Western and Chinese shame discourses acknowledge shame as sometimes positive and sometimes negative. Bradshaw (1990), for example, distinguishes "healthy shame" from so-called toxic shame, as does Resmaa Menakem (2017) and many other Western researchers. Even Bongrae Seok—whose philosophical commitment to advocating for a positive Confucian moral shame—acknowledges the ways in which the vast range of shame words in Chinese points to both positive shame or "modesty" (e.g., 廉耻 *lianchi* and 無耻 *wuchi*) and negative shame or "disgrace" (e.g., 羞耻 *xiuchi*, 耻辱 *chiru*, and 羞辱 *xiuru*). Disgrace, he thus notes, constitutes a form of "social shame" in which people "struggle to deal with potentially negative emotions (anxiety and fear) and disturbing or distracting action tendencies (hiding, fleeing, avoiding, and withdrawing tendencies) to protect their vulnerable interpersonal selves" (2017, 66). In the Chinese historical context, moreover, pathological shame has long been recognized in Chinese medicine as a form of severe suffering. As early as the Eastern Han dynasty (C.E. 25–220), for example, 卑谍 (*beidie*) appears as a syndrome in which people experience a desire to hide from the world, an intense fear, and a feeling of "apologies in the heart" (Pritzker and Yuan 2004, 9). While it is true that Confucius and other prominent Chinese philosophers articulated a moral theory of shame that was considerably more nuanced and detailed than that of Plato, the distinction between "good" and "bad" forms of shame in both settings thus calls the broad acceptance of the idea that "shame is good in Asian cultures" into question.

Second, I turn to researchers who have examined the ways in which shame and shaming have been variably shaped by sociopolitically entrenched gender ideologies that have prevailed throughout Chinese history. Women, as many scholars have discussed, have been shamed for being deceitful and potentially dangerous throughout multiple eras in China history, including the twentieth and twenty-first centuries (see, e.g., Hershatter 2004; Dai 2018; Bossler 2020). Gendered shame has not been limited to women in China, however. Everett Zhang, for example, discusses the ways in which impotence among men in contemporary Chinese society is often associated with "extreme shame" (2015, 11). Both cis-gendered women and men who have expressed or enacted same-sex desire have likewise been subject to persistent shaming throughout Chinese history (e.g., Wu and Stevenson 2006; Martin 2006; Wei 2020). Martin, for example, writes of "shame as a foundational injury that both inaugurates and fractures the tongxinglian [homosexual] subject" (2006, 178). The constant exposure to shaming likewise applies, throughout Chinese history, to those whose bodies or forms of expression push against the established gender binary (Sang 2006; Martin 2006). Overall, then, literature on gender ideologies in China suggests that shame is a powerful force with negative consequences for individuals presenting anywhere on the spectrum between "male" and "female."

Third, I turn to scholarship that takes an explicit historical perspective on shame in China. Stephan Feuchtwang (2013), for example, approaches the notion of what he calls "political shame" during the recent Chinese past. Specifically, he discusses how the pressure to express forms of "revolutionary ardor" during the 1950s and 1960s generated competition between those who were otherwise intimate, for example, family members and neighbors, and was often enacted as a continual form of shaming in China (2013, 226). Political shame not only fractured families and led to widespread suspicion among neighbors, Feuchtwang notes, it also generated a widespread and persistent "distrust" between citizens and state. Delia Lin likewise writes about how various forms of "coercive shame" persist in and across present-day society as a form of governance that hinges upon subjects' "fear of abandonment" to motivate compliance and behavioral change (Lin 2012, 174; see also Lin 2017). The notion of sociopolitically inflicted shame thus complements the distinction between good and bad shame as well as the gendered regulation of shame in particular individuals to call into question the flattened and simplified designations of "Asian" and "Western" shame cultures.

These ethnographic and historical perspectives bring us, I suggest, to one of the additional central *methodological* points made by Lo and Fung (2012). Shame, they suggest, ultimately must be considered in terms of specific interactions or "shaming practices" rather than simply in terms of real or imagined cultural differences. They suggest, in other words, that shame, or "shame-like" behavior or emotions, must be understood in relation to the discursive contexts in which they emerge. Here, then, it is critical to note my observation that conversations about shame at New Life, though often taking shape as a form of collaborative feeling and collective "remembering" that was heavily scaffolded by Western psychotherapeutic notions (as well as Indian spiritual philosophy and other retooled "foreign" ideas about embodiment, relationality, and selfhood), were also opportunities for collaborative theory-building (see chapter 4). Many New Life participants thus used embodied experiences of shame, whether framed as a cause of inhibition or arising as a result of embodied defrosting, to try to make sense of *why* certain painful experiences had occurred.

As both collectively and individual enacted projects of scalar inquiry, the linkage between shame and embodied political subjectivity becomes more apparent. Indeed, as demonstrated in chapter 4, such conversations also frequently involved discussion of how participants might better relate to both past and *present* practices, relationships, and institutional structures in which they experience or enact shame, as well as conversations about how they might intervene in transforming them. Shame, as I discuss below, was further often linked to the kinds of intergenerational trauma that Aileen invoked in our interview. Rather than taking shape around imagined or fictional experiences that they or their relatives experienced or enacted, finally, many of the historical inquiries that participants embarked upon here pointed to very real conditions and constraints affecting the lives of their ancestors and thus themselves.

In sum, then, throughout this chapter I forge a pragmatic rather than referential approach to shame and talk of shame. Such instances, I show, often reproduced and amplified reified ideologies of East/West. As discussed in chapter 4, however, such ideas were often not invoked as absolute realities but were drawn upon strategically and in different ways in order to discuss histories that were not only vague but often unknowable. Having experienced what Feuchtwang frames as the "transmission" of shame "in verbal or non-verbal and everyday ways" in intimate settings (2013, 223), in other words, it was a way to discuss what was rarely if ever explicitly understood but which nevertheless could be felt (Hillenbrand 2020). I thus embrace a simultaneously theoretical and methodological position toward the task of interpreting Ting Ting's and Sulin's references to shame and shame-like experiences and memories in relation to their descriptions of embodied defrosting. In so doing, my hope is to offer a perspective on how conversations about shame at New Life (and, arguably, in China more generally) suggest much more beyond simply an ideological process of subjectification (Foucault 1983) or interpellation (Althusser 2008).

THE HATE IN MY HEART

I met Ting Ting, a thirty-two-year-old woman who had just attended her fourth inner child retreat, at the 2015 extended inner child workshop with Teacher Jo, which she had attended with her mother. We met up just days later for a meal as well as an interview, which we conducted curled up on the couch in my tiny, center-city apartment. Given Ting Ting's diverse experiences at New Life as well as with a range of similar therapeutic settings, it was a long, nonlinear conversation. It began with her description of how she had first become curious about psychospiritual development.

Ting Ting's journey in self-development started, she noted, with a friend mentioning New Life and giving her a copy of Ekhart Tolle's *A New Earth* (2005). When she read it, she told me, she immediately recognized that, in her words, "there was a hole in my heart." No matter how much "good energy" she had tried to generate, as she put it, the hole seemed both immense and impossible to fill. She thus signed up for one of Teacher Jo's extended inner child retreats.

Everything about her first course, she laughed, had immediately turned her off. Recalling Aileen's critical stance, Ting Ting had particularly disliked the way people related to one another with so much seemingly feigned intimacy in the space. In the movement exercises, she said, she nevertheless struggled to understand the idea of "spontaneous expression." Paying attention simply to trying to "dance beautifully," as she put it, her body had been tight, and she could not comprehend what the music "wanted her to express." During a later exercise involving kneeling in front her "parents," however, she had a strange feeling, like she never wanted to leave. She had even shed a few tears, which had surprised her.

After that first course, Ting Ting explained, there had been a slight but significant shift, as if her body felt somehow *lighter*. It also seemed like it had suddenly become easier to let go of things that previously she would have "held on to," in her words. Recalling that Jo had said something to her about being "trapped," she decided to sign up for an ecstatic movement workshop with a German teacher. Still, she approached the course with skepticism and hesitation.

"How could just dancing help you with personal growth?," she remembered thinking. She gave it a try, however, and ended up having an experience of deep insight during the workshop. It was during an exercise in which they had been instructed to move with their eyes closed, much like in the "madhouse" exercise described in chapter 3. In this case, however, the teacher had them imagine that their eyes were on their hands, like sensors. At one point, Ting Ting had been lying down, and someone had come over to her, taking her hand and holding it for a moment. Her touch, Ting Ting explained, had felt wonderful. Suddenly, however, her new friend jumped up and left, and Ting Ting felt hurt, as if she had done something wrong to drive her away. She opened her eyes and peeked at the woman then, later addressing her directly about what had happened. The woman was surprised to hear that Ting Ting had been offended.

"She had just wanted to stand up and keep dancing, and since I was lying down, she figured she would just go find someone else to work with her," Ting Ting explained. "And suddenly I understood—I realized that it wasn't that I was good and she wasn't or vice versa. We just didn't *choose* each other. We weren't suitable together at the time." Suddenly, she continued, she understood that intimacy is not supposed to be reluctant or *forced*. This prompted her to let go of a lot of "stuff," including her constant concern with the ways others saw her.

Describing them one after another, Ting Ting went on to detail multiple insights that she had gained in particular workshops, many of which—like the above example—involved an embodied, relational component as well as a particular moment of sudden insight. She noted how her experience in a drumming workshop, for example, had helped her to maintain her own "heart rhythm" while simultaneously "integrating" with the hearts of others. Pointing to the ethical-relational implications of the extended *dawo* or

"Great Self" at New Life, as described in chapter 3, Ting Ting's reflections here suggested that drumming had offered her an embodied experience of a novel form of relationality that was simultaneously "individual" and "collective" (see also C. Huang 2016). One of the most deeply moving and pivotal experiences she had ever had, however, was during a course on music therapy, a workshop offered by a mind-body-spirit organization like New Life. At one point, participants were asked to sing a song that represented their heart, but Ting Ting had struggled to come up with a song for herself. She overheard another participant singing a song, however, and was struck with the revelation it afforded.

"She was singing something like 'you know how long I've waited, looking out of the window for you' and I just immediately came to life," she said. Heavy tears had formed in her eyes and she began having intense flashbacks of being in kindergarten, looking out the window and waiting for her parents. They had very rarely come to see her at the K-12 boarding school that she had attended. Ting Ting went on to describe, here, how the music, the setting, and the flashbacks had immersed her in an affective-embodied experience of her "child-self," as she described it, offering a "sudden" but deeply impactful realization.

"I just suddenly realized: *this* is where all of my *hate* (恨 hen) comes from—this hate right here," she said, pointing to her chest. "I did not understand, at the time, why my parents left me. I thought they didn't want me, so from that moment on, the hate was here."

Ting Ting's lasting sense of "hate," she further noted, was not only directed toward her parents. For many years it was primarily directed at one of her primary school teachers, who, she felt, had rejected her. As a result of her enduring feelings of resentment, she had developed the capacity to be "distant" and "critical." Noting that she had been *proud* of such a capacity, she told me she eventually become so "cold" that people had often been afraid of her.

"I was like a hedgehog before! If you spoke to me, I would immediately tell you everything that was wrong with you," she laughed, chronotopically highlighting the ways in which self-development had emerged as an embodied process of learning to love. The opening that occurred suddenly in the workshop, she noted, had constituted the first step toward her embodiment of a demeanor that was drastically different from a hedgehog (an observation I can corroborate based on my own experience of her). The experience of embodied defrosting had helped her, in her words, to develop relational "warmth" where she had been "cold" before. As she had cried and laid on the dance floor that day, moreover, she had further begun to understand that the feeling of "hate" that had seemed to perpetually seethe under her sternum area was actually what she described as a kind of "emptiness" related to not feeling *safe* in the world, and not feeling loved.

"I didn't know that, in my heart, I just really didn't feel safe. I really thought my parents didn't want me," she said, speaking in the past tense. Her eyes began to glisten, however, as she switched to the present tense, "but that isn't necessarily true."

Pointing to the ways in which shame-inducing traumas "break apart safety, connection, and dignity, leaving these needs at odds with one another, leaving us more compartmentalized and separate from each other" (Haines 2019, 318), Ting Ting's shift from "cold" to "warm" here suggests how her experience of embodied defrosting, in this case, *moved* something within her such that she realized that it was not, indeed, the case that she had been unwanted. Ting Ting described the shift as instant and overwhelming, but she also took care to mention that it had not been until she attended a later course that she had learned how to *forgive*. She could not recall the name of the workshop nor the specific method it had conveyed, but she described it multiple times as "experiential" in that it involved very little explicit dialogue.

"The one thing I learned there," she said, "is that, in forgiving others, you can accept yourself more." In a single moment during that workshop, she had thus decided to forgive her primary school teacher. "Because she did not—she was not perfect. She had just graduated from college, she didn't understand. Even though she hurt me deeply and caused a lasting injury, I feel now that I forgive her."

Going on to explain that she now sees how she had turned her teacher into an alternative "mother figure," the notion of forgiveness here points to the affective, embodied, and relational expression of the kind of "defrosting" that, according to Arendt (1971), also constitutes a relentless form of inquiry. It also, however, bears a resemblance to Arendt's perspectives on how the act of forgiving another—regardless of whether it also entails "forgetting"—generates new possibilities for the future (Arendt 1958). The act of forgiving, writes Arendt, releases both parties from "the predicament of irreversibility" that obtains when individuals are essentially locked into what she describes as a relational *confinement* tracing back to "one single deed from which we could never recover" (1958, 237). Ting Ting's decision to forgive her teacher was, in this sense, enacted as an agentive kind of anticipatory mode in which different possibilities began to take shape on the horizon. It also underscores the ways in which "healing shame," as Haines suggests, "allows us to imagine a positive future for ourselves and others, to reconnect authentically, and to take action toward what we care about" (2019, 300). While Ting Ting's teacher's perceived rejection had caused her to feel shame, in other words, the sudden and unspoken experience of embodied defrosting that occurred in the workshop motivated her forgiveness not as a form of forgetting but as a process of healing.

In attending to the role of critical reflection on the politics of shame, however, Haines further notes that "when someone is healing shame, we need to have enough conversation, offer enough *political education*, so the person has grounding to know what is their responsibility (their actions) and what is not" (2019, 302–3, italics mine). None of this, as I have discussed throughout this book, was explicitly included at New Life. Nor was it, at least in my experience, a known component offered by other similar centers. Notably, however, Ting Ting described the scalar links she had made and which had seemed to arise spontaneously vis-à-vis a series of *unspoken* interactions.

When it came to forgiving her parents, Ting Ting then went on to detail, the process had been—and indeed still *was*—exceedingly more complex. This involved many realizations about the ways in which, underneath his "coldness," her father loved her deeply but only expressed it by offering her financial support. Despite the relative closeness that she had always felt with her mother, moreover, Ting Ting had recently realized that she had always slightly distrusted her. Both of her parents would frequently reproach and scold her, she explained, often using physical violence to drive their message home. Pointing to the ways in which embodied defrosting often offered people insight into the ways *being* shamed had affected them, Ting Ting explained how her mother's sudden shifts into scolding and violence had generated a great deal of fear and distrust.

"I began to distrust her. I just felt that she was unreliable, that I couldn't count on her," she said, noting that she had only come to fully understand this in the recent workshop that her mother had also attended. I asked her how that felt, to be having such a realization in a space she was sharing with her mother. She had been worried about it, she laughed, and she was certainly not sharing this particular insight with her. Quoting Teacher Jo's consistent guidance, offered at the close of every workshop, she highlighted her understanding of why it is important to postpone trying to "process" specific insights with particular friends or family members because of the ways it which it might "land" upon them.

"If I told her this," she explained, "she wouldn't necessarily be able to digest it, to absorb it. It might impact her negatively. This is *my* homework (功课 *gongke*)," she said. Laughing, she went on to explain that she had originally hoped, back when she first started on her journey to become mature, that the process would involve learning how to better *critique* her mother. She felt like she no longer needed to do so, however, and was simply glad that her mother had attended for her own personal development.

Here, Ting Ting switched tracks, becoming reflective about how she had begun to see, in many workshops, that her own childhood experience of longing for her absent parents was far from unique. Indeed, as many scholars have noted, it is extremely common for children, across multiple generations, to be separated from their parents in China (e.g., Evans 2008; Johnston 2013).[3] Ting Ting's memories here reflect what I found to be a relatively ubiquitous experience in the past at New Life. Discussion about the long-term psychosocial *implications* of separation from one's parents was thus a common theme that often arose in the center, especially in connection to discussions of shame. Pointing to the ways in which embodied defrosting often entailed or at least afforded an intimate form of scalar inquiry that extended far beyond the "self," Ting Ting also learned about the ways in which her own exposure to shaming and violence from her parents—when they were around—was similarly common among attendees in her age cohort and beyond. This had moved her, in fact, to conduct a broader investigation of the Chinese past, particularly the ways in which past social, economic, and political pressures persisted within her own and others' bodies. Despite her own aspirations to become a teacher in psychospiritual self-development, which she mentioned several times over the course of our interaction, she thus noted that she had decided that—at least for now—she would only take classes from foreign, predominantly Western, teachers.

"Because Chinese teachers," she said, "if they grew up in situations where they weren't loved, the best they can do is imitate the content of the course. But they can never have a great love." Based on her observations of the ways in which Chinese students in the various courses she had attended all grappled with the same childhood wounds that she had discovered in herself, Ting Ting here crafted an expansive cultural chronotopization centering around the affective capacity to feel and give *love*. The Chinese past here limited Chinese teachers to a form of "imitation" and precluded the development of what she called "a great love." Ting Ting stopped here, however, offering a qualification of her assertion and very quickly going on to explain that she recognized that not all Westerners necessarily had the kind of "great love" that she was talking about.

"But Chinese people," she nevertheless reiterated, "especially the previous generation, the generation of people who are teachers now—people in their forties, fifties, sixties—they grew up under [a system of] criticism (批判批评下长大 pipan piping xia zhangda). There was a lot of chaos (乱 luan) that they experienced. It was neither an easy nor a comfortable time. So I don't take their classes. Some of them," she then added, "even the look in their eyes (眼神 yanshen) is sharp (犀利的 xili de), a kind of sharpness that is itself a kind of criticism."

Ting Ting's comment here echoed what Aileen had once said about how the central role of criticism and shaming across sites in the interconnected Chinese systems of education, family, and governance often led novice Chinese teachers to perpetuate harm within courses on self-development. Indeed, Aileen had explained that this was why she tended to hire *Western* teachers without much concern while she required extensive, multiyear internships for aspiring Chinese teachers before letting them lead. Like Ting Ting, Aileen thus situated sensitivity in response to criticism as well as the tendency to *be* critical when placed in a position of authority as a "cultural" characteristic that was grounded not in reified notions of so-called Chineseness, but rather in her own embodied experience as well as her many years of observing courses at New Life.

Ting Ting's preference for Western teachers, this comment suggests, was arguably rooted in a more direct engagement with the particular shapes that oppression took on in the recent Chinese past. Notably, then, the "chaos" and "system of criticism" that Ting Ting referred to points directly and unambiguously to the Maoist period in China, which spanned from the 1950s through the 1970s. Though arguably collapsing this history into a simplified or "flattened" narrative of oppression corresponding to the discourse of victimization that is upheld by the Chinese state (Rofel 2007; Hillenbrand 2020), I suggest that Ting Ting's framing engaged with a more nuanced focus on the ways in which "love" during the Cultural Revolution—though continuing in many ways—was also inhibited by an affective atmosphere within which "political shame" and "distrust" were not only pervasive, but intimate (Feuchtwang 2013). Ting Ting here demonstrated her understanding of the ways in which this political-affective environment had left a lasting affective-embodied orientation that was not only "personal" but also inhered in the ways that most Chinese people who had grown up during this time engaged with others.

In a vivid description of how "even the look in their eyes"—translatable also as "eye spirit"—was "itself a form of criticism," Ting Ting thus described how she had come to see how the traumatic political past endured in the present, moving *across bodies* within interactions at home and in the classroom. This further drew attention to the way shame was often discussed at New Life as a historically situated yet lasting embodied, relational, and affective experience. Ting Ting's analysis, specifically, hinged upon the strategic deployment of various spatiotemporal scales in order to translate what are often considered to be "public" events into what could be considered "personal" experience. Her framing, in other words, underscores the ways in which particular structures of governance in China *become intimate* within and across the body-selves of citizens. Pointing to the ways in which public secrecy in China is often experienced as "an active wedge driven between family members" (Hillenbrand 2020, 182), Ting Ting's description of the "sharpness" in the eyes of teachers affected by this history underscores how this wedge is further driven forward in interactions beyond the family. Ting Ting's experience thus seemed to have motivated an intimate scalar shift in her relationship to her own body as well as a cultural past that she had not previously considered.

This was not any particular individual's fault, she then clarified. "There was nothing anyone in the family could do," she said matter-of-factly. "The conditions (条件 *tiaojian*) just weren't there."

Situating the "systems of criticism" she invoked as an external force impeding the agency of families to enact love in ways they may have wanted, Ting Ting offered a kind of compassion toward those whom she characterized as lacking "a great love." Without enacting the kind of "historical forgetting" that Rofel undergirds the narrative of China's Maoist past as "nothing but a life of sacrifice" (2007, 118), Ting Ting here seemed to be expanding her capacity for forgiveness, described above in primarily interpersonal terms, at a much broader socio-spatial and temporal scale. Such expansion highlights the ways in which, within the intimate visceral geography of New Life (and in this case, other similar centers), *group* experiences of embodied defrosting afford more broadly scaled forms of inquiry. Notably, Ting Ting went on, here, to further expand her analysis to include herself and others in her age cohort.

"We all live with so many scars (伤痕 shanghen)," she said. "And we were raised by parents who also have many scars. There is just so much that needs healing." Engaging in what might be called a kind of hauntological genealogy in which personal pain is experienced as an ongoing form of embodied intergenerational trauma (Menakem 2017), Ting Ting paused here, seeming to reflect on the enormity of the task of healing the "scars" that persisted across generations. Such healing, she then noted, was especially complicated by recent Chinese society's emphasis on material, economic wealth rather than spiritual growth.

"Nowadays, moreover, all we have is material things. But there is a void (虚渺 xumiao), and so many people [still] don't have any love." Upgrading her assessment of the urgency inherent in the need for healing, she continued. "We really, really need this," she said. Extending her analysis of the political past to a socioeconomic present, Ting Ting thus noted that a "void" seemed to persist in Chinese society, giving rise to a shared form of suffering that demanded healing. Given Ting Ting's ambitions to become a teacher *herself*, however, the question remained as to whether and how she considered the possibility that, being Chinese, she might ever be able to overcome what she framed as a deeply entrenched and enduring set of cultural conditions.

"You want to become a teacher, correct?," I asked, bringing the question to the fore.

Ting Ting nodded.

"Do you think of *yourself* as unable to do it because you are Chinese?"

She laughed heartily here, as if she had already extensively considered this question. She then admitted that she frequently imagined how, one day, when she had overcome all of her own deeply entrenched blockages and wounds, she might be ready to teach. She realized, however, that given the processual nature of healing, such an ambition was arguably untenable. Switching into a more subjunctive mode, she then suggested that maybe she would *not* actually ever feel ready to become a teacher. She then amended her proposal yet again.

"Maybe in the future," she said. "Well, I dare not say what might happen."

Suggesting how her previously articulated cultural theories were the result not of reified forms of cultural determinism but existed more as a tentative process of inquiry, Ting Ting's expressions of unwillingness to say "what might happen" in the future here seemed to suggest that her theories had shifted multiple times in the past and *would* expectedly shift in the future. Though she seemed to embrace rather reified chronotopic (though intimately scaled) notions of East and West in crafting these theories, moreover, it is important to recognize how they served the pragmatic goal of making sense of a particular Chinese history that endured in the present. Here, in theorizing her own suffering as exclusive to Chinese body-selves, one might even suggest that Ting Ting was enacting a mediated form of scalar intimacy that arguably drew her closer to her Chinese "compatriots" precisely by investigating the unspoken yet deeply felt forms of oppression that continued through the generations (Feuchtwang 2013; Hillenbrand 2020), even while her desire was targeted toward the embodied knowledge and "love" of Western teachers. In the indeterminacy of her theories with regard to their potential to restrict her aspirations to become a teacher herself, however, I want to close by offering the perspective that, rather than idealizing Western knowledge, Ting-Ting was attempting to make sense of the ways in which her multiple experiences of embodied defrosting and scalar inquiry had led her, perhaps unexpectedly, to shift from "cold" to "warm" and to thereby remake the ways in which she related not just to other people but to a range of collective experiences as well.

"THOSE THINGS THAT ARE COLLECTIVE"

At the outset of chapter 1, I briefly introduced Sulin, noting how losing her marital home caused her to feel like she had lost her "self." As she described to me during an interview five years after the fact, the divorce had been almost unbearably disorienting, causing her to feel like she had lost touch with the sense that she was either valuable or "worthy of love" (指的爱 zhide ai). Sulin had, at the time, already undergone multiple years of suffering in relation to her (apparent) infertility.[4] The drive to heal had thus become urgent, eventually becoming a near-daily affair that led her to participate in courses and groups in everything from the Satir method to *jiapai*, neurolinguistic programming, hypnosis, the Enneagram,[5] pendulum therapy, and inner child work. In conveying her experience in self-development, which very much oriented toward the portrayal of a metamorphosis through which she had at least begun to learn how to love, Sulin notably shifted back and forth, repeatedly, between different spatiotemporal frameworks for interpreting and narrating her experience.

In one framing, for example, Sulin talked about her own life, using what Woolard (2013) might refer to as the chronotope of "biographical time." Sulin here placed her experience along a continuum of "adventure" that began with her youth, took an unexpected turn with her inability to have a baby and the start of a still-ongoing affair with the man who was later to become her second husband, and hit a crescendo with the demise of her marriage. Her story had ended—at least at the time we spoke—with the near-total restructuring of her life. Sulin also, though, frequently spoke in terms of the much larger, less personal framework of "socio-historical time" (Woolard 2013) or what Parmentier (2007) calls "cultural time" to chronotopically situate herself in relation to a thousands-year-old collective past. Like Sulin and Ting Ting, in other words, Sulin thus crafted multiple chronotopic formulations that situated her embodied experience within historical as well as ongoing forms of oppression.

It had all begun, Sulin recalled, with a dance class where, at least in the beginning, she was often ridiculed for being "stiff" and inflexible. Her instructor had made a comment that impacted her deeply, however. She had suggested, specifically, that people who danced stiffly had "lost touch with their own bodies." Sulin, who had been known for her fluidity and grace in college, immediately began focusing wholeheartedly on loosening her tightened muscles, intent on regaining that sense of contact with her body. As she did so, however, she had the distinct sensation that all the emotions, sensations, and knowledge that she had previously been unwilling to face would "come up" (饭上来 fanshanglai) in an immense and overwhelming wave of sensation that often, quite literally, took her breath away. It was at once a liberating feeling and one that felt like an enormous burden and unsolvable set of dilemmas that all seemed to lead her further into a dark and impossible labyrinth of sorrow and futility. She persisted, however, and over the years she had begun to realize that her own and others' everyday experiences of suffering were often infused with what she called *"those things that are collective"* (人共同的那些 *ren gongtong de neixie*). People were variably "bound" (束缚 *shufu*) by things that have taken shape over the past five thousand years of Chinese history, she said here. Without mentioning anything specific, she went on to emphasize how the collective effects are amplified by the conditions of *silence* that have often prevailed (and which often persists) in Chinese society.

"There was so much pain you couldn't talk about in the past," she said. Pointing to the ways in which public secrecy, as described numerous times throughout this and previous chapters, affects one's most intimate relationships and deepest embodied experiences, Sulin had thus begun to think of the ways in which collective and often *unspoken* trauma in China's past had given rise to not just her own but so many others' suffering. This silence had, she moreover noted, resulted in the ways in which specific information contained within the intimate embodied space of the collective subconscious was often opaque and difficult to access.

"The kind of pain I'm talking about is often from things you don't remember. It isn't something you can recognize yourself. Maybe you can recognize about 10 percent. But there's no way for you to directly grasp the rest," she said, chronotopically situating "collective things" within the obscure space-time of the personal, embodied unconscious.

Sulin's (re)chronotopization of her own experience vis-à-vis a more broadly shared, intergenerational experience here mirrors the descriptions offered by Aileen and Ting Ting. Like these other women, moreover, Sulin also narratively traced it back to an initial experience of embodied defrosting, for example, the "opening" she had experienced in the dance class. Unlike the others, however, Sulin did not situate her specific awareness of the collective unconscious in a particular moment, movement, or experience. Framing it more as a gradual process of learning to love or "becoming conscious," in her words, she did not offer any specific sense of how or when this perspective had arisen. She did note that it had been informed, in particular, by her experiences doing constellations as well as in Satir workshops. Sulin's depiction of her understanding of the collective was, furthermore, unlike Ting Ting's in that it lacked details with regard to the ways in which forms of explicit knowledge (e.g., about safety, forgiveness, or history) related to specific moments of relationally situated embodied defrosting. Reflecting the kind of generalized ambiguity in Aileen's description of the "heavy burdens we carry from our ancestors," Sulin nonetheless emphasized, at several points, how her process of learning to *live* in "the conversation, the company, or the companionship . . . of ghosts," as Derrida might say (1994, xvii), had led to a number of specific insights that had ultimately added up to an ongoing process of learning to love.

Sulin highlighted, for example, how conditions of *silence*, whether chosen or enforced, had perpetuated the suffering of children, in particular. She noted, here, how violence and various types of shaming directed at children had never been questioned as harmful. She further underscored her growing awareness of the ways in which long-standing patriarchal ideas in China had not only harmed many women but also persisted in many of the norms and expectations that shaped her own experience as both a child and an adult. Without using the explicit terminology, Sulin further described how she had, in fact, recently become attuned to the ways in which her suffering was entrenched in a long history of patriarchy in China. Persisting as a vital, intimate force in the present, Sulin described how she saw patriarchy as informing accepted ideas about who is a "good woman," for example: a wife to a successful, handsome man, a nurturing mother, and a loyal and obedient daughter, to name a few. Sulin had thus slowly began to recognize how deeply entangled her very sense of self-worth had been with what she described as the "labels" that society uses to judge the value of women. She saw, for example, how she had previously considered her husband, her home, and her job a kind of evidence that she had value and was worth loving.

"You have a husband who appears very honorable," she explained. "It implies you are a successful person. And then you have a seemingly pretty good home, so it appears you are a successful person." As a result of these realizations, Sulin had increasingly begun to distance herself from what she framed as the "labels" offered to her by society as well as the expectations of others.

"There are the people around you who have expectations and desires for you. Now I feel I just don't care about any of that—or I feel that I definitely don't *want* to [care], regardless of the results."

Sulin was beginning to understand the ways in which the expectations of others, though often expressed as a kind of care or concern, were rooted in a range of deeply problematic gender ideologies and social hierarchies. Much like Ping (in chapter 1) or Old Hong's daughter as well as Lan in the opening vignette for chapter 4, Sulin increasingly saw such expressions of concern as a form of *control* rather than care. Sulin thus began to scale herself differently in relation to many of the ideals and ideologies that she had previously taken for granted. Underscoring how she understood her new relationship to the collective unconscious as a form of *healing*, Sulin chronotopically articulated the importance of how such healing demanded a continual willingness to turn *toward* rather than *away from* emotions, sensations, and embodied experiences as they arose in the context of her everyday life. This denotes, I suggest, the ways in which embodied defrosting—though perhaps sometimes traceable to a specific event—constituted a continuous process of turning simultaneously "inward" and "outward." She admitted to the ways in which such a stance, rather than providing easy solutions, often generated more uncertainty. She was confident, however, that any kind of healing or transformation was made possible only in the willingness to directly confront or (more aptly) *embrace* the ways in which the social past had accumulated as an affective-embodied, relational way of being in the world.

The demand to engage in this way, furthermore, often arose for Sulin unexpectedly in a range of situations far beyond the space of particular workshops. In her current romantic relationship, for example, Sulin often recognized that she was getting "caught up" in what she described as the drama that had and continued to unfold in her partner's estranged marriage. Speaking to the salience of shame throughout this chapter, Sulin detailed how her partner would sometimes experience intense bouts of guilt and self-blame with regard to his "abandonment" of his family. In order to support him, Sulin explained, she had to continually work on "letting go" of his experience and had become increasingly capable of doing so. Here, she also mentioned her nascent but growing ability to resist the "advice" that her parents constantly offered. During her marriage, Sulin here recalled, they had continually advised her to control her temper, to avoid making her husband angry. Now that she had connected with a new partner, they further insisted that the couple quickly remarry. While she had heeded their direction in the past, she noted, she no longer did so, though it was not always easy.

Though sometimes related to a specific situation, Sulin also took care to explain that there were other times when she was simply overcome with intense emotion that did not seem to relate to anything specifically. Whether she was clear on the "cause" or not, she noted that she had been approaching her suffering systematically through the intentional, embodied cultivation of deep inquiry into "what it really is," in her words. Inquiry here supported Sulin in discerning the underlying causes of her suffering, but it also served as a strategy for diffusing it. She frequently used tapping therapy, for example, a method where you repeat a statement while continuously tapping on particular points of the body, to confront and hopefully shift both her immediate experience as well as whatever culturally situated beliefs and orientations lay beneath the pain. When she felt insecure, for example, she would tap her arm and repeat the words "I love myself" to combat her experience or perception of self-hate. The process of "discovering herself" in this way, as she put it, ultimately restructured the way in which she engaged with others and the way she acted in the world. It had taught her, in my framing, to both entangle and to love differently. Here, however, Sulin expanded her scope of the kinds of suffering that affected her, further mentioning the ways in which she was challenged by what she characterized as a "a social environment of injustice" (不公平的社会环境 *bu gongping de shehui huanjing*) prevailing in Chinese society.

"It is an extremely complex environment," she said, detailing how, in 2015 China, one was forced to endure the almost daily stress of continual *uncertainty*. Here, she mentioned relationship problems and—like Sylvia in chapter 4—problems related to parenting under the grueling and competitive conditions that prevailed, especially in urban centers (see J. Xu 2017, 2020). She also notably mentioned the stress of living among the kinds of constantly shifting "hidden rules" (潜规则 *qian guize*), which made it constantly difficult to plan and enact one's goals in the most mundane as well as the most consequential ways (see J. Yang 2015). In this regard, she further noted, if one did not have the right status or connections (关系 *guanxi*), it was often essentially impossible to succeed. Finally, bringing up the ways in which the lack of religion or "spiritual beliefs" (信仰 *xinyang*) presented a serious problem in China, Sulin observed how contemporary society often guided people toward equating money, power, and material sucess with a sense of safety in the world. These were all substitutes for a deeper form of spiritual connectedness, she observed, and often just perpetuated the kind of inherited pain that affected the personal as well as the collective psyche or spirit (精神 *jingshen*).

Sulin did not suggest that her engagement with the collective unconscious could contribute directly to the transformation of these more widespread forms of injustice, as she had described them. Much like Ting Ting had drawn attention to the impossibility of addressing the "hole in her heart" simply with "good energy," Sulin here quickly cast aside hegemonic discourses promoting "positive energy" (正能量 *zheng nengliang*), often presented in public discourse as the key to "speedy success" (Hird 2018, 111). Indeed, she was emphatic in her assertion that, under the circumstances of contemporary Chinese society, just having "energy" (能量 *nengliang*)—or even skill—was never and could never be enough. All she or anyone could do, she had realized, was to try to cultivate the ability to tolerate discomfort, continually probing one's subconscious for possible ways to transform the inherited conditions that had given rise to the kinds of injustices that prevailed in the present. Sulin had nevertheless come to think of this as a form of subversion, of sorts. While not the kind of subversion that inspires vast social change, Sulin's approach here served as the foundation for what she described as a new sense of being "home" within her own body. Sulin thus seemed to equate the notion of "being-at-home-in-the-world" (Jackson 1995) with the process of learning to love. Her rechronotopically cast notion of home as an embodied sense of direction and morality that strived for even if it did not always attain freedom from the past furthermore underscored how her investigation into the ways both the injustices of the past and the present permeated her body-self was also a form of *hope* for Sulin.

I hesitate to link such hope, however, to so-called optimism. Like both Aileen and Ting Ting, Sulin not only appreciated the immensity of the task of healing what she understood as thousands of years of (ongoing) injustice. She also, notably, expressed a great deal of skepticism with regard to the ways in which the psychospiritual development "scene" often contributed to people's narcissistic endeavors to constantly "transform themselves." Many courses in self-development thus often seemed to Sulin to cater to such desires, perpetuating such narcissistic obsession with "self-transformation." She noted, finally, how this capitalist configuration often encouraged what she observed to be many (if not most) participants' lack of commitment to sit with any form of discomfort for more than a brief time. Sulin's reflections here notably mirror an anthropological point of view on the role of capitalism in crafting both the desire that often leads people to centers like New Life and the marketing and enactment of such programs (see, e.g., Rose 1996; Illouz 2008; J. Yang 2018a-b; L. Zhang 2020). Our interview thus ended with her discussion of how difficult it often was, even for her, to find the strength or capacity—the *willingness*—to dig deep enough within oneself to really shift the gendered, historical, and social trauma that she ultimately saw as the only way out of the "mess" that people often found themselves embedded within.

CONCLUDING REFLECTIONS

I began this chapter with a description of Aileen's response to one of the standard questions I asked of all participants in this research: whether and how the knowledge, practice, or community at New Life was particularly relevant in China. In responding, Aileen drew upon the example of Bao, who had collapsed during an exercise involving the enactment of a happy nuclear family. She then proceeded to detail how her *own* embodied experience of "defrosting" after her initial inner child workshop had engendered a simultaneously embodied, affective, and relational "metamorphosis." Here Aileen underscored how, for her, this constituted a kind of scalar state change that afforded her uptake of Bao's extreme reaction as an index of an enduring "burden" that was linked to time, space, and history and which stretched across women's bodies in the space of the center and beyond. Though the details were different, I further demonstrated how Ting Ting and Sulin had multiple experiences of embodied defrosting that afforded, over time, a similar form of ongoing scalar inquiry investigating the ways in which both historical and present structures of power and social injustices had become entrenched within their own and others' body-selves.

Throughout the chapter, I further emphasized how shame, in particular, was invoked as an enduring assemblage of broad historical events and more particular relationships that continued to affect their experiences of themselves as well as others. Here, as I suggested at the outset of the chapter, shame was not only an index of oppressive relational practices and institutional structures, but an *embodiment* of them that posed a continual challenge both as a personally experienced or intergenerational transmitted experience and as an enactment of suffering. With both Ting Ting and Sulin, I thus offered a "long view" narrative perspective underscoring how the process of "healing shame," according to Staci K. Haines, "takes place in phases and over time" (2019, 302). Their stories of shifting their experience, enactment, and overall relationship to shame, if not necessarily fully "healing" it, underscored the process as one of ongoing, dialogically situated (re)chronotopization that was both embodied and intimate. Their extended narratives further demonstrate, I suggested, how such scalar inquiry constituted an ongoing, uneven, and often nonlinear process of uncovering. It was not, in other words, a one-time, absolute experience of "transformation," as perhaps suggested in the chronotopic formulation offered by Aileen at the outset of the chapter or within the stories of "personal transformation" often put forth in global self-help and psychospiritual literature (e.g., Woodstock 2005; Jain 2020). The unevenness of their narratives rather pointed to a continual experience of uncovering that, at least for these women, moved them to engage less with their personal drama and more with the ways in which historical forms of oppression and injustice were entrenched within their bodies.

Despite sometimes taking up relatively reified or simplistic notions of "culture," moreover, the cultural "theories" developed here, importantly, suggested at least the possibility of an openness to continual refinement. This resulted in what can only be understood as a fragmentary process of remembering the past as what Jie Li calls "a palimpsest process" constantly mediated by "texts and images, objects and places" as well as through "interpersonal communications between sentient bodies" (2020, 7): the "sharp gaze" Ting Ting noted among teachers who had lived through the Mao era, for example. Such openness was undoubtedly constrained by the reality that many of the specifics of the Chinese past, as the women understood well, were murky, unspoken, and only partially understood. I have nevertheless suggested that experiences of embodied defrosting served, at least for these women, as a kind of "pathway to the collective."

Aileen, Ting Ting, and Sulin thus variably portrayed a kind of spontaneous, relationally situated process of developing the kind of "critical consciousness" that, as Daniel José Gaztambide (2019, 164) describes, "brings into sharp focus how experience arises from the sociocultural systems that impact our collective well-being, and our individual role—even complicity—within those systems." Pointing to a long-standing yet often-neglected lineage in psychoanalysis, which led from Freud to Fanon to Freire and to the marginal but enduring practice of liberation psychology, Gaztambide thus argues, psychoanalysis has the capacity to open up (if not, in this case, encourage) intimate and, importantly, *scalar*, inquiries linking the personal to the political. To the extent that psychoanalytically framed self-examination, especially when enacted in a group setting, might unsettle what Rosa (2020) might call *the indexical disorder* within society, Gaztambide thus writes about how the connection between psychology and critical consciousness constitutes "an intentional process that is constantly revealed through relations with the world and with others" (2019, xxx). What I have discussed here, on the other hand, is arguably vastly unlike the kinds of explicitly politicized forms of liberation psychology that Gaztambide describes. Nor does it resemble the clearly articulated practices, within the emerging field of embodied social justice, for understanding somatic openings as a pathway to the transformation of entrenched forms of injustice as well as to the enactment of *justice* in the world (e.g., williams et al. 2016; Menakem 2017; Hicks Peterson 2018; R. Johnson 2018; Haines 2019; Hemphill 2020; Fikes 2021a-b; King 2021). Indeed, the lack of explicit scaffolding or education encouraging such linkages and bringing them into the space for further discussion is one of the primary limitations of the politics of the center. As I have repeatedly emphasized, moreover, the ways in which New Life constituted what I have been calling a heteronormative "Hantopia" posed a set of problematic limitations upon the salience of whatever forms of critical consciousness did happen to emerge in relation to participants' experiences at the center.

In closing, however, I want to reiterate that I do not, here, seek to attribute any kind of political or even social intentions to the material or to the center. Here, then, I return to Aileen's insistence that New Life had no ambition to politicize participants, nor even to support them in developing critical consciousness. Their goal was to provide them with a temporary space-time of "comfort" in an increasingly stressful society. In this sense, especially alongside Sulin's critical observations on the way capitalism-driven narcissism often lay at the heart of the self-development scene in China, what I have described here arguably points to Mattingly's notion of the "perplexing particular," which "not only surprises, in the sense of striking unexpectedly, but also eludes explanation" (2019, 13). I discuss these issues further in the conclusion to this book. Before doing so, however, I offer one final data-driven chapter that, like this one, examines the experiences of two longer-term participants specifically in terms of the ways in which their experiences at the center, over time, afforded them the opportunity to "tinker with the patriarchy" in numerous ways.

7

Tinkering with the Patriarchy

In practice... seeking a compromise between different "goods" does not necessarily depend on talk, but can also be a matter of practical tinkering, of attentive experimentation.
—ANNEMARIE MOL, INGUNN MOSER, AND JEANNETTE POLS

Permeability points... clearly to the idea that, being open (and therefore permeable) beings, we are all mutually affected by each other and the world around us, which in turn, is permeable as well.
—LETICIA SABSAY

At the outset of a *jiapai* salon in 2016, a woman named Dee introduced herself and her mother, who sat beside her. The pair had attended several of the longer workshops together, and their relationship had been transformed, Dee claimed, as a result. They no longer squabbled over small things, for example, and they had become much closer as they engaged together on their quest to understand their family's past.

While Dee spoke, the rest of the group looked on in admiration. Later, during a short break, a spontaneous discussion began when another participant posed a question about whether it was possible to develop oneself, or "become mature," without bringing one's parents to attend at least one course at New Life. Several newcomers expressed doubt in the possibility of transforming their relationships with parents who had not experienced the center firsthand. Recalling Old Hong's narrative in chapter 4, they were also skeptical, however, that their parents would be willing to come. Nor were they enthusiastic about the possibility that their parents would accept or understand the material or ways of relating in the space. Dee emphasized how, prior to bringing her mother to New Life, she had thought the same way.

Another longer-term participant—a woman who appeared to be in her thirties named Min—here moved over to join the small circle of women sitting in the middle of the room and inserted herself into the conversation. She said that, actually, there had been an enormous shift in her relationship with her mother over the past year she had been coming to New Life, despite the fact that here mother had never accompanied Min to the center. Nor, of course, had she come on her own.

"In traditional Chinese culture," she then said, "the concept of 'obedience' means that we suppress our own thoughts and feelings—we do what our parents want. Parents don't even have to say anything—they control us invisibly!"

Her description evoked laughter in the group. But Min then grew serious, and lamented that, even once she was an adult with her own child, her mother had continued trying to control her, often "indirectly" through various kinds of shaming and scolding.

"My mother is a teacher, so she has a very severe occupational disease," Min then joked, again generating laughter from the group. Everyone was listening intently, however, waiting for Min to continue.

Here, she began talking about her own shifts over the course of the year or so that she had been attending workshops at New Life. Before, she said, she would either try to tolerate her mother's control, get extremely angry, or try to "escape" (逃避 *taobi*) from the feelings of resentment that accumulated as a result of the ways her mother constantly "managed" her. Min noted, however, that after diligently attending *jipai* workshops, in particular, she had become capable of facing her own feelings. This was a deeply personal process, she noted, but as a result, she also took care to explain, she had gradually begun to learn how to express herself "in a proper way" with her mother. She had learned, for example, to say "no" kindly and in a way that her mother seemed able to accept. In sharing this relational shift with us, she drew upon a chronotopic contrast between the past and the present, highlighting how, prior to her engagement at New Life, her mother would systematically refuse to accept anything other than what she wanted to hear. As she had grown, however, her mother had, seemingly miraculously, *changed*. Her mother had even begun to encourage Min, in her words, "to do whatever I need to do without complaining that it is wrong or should be done her way." Perhaps even more surprisingly, her mother had recently begun to express interest in doing *her* own things, without Min.

"From the bottom of my heart, I can say that we are now equals," Min concluded, "and it feels much more peaceful."

By now, the group was enthralled. Mostly silent with jaws hanging slackly, there were a few women who, in response to Min's conclusion, began probing her for further details. Asking how she had done it, how it had transpired, how long it had taken, and more, they remarked several times upon how miraculous it was that it had happened without Min's mother having attended New Life herself. Min did not, however, offer the kinds of specific guidelines and recommendations that they seemed to crave. Instead, she repeatedly stated that we all just needed to learn to "speak out."

"We all have so many words in our hearts that we don't share, feelings we don't express. This actually hurts us, and it hurts others," she said, noting further that she felt confident about the ability of most people, including those in older generations, to "handle it all" more adeptly than one might expect.

"But when we just suppress it all," she concluded, "everybody suffers."

THE PERMEABILITY OF PATRIARCHY

The interaction described above underscores the ways in which the intimate psysociality at New Life often afforded multiple opportunities, outside of formal workshop exercises, for participants to discuss their desires and dreams as well as their concerns. Such interactions were notably often inclusive, allowing for the fluid incorporation of participants positioned variably as "ratified overhearers" rather than central interlocutors (Goffman 1981). The short interaction further demonstrates—alongside many of the examples I have shared in previous chapters—how "relationship talk" constituted the bulk of both formal and informal interactions at the center. As in other sites where the "inner revolution" is enacted in China, psychospiritual self-development at New Life was thus often intensely focused on a situated process of learning to love that involved the practical transformation of particular interpersonal relationships (L. Zhang 2020, 177). In this case, alongside numerous other examples presented in earlier chapters, it further reflects the *urgency* of conversations that focused on mother-daughter relationships in this setting.

Pointing to the ways in which generational hierarchies constitute a critical component of patriarchy in China (Santos and Harrell 2017), the interaction here reflected the intense desire that many participants had to shift patriarchal relational modes and to move toward the kind of "intergenerational intimacy" described by Yan (2016). The interaction suggests, finally, how the so-called transformation of patriarchy in China (Santos and Harrell 2017), as it emerged at New Life, often constituted a situated "care practice" in which "different 'goods,' reflecting not only different values but also involving different ways of ordering reality, have to be dealt with together" (Mol, Moser, and Pols 2010, 13). Involving a near-constant process of ethical-relational reflection and experimentation that gradually affects particular relationships, such conversations underscored how "transformation" emerged as distinctly less dramatic than what one might associate with the notion of "smashing" or "dismantling" the patriarchy. Throughout this chapter, I thus draw upon the notion of "tinkering" to engage with the gradual, situated process of attempting (and sometimes succeeding) to shift long-standing patriarchal relational patterns, within both generational and gendered relationships, at New Life.

"Tinkering," explain Annemarie Mol and colleagues, constitutes a kind of "attentive experimentation" that is both pragmatic and particular (2010, 13). The authors thus offer a novel definition for the concept of "good care," situating it as "persistent tinkering in a world full of complex ambivalence and shifting tensions" (2010, 14). Tinkering at New Life, as I discuss it throughout this chapter, was similar in terms of its persistence and relation to the kinds of "shifting tensions" mentioned by Mol and her coauthors. Here, however, I further attend to the ways in which tinkering occurred in multiple yet often-overlapping ways both within and beyond the center. First, to the extent that it involved concentrated periods of "disentangling" within which participants were situated within the unusual and distinct socio-emotional space of the center (L. Zhang 2020), tinkering at New Life involved the kinds of scalar inquiry and the subsequent development of various provisional rechronotopizations that tentatively rescaled normative cultural ideas, behaviors, and practices or "codes" in relation to particular participants' personal relational challenges (see Karimzad 2020; Karimzad and Catedral 2018, 2021). Always occurring within conversations that involved a varying number of long-term clients and newcomers, moreover, what might be called "tinkering with Chineseness" or *cultural tinkering* in this case emerged as a form of "co-operative action" (C. Goodwin 2018) that included the body-selves, narrations, and sometimes even actual parents or partners. Tinkering, from this perspective, constituted a collaborative project involving the interrogation and reevaluation of shared moral-relational chronotopes and the tentative or scalar repositioning of oneself in relation to them.

As part of what Daniel Roberts identifies as the ever-present ethical conversations, in China, addressing "the gap between how things should be and how they really are" (2013, 15), cultural tinkering here constituted a form of scalar inquiry or what I have discussed as "entangling differently." It also, however, underscores the ways in which subtle adjustments in the kinds of scalar intimacies that prevail within bodies who have been socialized into patriarchal ideologies reflect not only personal changes but also more broadly yet often minute shifts in "culture" that blur the boundaries between so-called "high" and "low" forms of justice (Lee 2023). Though small and not necessarily carrying any capacity to transform collective practice at a broad scale, such shifts emphasize the ways in which, as Leticia Sabsay notes in the epigraph to this chapter, mutuality and permeability in interaction underscore how, in her words, "the world around us ... is permeable as well" (2016, 286; see also Pritzker and Perrino 2020).

After fluidly inserting herself into the ongoing conversation with a brief comment about how it had not been the case that she needed to bring her mother to New Life in order to shift their relationship, for example, Min switched to an inclusive "we" framing that emphasized shared cultural experience. Situating herself and those who were co-present within the shared chronotope of "traditional Chinese culture," she thus issued a comment highlighting the meaning of "obedience." Specifically, Min defined obedience as it related to a combination of parental control and the suppression of "our own thoughts and feelings." Maintaining this generalization, she further invoked the ways in which affect and embodiment inhered in the presumably shared experience of parental control, which she noted was often "invisible" ("they control us invisibly!"). Min then offered a chronotopic depiction of her mother that she seemed confident would be familiar to her interlocutors, describing her mother as a certain kind of moral person-type: a teacher. The indexicality that such a characterization has, within what I have discussed as the "trifecta" of education, family, and governance in China (Lin 2017; see also chapter 4), afforded laughter in response to the remark she then made regarding how her mother, as a teacher, suffered from a severe "occupational disease."

Zooming in to offer a more personal perspective on her experience with her mother, Min's narrative then invoked what I discuss here as the second interrelated component of "tinkering with the patriarchy" at New

Life, within which participants applied insights gleaned at New Life within particular relationships with parents, spouses, and children, as well as with colleagues and friends. Here, Min proceeded to construct a series of chronotopic contrasts between the past and the present. In a personalized framing of the ways in which parental "education" in China is formulated as a form of governance or moral guidance issued over the life course within the hierarchically structured family (Kipnis 2011; Santos and Harrell 2017), Min here depicted the ways in which her mother had always demanded compliance, even when Min was grown and had a child of her own. Framing this dynamic as having existed in the *past*, however, Min went on here to illustrate the ways in which she had changed over the course of the year. Whereas her reactions to her mother's "management" had previously always evoked some combination of tolerance, anger, resentment, and the desire to "escape," she detailed how her gradual development of the capacity to face her own feelings had resulted in a relational capacity to express herself "properly" with her mother. Min proceeded to depict the intimacy that had emerged, seemingly organically and even miraculously given the fact that her mother had never herself attended New Life events, between her and her mother. Drawing upon a moral-relational frame in which various forms of equality, respect, and freedom rooted in honest dialogue prevailed across time as well as space, Min thus cast their relationship as existing, in the present, within the contrastive chronotope of "equality." In this sense, Min offered a relatively concise narrative of "transformation" or "metamorphosis" (Bakhtin 1981) within which she, as well as her mother and her relationship with her mother, had become radically different as a result of Min's engagement at the center.

As demonstrated by the rapt attention of Min's listeners, as well as the way they rapidly fired questions at her upon the completion of her brief narrative, Min's metamorphosis story also invoked what I discussed in chapter 2 as the "horizon chronotope." Upon hearing about the positive changes in Min's relationship with her mother, in other words, a new horizon of possibilities suddenly came into view for other attendees. Speaking to the possibility that her story reflected the recasting of shared relational chronotopes, Min responded to their questions by switching back to a generalized "we" voice. Referring to her previous characterization of the Chinese family, Min thus noted how the accumulation of unshared feelings, thoughts, and "words," in her framing, caused both personal and *relational* harm. Her conclusion, in which she offered an optimistic outlook on the potential for (even) older Chinese parents to "handle it," notably tied her entire narrative back to the skepticism that several of the women in the group continued to express.

Although Min arguably offered a fairly "tidy" and most likely simplified transformation story here, the overall interaction, I suggest, underscores the ways in which the so-called transformation of patriarchy in China took place, at New Life at least, as a continuous dialogic process of interrogating, experimenting, and "tinkering," often simultaneously, with cultural concepts as well as particular relationships. Such conversations only rarely, however, involved the kind of complete and total metamorphosis that Min depicted here.

Much like the ways in which experiences of embodied defrosting generated an ongoing process of inquiry and uncovering rather than simply transformation, the project and process of tinkering with the patriarchy often involved a near-constant back-and-forth between minute shifts and new challenges that emerged as a result of such shifts. Another brief example that, aptly demonstrates this overlap unfolded during a break at Teacher Jo's 2016 inner child retreat, when I was seated with a group of six participants. We had collectively decided to conduct an impromptu group interview and had been chatting amicably for fifteen minutes about what had brought people to the workshop. The conversation quickly turned into a focused discussion, however, when Chen, a fifty-year-old woman dressed in the draping attire of the time, told us about a difficult phone call she had had with her daughter just the night before. Her eighteen-year-old daughter, Chen told us, had called to disclose that she was a lesbian and was going to turn down the full scholarship she had received to a European university because she was going to stay in China to live with her thirty-year-old girlfriend.

"She was calm when she called and told me," Chen told us. "And I pretended to be calm, but I was very sad. I said that if you feel happy, it's fine, but I am very sad."

Chen then admitted to us that she felt both overwhelmed and angry. She was having trouble discerning if her usual stance of openness and acceptance toward homosexuality was, when it came to her daughter, not indeed open at all. She could not tell, however, because of her simultaneous anger regarding her daughter's choice to drop out of college, as well as the age difference between her daughter and her girlfriend. We all settled in to listen to Chen, who quickly began shedding tears. As this was the first and only time I heard any discussion of nonheterosexual relationality at New Life, I made a note of my own feelings of defensiveness and readiness to jump in should any of the participants respond with condemnation based on Chen's daughter's sexuality. Beyond what I discerned as a little bit of surprise from one of the younger members of our group, however, there was none. There was no clean resolution, however, perhaps not surprisingly given the immediacy of Chen's suffering as well as the fact that we were on a short break. Several members of our group did offer their perspectives, however. The only male among us, a thirty-five-year-old K-12 teacher, for example, inquired about the historic dynamic between Chen and her daughter, posing the possibility that her choices—particularly the choice to drop out of school—might have been made purposefully to raise Chen's hackles. A woman the same age as the teacher cut in, here, focusing instead on the details of the phone call. She asked specifically what Chen had said in response to her daughter's announcement. When Chen told us that she was "honest" about her anger with her daughter, the woman replied with direct advice:

"Older Sister," she said "I think when you express your own thoughts, you have to do it selectively. You must first pay attention to your daughter."

Chen nodded. Before we knew it, however, Teacher Jo came back into the room. Chen then flagged him down and they proceeded to move into a corner to chat privately. I did not get the chance, unfortunately, to follow up with Chen, though I tried to find her before the end of the workshop to give her my contact information. What I want to emphasize here, however, is not the "outcome," but rather the ways in which the conversation reflected the ways in which "relationship talk"—here between mother and daughter—constituted an emergent opportunity for participants to engage in collaborative theorizing that simultaneously addressed and even tinkered with complex cultural notions such as parent-child relationality (and, in this case, same-sex relationships) as well as particular relationships (e.g., Chen and her daughter). As in the previous chapter, however, I adopt a "long view" perspective in this chapter, focusing on the experiences of two women, Gracie and Ning. Before doing so, however, I begin with a short section specifically addressing the ways in which tinkering with the patriarchy was also considered "men's work" at New Life. I then introduce Gracie, New Life's administrator during my first year of fieldwork, and Ning, who I met only once during a 2014 evening salon. The section devoted to Gracie, whose narrative was recorded in a long, semiprivate interview, examines the complex ways in which "tinkering with the patriarchy" often constituted a spatiotemporally dynamic set of relational experiences within which "generation" and "gender" cannot be fully separated. Indeed, as Gonçalo Santos and Stevan Harrell write, gender in China "is so entangled with the generational axis that we cannot understand it thoroughly without taking into account the whole shifting patriarchal matrix in which it is embedded" (2017, 26). Ning's section, which is based on detailed fieldnotes collected during several group interactions that occurred over the course of a two-hour salon, demonstrates the ways in which ongoing experiences of "transformation" often presented simultaneously generational and gendered challenges. Throughout both sections, however, I emphasize the interrelated ways in which learning to love, as a simultaneously relational and cultural tinkering, emerged such that it was not only particular relationships and relational practices that became permeable, but indeed, in some small way—following Sabsay—the world did as well.

MEN'S WORK

Discussions of the ways in which the gender binary itself constituted an oppressive ideological structure that excluded all but those willing to embrace a cis-gendered life as a woman or man, in my experience, were entirely absent at New Life. The unsettling of gendered patriarchal ideologies within particular relationships—the notion, for example, that "men are superior to women" (男尊女卑 *nanzun nübei*) or its attendant socio-spatial mapping within which "men are in charge of outside, women are in charge of inside" (男主外, 女主内 *nan zhu wai, nü zhu nei*)—was, however, a frequent topic of both spontaneous interactions as well as specific exercises. Here, as the following section details, both women and men often engaged in an examination of the ways in which traditional gendered expectations for both men and women variably inhibited the expression of authentic emotion, further contributing to the kinds of "suppression" and "accumulation" that Min described.

Although most participants took care to acknowledge the ways in which patriarchy had harmed women far more than it harmed men, the unsettling of gendered patriarchy at New Life, though ultimately requiring effort from both men and women, was also often approached specifically as "men's work." The ways in which patriarchy constituted a unique and challenging form of "bondage" (*shufu* 束缚) for *men*, however—to borrow the term used by Gracie, whose story I detail below—was thus a frequent topic of both formal and informal interaction at the center.

Recall, for example, Chao's description of his first encounter with his inner child, detailed in chapter 3. After telling me how moving such an encounter had been, then, Chao had engaged in a scaling project that linked his own embodied experience to men in China more generally. Here, Chao noted how his own embodied experience of seeing the "dazed" look on his inner child's face—a look that he had interpreted as conveying his young boy-self's desperate desire for intimacy—informed the ways in which he had trained himself to attend constantly to participants' (especially *male* participants') subtle embodied expressions. Chao offered a rich depiction, here, of the ways in which the Chinese gender discourse that Magdalena Wong (2020) calls the "able-responsible man" causes a *hardening* of a man's body.

"Men in China have more armor (盔甲 *kuijia*), more defensiveness (防卫 *fangwei*) in their bodies," he said. "Because if you are a man, you have to support your family, you have to make ends meet. When a boy becomes a man, when there are so many burdens pressed upon him, he learns to cover his body with armor, how to have strength, how to support oneself. 'I don't cry, I'm not allowed to feel tired'—Chinese men are often like this. The walls of his heart and his spirit become thick (厚 *hou*) as the callouses on his hands become thick."

Constituting a "hegemonic ideal" in China, as the name suggests, the notion of the "able-responsible man" points to the expectation that men in contemporary China are expected to be strong, capable providers for their wives, children, and parents (2020, 130). Able-responsible men are thus expected to only very rarely (if ever) become overcome with emotion or weakness. Reflecting shifting ideals with regard to masculine "toughness," which is increasingly devalued in favor of a more "caring," "sensitive," and "soft" masculinity (E. Zhang 2015, 21), the ideal of the able-responsible man further represents a shift away from "a masculine model dominated by money" toward one emphasizing "ethics and responsibility" in ways that actually benefit women (Wong 2020, 137). Indeed, women often "fertilize" the notion of the able-responsible man, writes Wong, "through direct compliments (to those who are able-responsible), complaints (to those who are not), and by making comparisons between men" (2020, 69). The resulting tension leads men, according to the group of life coaches introduced in chapter 4, to be especially "*mensao*" (闷骚). A colloquial expression describing someone who appears meek or even shy but who is actually deeply passionate, *mensao* might be translated into something like "still waters run deep." As one of the younger coaches argued, however, the ways in which *mensao*-ness is often associated with repression and fear makes it uniquely Chinese. The group thus agreed with Lao Fei (quoted in detail in chapter 4) that, although *all* Chinese people struggled with expressing emotion, it was men who were particularly challenged. Chao thus offered a rich portrayal of the ways in which men's bodies are seen (and, in his case, experienced) as "bound" by patriarchal ideals that, as Everett Zhang notes, further give rise to "a crisis of masculinity" in which it is often unclear how to balance strength and sensitivity (2015, 21).

As a teacher-in-training, Chao thus explained, his recognition of his own inner child's sensitivity had been extremely valuable. It had taught him specifically how to attend differently to the men in class. "Watch his body movements," he said. "Maybe his face is numb—no feeling. But you might find that his hand is slightly clenched—his anger, his emotions, they manifest in many parts of the body."

Men's sensitivity is *there*, Chao insisted, just like it existed within himself. It often required a sensitive facilitator who had experientially developed what he called a kind of "antenna," however, to be recognized. Suggesting his understanding of the ways the "able-responsible man" (Wong 2020) is entrenched in men's bodies, Chao seemed to suggest here that he had come to see this ideal as a handicap within the space of New Life, at least in comparison to women, who he described as more "sensitive" (敏感 *mingan*) than men. Notably, Chao went on to suggest that women were also more flexible in accepting the "mysterious" ideas and relational configurations often conveyed at New Life.

"With this stuff—you can call it New Age or body-mind-spirit or whatever—there are some fundamental conflicts with ideologies (意识形态 *yishi xingtai*) in China," he noted. "Because China teaches belief in terms of Marxism—everything exists without anything spiritual. Everything is just material. But these things here, they teach that you have a consciousness, and your consciousness has a higher purpose/pursuit (追求 *zhuiqiu*). It teaches that the realm of the spiritual actually exists."

Indicating that he considered political socialization in China to impact men more so than women, or that it somehow made it more difficult for them to move beyond the ideologies of Marxist materialism, Chao actually interjected his own narrative here to object: "Well, this is for both men and women," he said.

Chao's shift, mid-speech, to redirect the argument he had been starting to make demonstrates what I have discussed as the constant cultural *theory-building* that I witnessed occurring at New Life (Rosa 2019; see chapter 4). His theory regarding the ways in which the ideas at New Life challenge deeply rooted cultural and ideological orientations, however, speaks to what Lina called the "mysterious atmosphere" at the center. Underscoring the ways in which New Life exercises often pushed participants well beyond their conventional ways of thinking, relating, and being-in-the-world, it also contextualized the ways in which the very idea of the extended *dawo* was often difficult to embody. Alongside his observations of the embodied, relational, and affective effects of masculinity, in other words, his reference to the ways in which political ideology became entrenched within the body-selves of participants speaks to the ways in which the extension of the body-self in various configurations at New Life took shape as an embodied experience that indexed shared histories. Events, practices, and policies of the past and present were often mapped as occurring both outside and inside of the body.

Men were thus frequently approached as having significantly more "work" to do than women when it came to developing self-awareness, becoming mature, and learning to love. Indeed, when they came to the center, they were often warmly welcomed, and sometimes explicitly praised, by instructors and other participants for having the "courage" to attend. One evening at an inner child salon during my first summer of fieldwork for this research, for example, for example, a man—one of only a few that evening—introduced himself during the opening circle.

"I'm this lady's husband," he said, pointing to the woman beside him, smiling and prompting the hearty laughter of other participants, who, aside from Teacher Du, were mostly cis-presenting women. Going on to describe how she had urged him to come, the man listed the numerous retreats and workshops he had attended. He'd begun to "return" (回来 *huilai*) as a result, he noted, concluding with a simple comment regarding the fact that he still had much more to learn and was glad to be there that evening.

"We especially welcome men," responded Teacher Du with a great deal of enthusiasm. He then noted that there were only a few men in the room that evening. "But" he noted, "if we keep attending these kinds of events, and if we can support one another, encourage one another, see one another's process, it's a great help. So you are very welcome here."

This brief exchange stood out immediately to me, not least because of the way the man introduced himself as "the husband" to a female attendee but also because of the way he went on to situate her as his "leader" in guiding him to the center. His introduction thus seemingly inverted—or at least engaged playfully with—normative gender hierarchies in a format that, indeed, afforded laughter. Here, however, it is relevant to revisit the common chronotopic mapping of New life vis-à-vis the chronotopes of "home," described in detail in chapter 2. Though technically a public space, the formulation of the center as "home" thus situated it as a distinctly feminine space within which participants engaged with affect, embodiment, and other domains traditionally associated with women. Indeed, writes Li Zhang, many men in China "see talk therapy as a feminine sphere that can potentially undermine their manhood" (2020, 70). This gendered chronotopization of the space—despite the fact that many of the head teachers and interns (at least during my time at the center) were, in fact, men—undermines the notion that this participant's apparent deference to his wife constituted a true "inversion" of gender norms. From this perspective, his self-positioning here might be seen as perpetuating gender inequality by recognizing and endorsing the gendered division of labor as well as space. As governor of the "inside," women's role in contemporary China is not only (and not always) associated with the mandate to remain physically in the home, but rather extends to the labor of nurturing and caring for the emotions of others, especially their husbands.

From this vantage point, one might further note that Teacher Du's response, in which he enacted a kind of male exceptionalism by noting that "men are especially welcome," served to entrench these normative gender hierarchies. The participant's acknowledgment of the (relative) importance of developing self-awareness and, in his words, "learning to face emotions" nevertheless *did* situate him as an outlier. His mere presence, indeed, implied a contrast between *this* man and the other men in the world who had refused or who would refuse if asked (by anyone) to come to the center. In this sense, the enthusiastic response that he received from Teacher Du reflected the ways in which participants, generally speaking, deeply valued the willingness of men to participate.

The paradoxical, both/and nature of this brief example, I suggest, underscores how "tinkering with the patriarchy" at New Life often involved a simultaneous unsettling and reentrenchment of dominant (cis)gender ideologies. While the notion of "men's work," for example, tended to overvalue men in relation to women within the space, it also acknowledged and interrogated the very real suffering of both men and women under the regime of male dominance.

"THAT HOME IN YOUR INNER HEART"

In 2014, my days at New Life were long and included many hours of downtime between events and sessions. I thus often spent time "hanging out" with Gracie, a woman with whom I had formed an immediate bond of recognition. She would often bring her young son to work, and we would sit and watch him toddling around the space carefully picking things up, examining them, and moving on, or simply running around in circles. As we watched him, Gracie and I often discussed the numerous joys and (possibly more numerous) struggles involved with being working mothers with young children. Often in connection with such conversations, we also discussed spirituality, culture, relationships, and how to relate ethically to capitalism while also cultivating a sense of beauty and style.

About a month into my fieldwork that summer, when Gracie and I had not yet set a time to conduct a formal interview, I was on the balcony formally interviewing several of the male students of Dr. Yu, New Life's resident Chinese medical physician at the time. Gracie joined us, comfortably inserting herself into the ongoing conversation. As she responded to my queries, building upon many of our previous conversations, she began talking about how she had always been a kind of "lone wolf," a tough girl who had never dreamed that she would ever marry, let alone become a mother. She had decided when she was young that, despite being Chinese, she neither needed nor had the capacity for the "drama" of family. She had too many "bad emotions" (情绪不好 *qingxu buhao*), she admitted candidly, and she also had a terrible temper.

"When I would get angry, I would just explode and leave," she said.

"Beautiful women are all like that," one of the men said quickly in response, invoking a common moral chronotope that situated "beautiful women" as especially unruly. The other men smirked. Gracie immediately protested, however.

"No, actually it goes back a long time, to my childhood," she said in a dry tone mediated by a feeling of honest, heartfelt refusal.

In response, the man who had spoken attempted to make another joke, but it fell flat. Meanwhile, Gracie and I moved on, beginning an intense conversation that lasted several hours. Very quickly after the previous interaction, the men I had been interviewing slowly began to drift away, one by one standing up and all but tiptoeing off the balcony. Gracie and I barely noticed their departure, however. She had begun telling me how she had come to understand the ways in which her "bad temper," as well as her overall attitude toward family, had been shaped by her early experience as a child.

When Gracie was growing up, for example, her father had worked long hours as a truck driver, for example, and had often been gone for days at a time. When he did come home, he was often violent. Whenever she cried or made any other sounds at night, she recalled, he would beat her, scold her, and "toss" her out into the courtyard alone.

"It was so dark . . . and I was so terrified," she remembered, shuddering. To this day, she swore, she slept as if she was wearing a straitjacket, never daring to move or utter a peep lest she disrupted others.

Her mother, she then noted, worked alternating day and night shifts in a local factory. Like her father, she had rarely been "around," even when she was home. Before Gracie had been born, she explained, their town had experienced a huge earthquake that had caused their family home and the homes around them to collapse. Her mother, who had been home at the time, was crushed by the falling structure. She was eventually rescued, but the rest of her family had all died in the quake, including both of Gracie's grandfathers, her grandmother, her mother's sister and brother, and their three children.

"After that, although she remained alive and with me for many years, her heart was focused on the dead. So she had very little of that so-called 'mother energy' left to give me," Gracie shared. It was only once she had started working at New Life and attending the workshops that she had "seen" this, however. She went on to describe her insight that, because of the violence enacted by her father and the abandonment by her mother, she had never had the opportunity to develop a stable sense of *home*. She then stopped to clarify what she meant by "home."

"I mean that home in your subconscious (潜意识 *qian yishi*), that home in your inner heart (内心那个家 *neixin nage jia*)," she said, invoking the home chronotope but situating it *within* the body. Pointing simultaneously to the cultural chronotope of home in terms of kinship, intimacy, and closeness, Gracie's comment here also invoked the notion of "being-at-home-in-the-world" as a sense of connection and *agency* (Jackson 1995). Underscoring how cultural concepts like "home" are often interrogated at New Life in relation to embodied experience, Gracie reiterated the previous absence of any sense of home in her heart. "It completely didn't exist for me," she said matter-of-factly.

Gracie went on to describe here how her previously normative way of being-in-the-world—framed here as her previous attitude or condition/mode or *zhuangtai* (状态)—had been centered around the presumption that both people and relationships were inherently unstable as well as unsafe.

"With these family conditions, when you grow up, you feel that this family thing—if you don't have one, whatever. You can be free and easy in life (随时随地 *suishi suidi*)—if you aren't happy, you can just leave, right?"

Generalizing her experience here by using the pronoun "you" to situate her response as natural, Gracie went on to detail how much she had enjoyed a "free and easy" lifestyle throughout her twenties. She had experienced many relationships with different men, for example, moving quickly to the next once something displeased or challenged her. She assumed this would be the case when she had first met the man who later became her husband. They had made an organically good match, however, and somehow—she did not fully understand how—he had convinced her to marry him. Speaking to the ways in which women's personhood in China is often deeply intertwined with their marital status, she noted here that she had enjoyed the unexpected shift that being married conferred upon her socially. Throughout the first several years of their marriage, however, she had still secretly struggled with the idea of staying put in any one place for long enough to create a "nourishing home." When she became pregnant, the anxiety around this issue had skyrocketed. Because of her experience growing up with a father who was barely around and a mother who lacked any substantive "mother-energy," she reiterated, she had been skeptical and distrustful of her own ability to be a competent mother. Once her son had been born, moreover, she often felt like she was continually walking upon unsteady, dangerous terrain.

"Even though I had that the status of 'mother,' I didn't necessarily have the ability to be the kind of mother that could really give him love, the so-called 'competent mother'—I may have even been giving him *less* than I myself received."

Adopting a chronotopic framework that seemed to foreshadow a change or metamorphosis, Gracie spoke here in the past tense. Prior to describing "how she became other than what she was" (Bakhtin 1981; pronouns changed), however, she offered an example of a kind of "low point" that served to illustrate the depths of her so-called incompetence as a mother. When her son was little, she explained, whenever he would cry or fuss at night, Gracie had found herself feeling an uncontrollable rage.

"I would hit him and scold him," Gracie admitted shamefully, noting how she realized at that point that she was repeating behavior she had learned from her father.

About six years prior to our interview, however, she had experienced a kind of embodied defrosting that she framed as a revelation. It was during an exercise in Teacher Jo's inner child workshop. Participants were guided to imagine their parents and ancestors in an inverted pyramid behind them, their parents' hands on their shoulders, their grandparents' hands on their parents' shoulders, and so on.

"When I did that exercise, the feeling was very deep," Gracie recalled. "Although on one level, my mind maybe doesn't acknowledge it—I mean in my head I may know that I have grandparents, but maybe on an emotional level—because I haven't *seen* them, so I feel in my heart that I just don't have that position (位置 weizhi). But doing that exercise, I felt it so deeply, I had such great big emotions—actually the blood flowing through my veins is *their* blood."

As I mentioned briefly in chapter 3, classical Confucian ideologies of the Great Self often excluded women, who learn as girls that they "are not a part of anyone's historical past and seem to be irrelevant to anyone's future but their own and, they are told, to some known family in some unknown place" (Wolf 1994, 261–62). Boys, in contrast, are taught that they occupy a central place in "a long line of ancestors stretching into a distant past and an equally long line of descendants waiting in an unknowable future" (259). Gracie's story of abuse and neglect further contributed to the ways in which the knowledge that she had a "position" within an embodied, emotionally tethered lineage that stretched into the recesses of Chinese history struck Gracie as a shock. The "revelation" that she, too, was part of such a lineage—that the lineage, indeed, flowed through her *blood* and thus constituted a significant piece of her embodied being—underscores the ways in which encounters at New Life sometimes functioned, often without much explicit dialogue, as an affordance for intimate, embodied, and deeply expansive (re) orientations of participants' body-selves in space and time.

Chronotopes of "home" and "horizons," I further noted in chapter 2, often served as mutually generative orienting devices that opened up space for participants to consider alternative possible futures. Indeed, Gracie's newfound sense of connection to the past had inspired her to work more diligently on herself as an agent of a personal transformation but also as an agent of contributing to a more broadly social Chinese future. Her inner work at the center, which she had previously considered primarily as part of her work duties, thus began to take on more meaning. She shared, here, how she had finally had the courage to admit to Teacher Jo that she would sometimes find herself lashing out violently at her son. Expecting him to criticize her for reproducing the past or to offer explicit direction in terms of stopping her behavior, she had been struck by the way he had responded. Telling her that her participation in the courses was itself an intervention that would ultimately serve her son by cultivating awareness in his mother, he noted that her new forms of awareness would undoubtedly help her recognize more quickly when she was speaking or behaving in ways that did not align with her intention to create a loving environment for her son.

"After this class, he told me, 'You won't be perfect—it's impossible. But there will be this awareness,'" Gracie said, voicing Teacher Jo's words as if she had recorded them in her memory. She admitted that she had been confused by his response at first. Presenting Teacher Jo's remarks as an *ongoing* intervention, however, she described how his words would, indeed, "come to her" whenever she observed herself beginning to cross a line with her son. Situating the cultivation of awareness as an effort, on her part, to become more responsive and present, she spoke proudly here of the ways in which she had become able to recognize when she had acted or was about to act out inappropriately with her son. She had even, at times, been able to intervene in such moments in order to more quickly rectify her behavior and attitude.

As described in chapter 4, mother's "emotion-work" in China is often situated vis-à-vis a national dialogue that requires them to refine themselves in order to produce "quality" children. Pressures to do so, indeed, permeate the public landscape in media, government issued statements, and other propaganda (Fincher 2021). Again, however, it is important to recall the perspective offered by Teresa Kuan (2015), in which the same kind of emotion-work enacted by mothers might be reconsidered in terms of the related notions of *moral agency* and *ethical subjectivity* (see chapter 4). Specifically, Kuan details the felt experience of one mother's "self-blame" for expressing excessive anger toward her child not as an internalization of social expectations, but as a form of *ethical subjectivity* that emerged as "a perception of an incongruity between emotion and situation" (2015, 103). Though undoubtedly also entangled with national discourses of motherhood, Gracie's efforts to learn how to better "control" her emotions, like the mother in Kuan's ethnography, might thus be considered a form of "tinkering" that emerged in response to her recognition that her behavior was not only "inappropriate" by contemporary social standards but also disproportionate to the situation. Gracie's tinkering here, applied both to herself and within her relationship with her son, further underscores how previous intergenerational suffering often inspired a sense of desperation among many New Life participants, who were urgently trying to figure out how to create a future in which the past no longer *bound* them or their children to ideologies and practices they considered excessive or violent. Indeed, Gracie here went on to carefully distinguish the ways in which her own orientation to parenting diverged from the violence enacted in the name of love in previous generations.

"Our parents, that generation—or even our ancestors," she said, "they thought that this is love. Maybe now we can see that those perspectives are mistaken. But during that time, in terms of that information that they had received, they thought that was love. They thought if I beat you and curse you, it was good for you. But they—at that time, they didn't have any of this knowledge to nourish them. So it is also—we feel—we are sometimes—living in this time, we might think our air isn't as good as in the past, that our food isn't as safe as in the past, but on a heart-spirit level, actually compared to those people in the past, I've received much more nourishment. It's like my inner heart has become, little by little, more powerful."

As Perrino and I have discussed, Gracie's remarks here notably shifted between multiple proximal and distal deictics that positioned the present space-time as well as its occupants (e.g., "this," "here," "now," and "we") in contrast to the space, time, and peoples of the past (e.g., "that," "there," "then," and "they"). In doing so, we argued, Gracie continually worked to instantiate the distinction or critical *distance* between herself and her parents and "even" (her words) her ancestors. At the same time, however, we also noted that "her continuous comparison of herself to 'people of the past' intimately [bound] her to them in an imagined trajectory of spiritual development" (2020, 378). Underscoring how this progressive framing seemed to reproduce discourses of "development" in China, we further called attention to the ways in which it served to reinstantiate Gracie's position within a long lineage stretching back in time. Her careful construction of chronotopic contrasts, in other words, simultaneously afforded distancing while also preserving her newfound connection to her ancestors and allowed her to formulate her present efforts to transform her behaviors with her son as an anticipatory mode of *hope* as well as *nourishment*.

Beginning by invoking "our parents, that generation," at the outset of this segment, Gracie thus expanded her scope to include "even our ancestors," all of whom were then rhetorically positioned as distant with regard to what they "thought" was love. Again, distinguishing present from past by posing the possibility that "maybe now we can see" such mistakes, Gracie notably took care to attribute these mistaken ideas about love as being situated in the *knowledge* that was available to them at the time. Notably, Gracie did not, at any point, call either their love or their good intentions into question. Rather, she strategically situated their mistaken ideas (e.g., that violence was "good for you") in relation to their lack of knowledge. Formulating knowledge as "nourishment" here, she then shifted back into the present, adopting a "we" voice to chronotopically map the feelings and thoughts of those living in present society. Here, she self-corrected several times ("we feel—we are sometimes—") before proceeding with a depiction of the ways in which "we might think that our air/food isn't as good/safe as in the past." As Perrino and I noted, Gracie's parallelism—as a discursive strategy that often functions to make discourse "memorable, repeatable, [and] decontextualizable" (Wilce 2001, 191)—served to rhetorically "lock" her distinction of the difference between the past and present into place. Underscoring the ways in which such feelings invoked nostalgia in many people, Gracie's conjunctive "but" further instantiated her distinction. Without necessarily dismissing the validity of peoples' concerns regarding air and food—which, in 2014 China, were significant—her conjunction here did, however, dismiss the kinds of nostalgia people might feel for the past. Nostalgia dismissed, Gracie went on to craft an embodied and intimate chronotopic mapping of the ways in which she personally, while perhaps less physically secure in terms of air to breathe and food to eat, was nevertheless more *nourished*, at least on "a heart-spirit level," in comparison to those who lived in the past. Implicatively tying her statement back to the forms of knowledge that she had access to at the center, Gracie's conclusion foregrounds her own progressive development in which her "inner heart" had become "little by little, more powerful."

In the analysis that Perrino and I developed, we suggested that Gracie's fluid scalar movements between past and present as well as public and private here demonstrated how the dialogic enactment of scalar intimacy, though often serving to reproduce, reentrench, and reinstantiate long-standing cultural ideologies, also creates space for "slight modification[s]" (Pritzker and Perrino 2020, 382). Such shifts, even if slight, underscore how the kinds of "tinkering" that I have been discussing in this chapter were applied not just within relationships but also to cultural ideologies. In Gracie's case, for example, her numerous inquiries into her own past had moved her to engage in the kinds of intimate scalar inquiries that draw deeply personal experience together, instantaneously, with broader cultural concepts such as ancestry or lineage, marriage, motherhood, love, nourishment, and even relational gender norms.

Here, then, Gracie began to talk about how her husband had developed, in the past several years, an intense disdain for his work. He had become increasingly irritable, in fact, and was always tired. He had become, in fact, in Gracie's terms, *intolerable*, and Gracie herself was growing increasingly fed up with the situation. Just the day before, she had finally "hit a wall," so to speak. Underscoring the ways in which the gendered pressures upon men to enact the ideal of "the able-responsible man" (Wong 2020), she had realized that she was no longer interested in staying with someone who was continually sacrificing himself in order to enact what she referred to as "this ridiculous ideal of masculinity." She had thus called him, in the middle of the day, to issue a kind of ultimatum.

"I said I don't care about the work you do; I want to know about your feelings. I said that a person who does not love their own body, does not value their own feelings—even if you work harder, you just get recognition from others. People think you are worthwhile, and so you are satisfied. I said that actually these things aren't important. You come home every day and you can't even communicate with me, you just collapse. I said that if a person is living solely for responsibilities, for obligations, for his family and not himself, one day he will collapse. I said that if a person lives for love—and is better able to love him*self*—then he will be able to love his family, and the family will be better."

"In traditional Chinese culture," she continued, "a man lives for others, for obligations, for the family. But I told him I could allow him to rest for some time, so that he could be quiet and reflective."

She went on to explain her hope that the next few months would be a time when her husband could "listen to his heart" and let it guide him toward creative things that he *wanted to do* instead of things he was obligated to do. She thus expressed a clear sense of optimism that, despite her husband's initial resistance, he might eventually relent and quit his current job. If he did so, she noted, it might make him less of a pain to be around.

In offering to be the provider for her husband while he stayed home and "listened to his heart," Gracie was arguably enacting her own gender role as the "nurturer" in the relationship. Here, however, it is also critical to recognize the ways in which Gracie's offer constituted a true inversion of traditional gender roles that, not surprisingly, her husband had at least initially refused. Gracie thus expressed a great deal of pride with regard to the fact that, because she had a job that she not only loved but was lucrative enough to cover them for a while, she *could* make this offer. As I discussed above with regard to Gracie's efforts to become a better mother to her son, it is also important to note the ways in which her offer constituted a form of *moral agency*. Moral agency, Kuan writes, "is a variety of moral experience that has less to do with conforming to normative moral codes than with a kind of practical philosophy" (2015, 18). Attention to *situation* here underscores the ways in which Gracie's offer emerged directly in relation to the pragmatics of her own suffering, for example, her increasing inability to tolerate his constant fatigue and irritability in relation to his current job. As described above, she thus relayed the phone call by adopting an optimistic anticipatory mode. Here, moreover, she concluded this portion of her interview with a reflection that extended from her personal experience to a discussion of how patriarchal norms caused suffering for everyone.

"And this is why traditional Chinese men should transform the shackles that bind them—even the whole concept of 'male superiority and female inferiority.' It's stressful for everyone," she said matter-of-factly.

Gracie here engaged in the kind of theory-building and scalar inquiry that, I have suggested throughout this book, often invited participants to rescale their relationship to long-standing ideologies, practices, and structures. In her rechronotopization of Chinese patriarchy as "stressful for everyone," in other words, Gracie drew upon her own lived experience to construct a scalar argument that calls to mind the perspective of leading cultural critic Dai Jinhua, who notes her realization of the ways in which patriarchal ideologies oppress both genders, though often in different ways (2018, 161; see also Xie 2021, 131).

In this sense, her offer to her husband might be approached as a form of "tinkering with the patriarchy" that was informed by a longer-term and more broadly collective desire or hope. As detailed in the following section, however, in order to fully appreciate Gracie's offer, it is important to recognize the ways in which her fuller narrative underscores the ways in which "patriarchy" in China constitutes a complex spatiotemporal set of relational experiences within which "generation" and "gender" cannot be fully separated.

Drawing upon Leticia's Sabsay's notion of permeability, Perrino and I suggested how scalar intimacy—as a process through which people continuously *relate* to cultural notions, norms, and values as well as maintain them—underscores the role of vulnerability that inheres in the relationship between people and culturally salient ideologies and practices. "When people scale themselves as affective, embodied, cultural beings in particular interactions," we wrote, "they discursively enact what Sabsay refers to as 'the unstable (and always in the process of being negotiated) boundaries of the vulnerable 'I'" such that the world, as noted in the epigraph, "[becomes] permeable as well" (Sabsay 2016, 286, as cited in Pritzker and Perrino 2020, 381). We also took care—as I do here—not to equate such "tinkering" with the "smashing" or "unmaking" of cultural ideologies or practices at a broad scale. This gives us insight, I suggest, into Gracie's embodied political subjectivity in terms of the intimate ways in which she *related* to more broadly sociopolitical ideologies. I maintain here that her tinkering—with patriarchal notions of exclusionary lineage, for example, or with gendered norms in marriage—is nevertheless significant.

RETHINKING THE YIJING

One evening during an inner child salon led by Teacher Du in 2014, a thirty-two-year-old participant who I will call Ning introduced herself during the opening circle. Ning drew quickly upon the chronotope of metamorphosis (Bakhtin 1981) to tell us how, after attending many workshops, she had transformed in many areas of her life. Recently, in fact, she had finally discovered what she wanted to do with her life. The problem, however, was that the career she wanted to pursue would require her to leave China for at least a year for training in Europe. Pointing to the complex ways in which relational challenges at New Life were only rarely specifically focused upon either generational or gendered relationships, Ning went on to explain that this realization had led to further struggles, as she had a husband and young son that she would have to leave behind. She had pretty much already decided to leave, however, but there were still doubts in her heart regarding the ways in which her departure would be particularly harmful for her son.

"A Chinese mother needs to stay with her child," she said multiple times during her introduction. Though I do not know Ning's particular past, her repeated insistence that a *Chinese* mother, in particular, needs to stay with her child may very well have reflected the ways in which she had come to recognize the long-term effects of parent-child separation. As mentioned in the previous chapter, such separations were often discussed at New Life. Whether she personally had experienced a separation from her parents or whether she had adopted this moral perspective through witnessing others suggests how the moral-relational commitments lauded at New Life often become intimate orienting devices for participants, who—like Ning—struggle to make sense of them over time

When she finished speaking, Teacher Du did not respond. Instead, he turned to the rest of us in the circle, and, eschewing the usual participation framework of the opening circle, addressed us instead of Ning.

"We all experienced something different in hearing Ning's speech just now," he said. "It contained a great deal of information, much of which affected us directly in our hearts, in different ways."

Underscoring the ways in which, as mentioned above, "feeling-with" or "telepathy" was intentionally cultivated at New Life, he then asked us to comment on what emotions we "heard" in her narrative.

"This process can teach each of us what we feel and what is most important to us. But it can also teach her how much is going on for her, help her to get clear—so many different perspectives. . . . so what are the main emotions here?"

It was silent for a moment, but some of the other regular New Life attendees soon began to speak, calling out feeling-words, including "entanglement" (纠结 *jiujie*); "concern" (纠结 *qiangua*); "courage" (勇气 *yongqi*); "attachment" (执着 *zhizhuo*); "joy" (喜悦 *xiyue*); and "worry" (担心 *danxin*). As each answer was given, Du then repeated it. As the exercise gained momentum, several participants began calling attention to the temporal nature of Ning's dilemma. A man suggested "dissatisfaction with the present" (对现在不满 *dui xianzai bu man*), for example. A woman responded quickly here, adding "a kind of excitement about the future" (对将来的一种兴奋 *dui jianglai de yizhong xingfen*) to this kind of emotional-temporal tracking of Ning's experience.

Unlike the mirroring exercises described in chapter 3, in which we were given explicit time to reflect back to those who had offered us their felt experiences of us, we did not—at least at this point in the evening—have the opportunity to hear how Ning felt as she received our feedback. After the comments from participants began to wane, Du then shifted back into a pedagogical mode. The opportunity to hear the impressions others have of certain aspects of ourselves that we usually keep hidden, he explained, had the potential to help each of us become more aware of the nuances of our own emotional experience. Becoming aware, Du further emphasized, could help us "release" or "liberate" those feelings. This was a way of loving ourselves (爱自己 *ai ziji*), he insisted, clarifying here that the kind of self-love that he was talking about was not a selfish kind of individualizing self-love, but a self-love that would make us more capable of loving others and more available for connection *with* others.

The introductory circle continued from there. Later in the evening, however, we came back to Ning's dilemma. We were playing a "game" in which Du was "quizzing" us on our ability to differentiate emotions (情绪 *qingxu*) from judgments (判断 *panduan*), beliefs (信念 *xinnian*), thoughts (念头 *niantou*), events (事件 *shijian*), scenarios (场景 *changjing*), and standards/norms (标准 *biaozhun*). Du thus began by issuing several "I-statements," to which participants responded by calling out. At first, the statements were all clearly describing emotions (e.g., I am sad, I am annoyed). The quiz became a little more complex, however, once we got the hang of it. "I can't do it," for example, provoked debate. Du explained that it is a belief statement, but one that possibly points to underlying feelings of inferiority (自卑 *zibei*). The statement, "I'm at work and I'm going to go crazy," was similar: a *belief* about underlying *feelings* like suppressed anger. People's faces started to light up with recognition as they began to put it all together. Ning, however, raised her hand and admitted that the exercise was making her more confused about her situation. We learned a bit more, here, about the complexity of the relational aspects of her dilemma when she shared how her husband was actually adamantly opposed to the idea of her leaving for a year.

"Your husband doesn't want you to go. How do you feel about that?," Du asked her.

"I feel like I'm not a good wife; I'm not doing what a wife should do," she responded, chronotopically situating herself as a moral aberration vis-à-vis the person-type "good wife." A good wife, she seemed here to suggest, should not only obey her husband's wishes, but should herself desire to stay with him. As confirmed later in the evening, moreover, it also related to the gendered mapping of space, described above, in which a "good wife" was not supposed to leave the *home*.

Du turned to the group, "Are these statements she is making beliefs or reactions or emotions?"

Notably, Du did not, here, offer the option for participants to identify Ning's expressions as or in relation to standards or norms (标准 *biaozhun*), which he had originally suggested would be one of the classifications we could draw upon. An almost immediate consensus, however, formed around the fact that they were *beliefs*. Du concurred, turning to face Ning. Seeing that she remained confused, he called several members of the group to the center of the circle to stage a dramatic enactment of Ning's feelings, thoughts, and beliefs. As briefly described in chapter 3, four regulars hopped up and volunteered to embody Ning's fear, her excitement, and her anger. Proceeding to enter into a physical struggle, they eventually turned their backs to one another, remaining there.

Du asked Ning, here, if the scene felt accurate. She said that it did. She was still struggling, however. She was particularly concerned, she said somewhat ironically, that if she left, her child would one day have to seek out therapeutic workshops (like the one we were currently attending) in order to heal from the wounds that her departure had caused. The entire room—including Ning herself—erupted in laughter. The exercise eventually resolved, however, once Du guided the participants enacting Ning's inner landscape to "walk together." As they did so, he conveyed to Ning that the "reality" underlying all of it related somehow to her inner child. Her eyes then lit up and she said, somewhat mysteriously, that she had then suddenly "remembered." Exactly *what* she "remembered," however, remained unclear.

In a previous analysis of the exercises that evening, I reflected upon the ways in which this "resolution" seemed to elide any discussion of the ways in which Ning's dilemma was not only a personal experience but also an experience deeply informed by prevailing ideologies of gender (Pritzker 2016). Although the identification of her feelings as "beliefs" suggested that such a conversation *could* have easily emerged, for example, Du's explanation here seemed to explicitly discourage a conversation, among the group of us, about the systemic inequalities that permeated the Chinese social landscape.

Though still arguably the case, upon reviewing my fieldnotes, I discovered that I had left out a critical piece of Ning's story. It occurred during the closing circle. After several other participants had shared their experience, we came to Ning. She was quiet at first. When she spoke, however, she thanked us, explaining that she had received immense benefit from everyone's reflections throughout the evening and had "basically solved" her dilemma as a result.

"I feel like when we first began, I couldn't discern what was important or who was at fault," she said. "But before, it seemed like no matter what I attempted there was struggle—on one hand I was feeling a kind of bondage (束缚 *shufu*), while on the other I have my own thing that I have been working so hard toward for so long. Then tonight, it pushed me to understand that at least if I do it this way it isn't wrong, it isn't that I'm *bad* this way. Once this restriction was lifted, I felt like there are all these possibilities to achieve a kind of harmony in my life."

In this first segment of her closing comments, Ning began by drawing attention to the kinds of confusion and circumscribed horizons that, as described in chapter 1, often centered around a lack of ability to discern—in Ning's terms—what was important or *who* was to blame. Ning then offered a rich illustration of her embodied experience, which involved being caught between "her own thing" that she had been working toward and the "bondage" of her duties within the family.

In contrast to the genres of self-improvement that are specifically targeted at developing women's domestic sensibilities—for example, by inculcating the notion that women should be "nurturing and flexible in their marriage" (J. Yang 2018b, 137–38; see also Fincher 2021)—Gil Hizi calls attention to the ways in which young, not-yet-married women involved with self-development courses are often forced to reckon with the ways in which their inevitable future marriage places severe constraints upon their realization of the kinds of "self-mastery" and "autonomy" they are learning. He thus concludes that marriage (and motherhood) exist as "a predicament" that contradicts the kind of autonomy required for full self-actualization (Hizi 2018, 306). As noted by Leta Fincher (2021), feminists in China have increasingly chosen to remain single for precisely this reason. Framing the overall struggle as a form of "restriction" (限制 *xianzhi*) that had been "lifted" over the course of the evening, however, Ning formulated the total interaction as a kind of *alchemical* process within which she had begun to see a new horizon promising the possible "achievement" of future harmony.

Ning continued, offering an example that further underscored how this process had given her the opportunity to tinker with the ways in which she understood her relational, and *cultural*, self. Notably, she went on here to invoke the *Yijing* (易经) or *Book of Changes*, a classic Chinese philosophical text that warrants at least a brief introduction in order to better understand Ning's further comments. Originating somewhere between the tenth and eighth centuries B.C.E., the *Yijing*, as Smith (2008, 2) explains, is an "almost hopelessly complex" treatise whose meaning has been endlessly debated by prominent Confucian, Daoist, and other philosophers in thousands of interpretations over thousands of years and which has recently regained popularity as "a vehicle for the contemporary expression of a revitalized cultural pride, focused squarely on China's long and glorious past" (2008, 218). Specifically, the text is composed of sixty-four hexagrams that were (and indeed, *are*) seen as "the symbolic means by which to understand phenomena, including the forces of nature, the interaction of things, and the circumstances of change" (Smith 2008, 40–41). Within classical alchemical and divinatory practices within which "the goal was to align the body and mind with the cosmos," the hexagrams also served as "markers of time and space" (Smith 2008, 106) that worked alongside various substances and exercises to guide the often elaborate practice of internal alchemy (内丹 *neidan*). The specific meanings of the hexagrams, however, have been the subject of intense debates by hundreds of esteemed philosophers and cultural authorities. Indeed, the first two hexagrams, Qian and Kun—which are the ones that, as described below, Ning brings up—have perhaps been *the* mostly hotly contested figures in the text.

Very briefly then, Qian (the first hexagram)—with six solid lines (see fig. 7.1)—is understood to represent "Pure Yang." In contrast, Kun—with six broken lines (see fig. 7.2)—is known as "Pure Yin." These two hexagrams thus constitute the foundation for the Chinese correlative cosmology of *yin-yang* (阴阳). Like yin and yang, Qian and Kun are thereby often understood as complementary, mutually constitutive, and mutually transformative. The fundamental philosophical *equality* of Qian and Kun, in other words, arguably constitutes the core of the correlative logic they represent. When taken up by various scholars over the course of Chinese history, however, the chronotopic mapping of Qian/*yang* onto "Heaven" (天 tian) and Kun/*yin* onto "Earth" (地 di) contributed to the development of the kinds of gendered stereotypes, described above, that associate men with a superior positioning corresponding to honor, virility, creativity, strength, and activity and women with a "lower" position corresponding to humility, submissiveness, weak-

Figure 7.1. Qian, the first hexagram of the Yijing

Figure 7.2. Kun, the second hexagram of the Yijing

ness, docility, and receptivity (Smith 2008; Chen and Bo 2011). Within this socio-moral geography of gender, men (as Qian) are understood as suited for activity in the *exterior* or outside world of human affairs, while women (as Kun) are best suited for docility within the *interior* spaces of the home. Although many alternative readings of the hexagrams have emerged within the diverse and vibrant hermeneutics of Chinese classic text interpretation over thousands of years—many Daoist and so-called postpatriarchal Confucian interpretations, for example, eschew the notion that Qian is superior to Kun (Smith 2008; Nelson and Liu 2016), Ning's interpretation, however, invoked the dominant reading, which equates men with movement and exteriority and women with quietude and interiority.

"For example saying women are Kun (坤)—they all take the *Yijing* to tell me, to say women are Kun and cannot move around," Ning said, invoking the authoritative "they" who have conveyed the meanings of the hexagrams to her. "And me, I felt like maybe this is the state of my future, the goal of so-called harmony."

Going on to fluidly insert herself into the long line of authoritative interpreters of the *Yijing*, Ning continued: "But actually, before one can reach that goal, one should experiZence the hard work [of getting there]. And I'm going through that process now, and in this process I have become aware that my doing it this way isn't necessarily *bad*. At the same time, I now understand that maybe in the future, that harmony will be there, and maybe I will achieve it naturally. So that has helped me to relax and set down the worries I've had about my son. I feel like maybe he's even looking for me to be this kind of mother. Very possibly, he'll let me leave him for a short time, and that will cause him to become more mature. And I also know that my husband will take good care of himself. So it's really good."

Her struggle, Ning suggested here, had initially taken shape as a result of the ways she understood, or *scaled* herself chronotopically, in relation to national or cultural norms that required her, as a woman, to remain stationery and content within her marital home. Albeit through the lens of her personal drama, she thus explicitly presented or *topicalized* this culturally salient ideology in the space. Telling us how she had lived within a chronotope corresponding to dominant interpretations of the *Yijing*, for example, Ning highlighted the ways in which she had previously oriented to this interpretation as the "state of [her] future, the goal of so-called harmony." Invoking the state-supported chronotope of "harmony" as well as pointing to the kinds of circumscribed horizons that faced newcomers to the center,

Ning's testimony here further foregrounds the ways in which, even for long-term clients, learning to love or "becoming mature" constituted a cyclical process through which they were continually moved to question or interrogate long-held assumptions and orientations.

Ning's subsequent remarks, moreover, offer insight into how collaborative scalar inquiry and cultural theory-building sometimes emerged *implicitly* over the course of particular workshops at New Life. Beginning by stating "but actually," Ning thus went on to articulate an inversion of the dominant reading that she upgraded to the status of a truth deeper than that set forth by Yijing scholars. Whereas the authoritative reading hinged upon a gender binary attributing a fixed and enduring set of qualities and behaviors to "men" and "women," Ning's reformulation, in contrast, situated Qian and Kun in *temporal* terms. Specifically, she rescaled them as aspects of a "self" that included both genders over time. Qian, she explained, from this perspective represented the kind of "hard work" that leads, over time, to the stillness of Kun. Describing the "hard work" of Qian as the process within which she currently found herself, Ning thus notably set forth a rechronotopization of her life trajectory that pointed her, at least tentatively, toward a *different* kind of harmony in the future ("maybe in the future, that harmony will be there"). Something about the events of the evening, she suggested here, had helped her to "become aware" that neither she nor her choice to leave her husband and son in China while she went to study abroad were necessarily "bad." Underscoring the embodied shift this had evoked, she told us how this reformulation had helped her to "relax."

Highlighting Ning's embodied discovery of a new sense of agency in the world vis-à-vis traditional gender roles, her remarks further engaged a hopeful, even optimistic, anticipatory framework in which she had come to see, at least tentatively, how her departure might actually positively impact her son. Ning thus subjunctively repositioned her choice to pursue her passion as originating with the *desires* of the son, who might thereby "let" her leave and who might even "become mature" himself as a result. As a kind of afterthought, Ning closed by noting her confidence in the likelihood that her husband would "take good care of himself" without her there.

Demonstrating how unspoken yet intercorporeally enacted forms of cooperative action (C. Goodwin 2018) served as opportunities for participants not only to disentangle but also to "entangle differently" with culturally salient ideologies and practices at multiple scales, I suggest that Ning's reformulation of the *Yijing* here further constituted an example of simultaneous cultural and relational tinkering. The authority with which Ning ventured into her reformulation of the meanings of Qian and Kun, for example, suggests a kind of interpretive agency that was, in her case, bolstered by her previous embodied interactions with Teacher Du and others at the workshop that evening. Though we did not get a specific sense of "how" this had emerged for Ning at least explicitly, we might even understand it as a kind of alchemical process of co-operative action, through which scalar inquiry takes shape in interactions that are neither explicit nor referential but which nonetheless function as affordances for the kinds of shifts that Ning made during her closing comments. Perhaps this kind of "discursive alchemy," like the *Yijing* itself, worked allegorically in order to elicit or effect a *transmutation* of Ning's previous orientations to gender, harmony, and authoritative readings of the *Yijing*.

Ning's rechronotopization of the meaning of Qian and Kun in relation to the anticipated trajectory of her life as well as her expectations with regard to her son and husband's possible responses to her departure here accomplished a performative rescaling of what Judith Butler (2016, 18) refers to as "those citational chains of gender normativity." By noting her confidence that her husband would "take good care of himself" without her there to enact the role of nurturer, for example, Ning's reformulation here arguably "[made] room for new forms of gendered life" (J. Butler 2016, 18). Her overall reformulation and rechronotopization of the very notion of gender within this ancient text (as well as the notion of "harmony") might further be engaged, given her ultimate embrace of the decision to leave, as enacting a kind of feminist resistance centered around the (re)valuing of "individualistic emancipation" (Fincher 2021, 162). Ning's *temporal* reframing of the Qian-Kun dyad, however, in which her departure and self-actualization served as a basis for her *future* ability to (hopefully) "remain settled" *with* her husband and son arguably suggests that she was attempting to formulate a kind of middle ground somewhere between total resistance and total conformity. One might then suggest that Ning's experience that night did not necessarily move her to "transform" or "smash" patriarchal ideologies in China, but rather afforded her the ability to "tinker" with them such that new horizons began to appear.

Whether or not Ning was able to successfully convince her husband (or son) that her reinterpretation of the *Yijing* was acceptable, remains an open question. I did not, unfortunately, have the opportunity to follow up with Ning beyond this brief encounter. One might predict, however, that Ning's bright outlook on the positive ways in which she might maintain her connection to her family while pursuing her new career led to a new series of challenges within her family. As Xie (2021) notes, for example, under the current Chinese regime, even for women who recognize and even embrace a feminist-leaning approach, "resistance to the norms is deemed to be a costly and painful process" that makes it "'easier' for women to conform to a family-centered lifestyle than to embark on a lone struggle in a male-dominated public sphere" (217). Though readers might align with me in hoping that she prevailed, Ning's ultimate success (or not) with regard to her reformulation of gendered personhood does not necessarily negate the ways in which she experienced her participation that evening as a form of empowerment that afforded her a new sense of agency to tinker, simultaneously, with both generational and gendered patriarchy.

CONCLUDING REFLECTIONS

Throughout this chapter, I have focused on the ways in which New Life participants variably "tinkered" with the relationships and concepts of generational and gendered patriarchy in China. Occurring within both formal and informal interactions as well as in particular relationships over time, such tinkering, I suggested, involved a near-constant form of simultaneously personal and cultural interrogation. Scalar inquirty here included collaborative, multimodal investigations within the discursive, intimate, and affective-embodied practices at the center. Such inquires, I suggested—alongside specific or diffuse experiences of embodied defrosting—inspired at least *some* participants to "transform" or shift the ways in which they experienced, understood, and enacted their relationship to and within normative cultural ideologies and practices, while merely inspiring the curiosity and desire of others. The "tinkering" that I have discussed here, in this sense, was similar to the kinds of rechronotopizations and reformulations offered by Aileen, Ting Ting, and Sulin in chapter 6. As a specific relational process pointing both to adjustments in ways of relating to particular cultural forms as well as *people* (e.g., parents, children, and partners), the notion of tinkering constitutes an extension of my previous arguments further into the realm of what might be called "relational outcomes."

Gracie's narrative and Ning's reformulation of the first two hexagrams in the *Yijing*, to be clear, both lack the kind of long-term ethnographic perspective required to fully situate them as "outcomes." They nevertheless both underscore the complex ways in which generational and gendered norms overlap and inform one another within the culturally salient chronotope of patriarchy in China. They further demonstrate the ways in which "transformation" or "metamorphosis" at New Life—though sometimes presented in terms of a tidy and complete chronotopic shift—were rather uneven, emergent, and relationally situated processes of *"becoming other than what one was"*—to riff on Bakhtin's notion of metamorphosis as stories detailing the ways in which a character *"has become* other than what [they were]" (1981, 115). In a separate part of our interview that perhaps speaks to such a process, for example, Gracie invoked what she called "an old Chinese piece of talk" (老化 *laohua*) to explain why New Life had been so successful when many other similar companies had failed. The proverb she quoted is often translated as "biting off more than you can chew" (贪多嚼不烂 *tanduo jiao bulan*). Gracie adapted the phrase, however, personalizing it by adding the pronoun "you" (你 *ni*). She also shifted the first part of the proverb, which references excess greed or insatiable desire (贪多*tanduo*), such that it emphasized actual consumption or "eating a lot" (吃多*chi duo*). The resulting phrase (吃多你嚼不烂 *chi duo, ni jiao bulan*) might thus be translated as "If you eat too much, you cannot chew well." If you also eat it too quickly, she added using more colloquial speech, you won't be able to digest it. Though focused on the articulation of "expertise" when describing teachers, Gracie's adapted description pointed to the ways in which the intensive process of "becoming other than what you were" at New Life was not something that could be achieved overnight but rather required a long-term commitment to interrogating and tinkering with both cultural and relational structures.

Tinkering, in this sense, involved reflection on the past, both one's own past and the vast, cultural histories that had become entrenched in one's body as well as inscribed within specific relationships. It was also, however, enacted as a distinct anticipatory mode within which participants reformulated their visions of the possible future. Instances of "tinkering with the patriarchy," as discussed here, were thus often infused with optimism and hope. As they engaged with the permeability of the patriarchal relational world, if you will, both Gracie and Ning further hinted at the kinds of broadly scaled anticipatory modes targeted not just at relationships but at Chinese society more broadly.

Throughout the chapter, I have also remained clear on the limitations of tinkering to enact any kind of broad, transformational change in Chinese patriarchal norms or to shift anything beyond specific relationships. To that end, I have also maintained caution with regard to the ways in which particular instances of tinkering might have enacted transformation even within particular relationships. We do not know the outcome of Gracie's offer to act as provider for her husband, for example, nor do we know the result of Ning's decision in terms of her husband's (or son's) acceptance. Instances where people can be observed making nuanced adjustments or "tweaks" to their enactment of scalar intimacy, however, "if nothing else ... can help us better understand what Sabsay (2016, 295) refers to as the 'political space' opened up by momentary interactions not just to reproduce but also to problematize and contest problematic ideologies in ways that may have important consequences over time, for better or for worse" (Pritzker and Perrino 2020, 382). Such a perspective, which I discuss further in the following, concluding chapter, speaks simultaneously to the limitations of tinkering and poses the possibility of reconsidering such projects in terms of the ways in which they lay the groundwork, so to speak, for conversations that tinker explicitly with the embodied, intimate, and scalar formulations of political subjectivity and the often-violent consequences of conformity with state discourse in China.

Conclusion

By struggling through the web of lies to reach the other, we can begin to acknowledge—and mentalize—about the calamity we are both caught up in. In this way, we restore a sense of our shared humanity, and "connect the dots" to understand the world we must transform together.
—DANIEL JOSÉ GAZTAMBIDE

Throughout this book, I have offered a range of perspectives on the embodied, relational, affective, and sociopolitical project of *learning to love* at New Life. This began with an investigation of the complex ways in which newcomers were often suffering from a spatiotemporal disorientation, a sense of being "off" both *in* and *with* the world at multiple scales. Their suffering was often characterized, I demonstrated, by a tentatively circling around possible solutions within a circumscribed set of horizons (Heelas 2008). Often engaging with a number of culturally salient chronotopes, such as "home" (家 *jia*), "filial piety" (孝 *xiao*), and "happiness" (幸福 *xingfu*), participants here often underscored a feeling of "distance" from particular people or recognized cultural configurations of time and space. Their storytelling here constituted a narratively enacted expression of their *desire* to reconnect, find, or establish "closeness" with such forms. Such interrogations often generated more uncertainty rather than offering clear answers, however.

Going on to describe the ways in which interactions at the center did not necessarily confer an immediately formulated "new self," chapter 2 rather emphasized how new "horizons of possibility" emerged in the embodied, affective, and relational *atmosphere* that was enacted by people in interaction with one another as well as with a range of aesthetic objects at the center (Sumartojo and Pink 2019). In chapter 3, I then offered insight into the ways in which participants' body-selves were reconfigured in nonnormative and often deeply uncomfortable encounters that, at least sometimes, motivated a form of embodied scalar inquiry in which participants interrogated their fundamental understanding and enactment of selfhood, relationality, and "love."

Conversations and interviews, I further showed in chapters 4 and 5, often incorporated a collaborative mapping of culture, history, and memory. Here, I suggested, conversations among participants as well in unspoken encounters within which participants "wrangled with ghosts" took shape as collaborative interrogations of numerous structures of governance that scaled quickly from the state to the family and vice versa. Though not a study of "outcomes," I also showed, in chapter 6, how a similar process of scalar inquiry emerged in response to several participants' experience of *embodied defrosting*, which had motivated them to interrogate how they had been shaped by structural forces far beyond their individual or even their family's experience. Finally, chapter 7 engaged with the ways in which New Life participants variably "tinkered," in the context of particular interactions at the center as well as within particular relationships with parents and spouses, with the relational and socio-moral chronotopes that structure generational and gendered patriarchy in China.

Throughout my discussions, I have privileged a range of theoretical and methodological perspectives that attune to the many ways interaction at New Life emerged as a form of *co-operative action* within which the development of "intersubjective co-presence" involved language but also gaze, touch, gesture, and emotion as well as objects, texts, past experiences, and desires for the future (C. Goodwin 2018, 53). Within these interactions, I showed a number of culturally dominant chronotopes and shared scalar intimacies that were continually brought to life in both spoken and unspoken ways that variably reproduced or challenged them, but also often interrogated them. This book thus continually engaged with the ways in which the development and enactment of political subjectivity at New Life was never simply "subjective." I showed, rather, that it was deeply co-constructed in a collaborative, intercorporeal, affective, and simultaneously personal and social process of scalar inquiry in which participants interrogated and sometimes rescaled themselves in relation to dominan, normative ideas and practices.

Throughout this book, then, I have shown that New Life was—at least sometimes—much more than simply a site for "comfort" and "disentangling" (L Zhang 2020), but also offered an opportunity for at least *some* participants to *entangle differently* and thus to develop a form of embodied political subjectivity that I have also taken great care to distinguish from social action. To the extent that such rescaling or "tinkering" primarily focused on shifts within particular relationships, I could therefore quite comfortably conclude with a reflection, similar to Li Zhang's, that learning to love at New Life is "a form with its own limits" in terms of the particular ways in which it might transform Chinese society more broadly (2020, 129). To the extent that such opportunities were often implicit, moreover, they could often be "read both ways" in terms of how they simultaneously instantiated a range of hegemonic ideologies even as they challenged them. I could thus conclude with a critique about the unsystematic and thus haphazard ways in which this seemed to (sometimes) take shape as what Duncan and I have proposed is (sometimes) a "technology of the social" (Pritzker and Duncan 2019).

Here, however, I want to come back, yet again, to Mattingly's (2019) notion of "perplexing particulars" as pointing to the unique cases that deviate from expectations and thus undermine the hegemony of such expectations, which I have repeatedly emphasized throughout my analysis. Perplexing particulars, in this sense, are scientific in that they disconfirm a hypothesis or expectation. In this case, the particular ways in which they disconfirmed the hypothesis that "self-development" and other forms of "self-care," when practiced by middle-class Han or white bodies, *inherently* elide the political is thus at least somewhat relevant.

Perplexing particulars are not, importantly, either generalizable or predictive. Nor do they, at least in this case, afford the identification of causality. If my research question were framed, in other words, as "Does participation at New Life *cause* resistance or any kind of social action?," my answer would be an unflinching no. "Does it sometimes *prevent* it?" Possibly. "Does it *always* prevent it?" No. This line of questioning, however, leads down a precarious pathway in terms of the assumptions it makes about the role that any one type of activity, conversation, or technology has in determining, shaping, or productively rupturing the mundane enactment of complicity by people whose proximity to power often affords a violent form of "innocence" or ignorance. To this extent, it is important to further question whether the kinds of isolation and circumscription that characterized newcomers' experience of suffering when they first presented at the center is somehow better than the kinds of connections and interrogations (or connective interrogations) they participated in at New Life.

I acknowledge that all of this also may seem a bit like academic modernity chasing its own tail, so to speak (cf. Bauman and Briggs 2003). I mean this in the sense of the tautological ways in which academic discourse seems sometimes to wedge itself into a corner where arguments are formed in order to deconstruct arguments that themselves emerged out of debates about other arguments. Meanwhile, people are being abused, manipulated, and surveilled in ways that perpetuate the very oppressive systems that such analyses seek to decode. Acknowledging the futility of the whole matter is, in this sense, critical. I nevertheless want to return to the importance that both Arendt and Mattingly attributed to "defrosting" hegemonic concepts such as the linkage between "self-care" and the politics of inaction that has become such a reflexive argument in academia. Here, it is impossible to ignore how proclamations issued by academics condemning self-care practices themselves often reproduce a moral ideology that ignores the body in favor of "real social action" (R. Johnson 2018). Such discourse, as Savannah Shange observes, often generates kinds of social action that are either entirely performative or that exhaust the energy of activists in a never-ending *competition* within which "winning," as Shange writes, constitutes "the dominant logic of social justice work" (2019, 3). Following Shange's questioning, here, of "Who loses when 'we' win?" (2019, 3), I thus maintain my assertion that an attention to affordances as well as to both the perplexing and the particular is worth something, if not everything. If nothing else, the extremity of the Chinese case—where any real form of embodied resistance is met with social, emotional, or even physical death—might be supportive for thinking about, understanding, and further interrogating the role of interaction (whether among Han citizens learning to love or academic citizens writing largely for one another) and self-reflection in motivating positive social change.

PERPLEXING PARTICULARS IN THE ERA OF COVID

This book has focused on a concentrated study of events and encounters occurring between 2014 and 2016. In reality, the seeds of this project began in 2008, as detailed at the outset of this book. I also remained in close touch with many participants through at least 2019 and had further planned on a summer 2020 trip back to China to follow up on New Life workshops, instructors, and content. That trip, not surprisingly, was canceled with the onset of the COVID-19 pandemic in early spring 2020. Since that time, however, I have continued my investigation of scalar intimacy and scalar inquiry in China in other, online sites. Though not necessarily directly or even indirectly connected to New Life, these studies are nevertheless worth mentioning here because of the ways that they speak to the diverse ways in which both scalar intimacy and scalar inquiry take shape in different spaces consisting of a variety of more-or-less anonymous participants.

Beginning on February 7, 2020, for example, I began to track the massive online public reaction to the death of Li Wenliang, an ophthalmologist at Wuhan Central Hospital who died from COVID after being sanctioned by hospital authorities and local police for sharing a warning among friends and colleagues (see, e.g., Fang 2020; Kuo 2020; Li and Taylor 2020; Rudolph 2020). In an *Annual Review of Anthropology* article on language, emotion, and the politics of vulnerability finalized just week's after Li's death, for instance, I framed my discussion around the ways in which Li Wenliang's death "affected people in such a deeply personal way that even the most compliant citizens began to speak out" (Pritzker 2020, 141). Here, I examined the ways in which the public response in the hours following Li's death involved Chinese citizens' personal identification with Li, and consisted of a uniquely collective recognition of their vulnerability to both COVID-19 and the Chinese state. This vulnerability, in turn, motivated a uniquely affective as well as agentive collective response.

Throughout the following year, I continued to track this response on Li Wenliang's public Weibo page, which has famously become known as "China's Wailing Wall" (Fang 2020; Kuo 2020; Li and Taylor 2020; Rudolph 2020).[1] With over a million comments posted between February 2020 and the present, detailed analysis was foreboding, not least because the site is regularly swept by Chinese internet censors. Not long after starting this project, however, I began working closely with Tony Hu at *China Digital Times* (CDT), an organization dedicated to keeping detailed records of "content that has been or is in danger of being censored in China."[2] Beginning just weeks after Li's death, specifically, Hu initiated the long-term project of maintaining a stand-alone CDT archive of posts deemed at risk of being censored on Li Wenliang's Weibo page.[3] With an emphasis on "at-risk" posts, the CDT archive is far from a representative sampling of messages on Li's wall (Pritzker and Hu 2022). With over 10,000 posts preserved in their original form, however, the archive nonetheless constitutes "a kind of temporary community that formed in a quickly disappearing yet continuous conversation that took shape on the margins of Li's wall" (Pritzker 2023, 5) as well as "an index of a broader conversation that took place, over time, on China's Wailing Wall" (Pritzker and Hu 2022, 8).

A close collaborative analysis of posts within the CDT archive has thus led to two papers investigating scalar intimacy and scalar inquiry on Li Wenliang's Weibo page in the year after his death. Both of these analyses engage Li's death and a series of preceding and following events in China as well as globally as potential motivators of the kind of chronotopic rupture that I discuss in chapter 1 of this book. Such widespread and far-reaching events, however, emphasize how rupture on a collective, synchronous scale underscores how widespread disasters as well as ongoing atrocities and "absurdities" present people with the opportunity to *scrutinize* a range of "issues" that existed but often went unnoticed in so-called "normal times" (B. Xu 2017, 23).

The first paper, coauthored with Tony Hu, engages with the chronotopes that Chinese netizens posting on Li's wall drew upon to situate Li—and themselves—vis-à-vis culturally salient "figures of personhood" (Agha 2005; Park 2021) in China. Specifically, we discuss how participants enacted scalar intimacy by situating Li variably as a *moral hero*, a *kin member*, or a *deity* with whom they could engage in direct forms of address. Such positionings, we argue, "moved authors into a position of distance from hegemonic national chronotopes" in often novel ways that moved Chinese citizens to "grapple with shifts in their felt experience of nationhood and/or 'culture'" (Pritzker and Hu 2022, 22). Throughout our analysis, we were careful to distinguish the novel enactment of scalar intimacy in this context from explicit forms of collective social action. In an independently authored follow-up paper, however, I engage more explicitly with the potency of *questioning together* in posts that interrogated temporality, nationhood, and relational selfhood on Li's wall (Pritzker 2023). These interrogations, I suggest, constituted a unique form of collaborative scalar inquiry that arguably contributed—over time and alongside other semipublic conversations—to the November 2022 protests against COVID restrictions in China (Feng 2022; Hall, Horwitz, and Pollard 2022).

Both of the previously summarized papers, importantly, situate Li Wenliang's Weibo page as constituting an intermittent and temporary conversation on the margins of mainstream, heteronormative Han Chinese society. Participants in both spaces had at least previously enjoyed the privilege, in Ta-Nahesi Coates's terms, of "folding [their] country over their head[s] like a blanket" (2015, 11). Unlike ethnic, gender, or sexual minorities in China these were largely individuals, in other words, "whose bodies and everyday lives fell 'within the established rules of order'" (Fikes 2021b, as cited in Pritzker 2023, 3). Seeing others as the "same" here often worked therapeutically—like at the New Life Center—to usher (some) individuals out of intense experiences of isolation and anxiety, in addition to despair. It also provided a common ground for implicit, indexical communication. Rarely if ever, however, did it encourage an engagement with real difference in terms of social class, sexuality, ability, or ethnicity. I have suggested repeatedly that this points to one of the severe limitations of the otherwise liberally leaning, humanistic politics of the space, raising questions about where (and to whom) the "love" or "justice" ultimately "travels out." In a related yet separate investigation of a spontaneous conversation that emerged on the social media app "Clubhouse" in 2021, however, I examine collaborative scalar inquiry in conversations "beyond the Hantopia," so to speak, in China. Originally organized in presentation form (Pritzker 2021), the following analysis thus extends this book's argument about the ways in which New Life took shape as a Hantopia in which middle-class, Han Chinese citizens "learn to love" in a space of material as well as social comfort within which difference was frequently collapsed, flattened, or erased entirely such that it became, effectively, a form of nonknowledge.

"STAY WITH US"

You don't want to go back. Don't expect to return to your normal life before you knew all of this. You need to be with us moving forward. Don't forget this moment. Don't leave this moment behind.

—ANONYMOUS

On February 6, 2021—nearly a year to the day following Li Wenliang's death—a room entitled "Are there concentration camps in Xinjiang?" opened on the social media app, Clubhouse. Designed as a casual space for users "to tell stories, ask questions, debate, learn, and have impromptu conversations on thousands of different topics," Clubhouse—which experienced a brief period of global popularity in 2021—offers a unique voice-based interface in which users can participate in "casual, drop-in audio chats" occurring within variously titled rooms.[4] Clubhouse users can move in and out of open rooms, many of (or each of) which are moderated by other users who control access to the "stage" during conversations, which are often limited to only a few users and are often short-lived. Running for nearly eleven hours and accumulating nearly five thousand participants in China, the United States, Canada, and other international locations, however, the concentration camp conversation unexpectedly drew a great deal of global media attention.

The unexpectedness of the encounter was due in large part to the fact that the originators of the room—a group of Han-identifying Chinese citizens—quickly turned moderation over to Uyghur and Kazakh participants who had joined (Kuo and Goldkorn 2021). In an inversion of normative frameworks for interaction in China, the conversation thus situated Uyghur and Kazakh participants as "speakers" and Han participants as "addressees" or "recipients" (Pritzker 2021b). The initial four hours of the conversation thus constituted an unprecedented privileging of Uyghur and Kazakh voices. The inversion of the normative participation framework for interactions across ethnic difference in China also afforded a rare opportunity for non-Han participants to offer intimate, scalar chronotopic depictions of the lived experience of suffering in a system of oppression in which one's own body is situated as deviant (Pritzker 2021b; see also Fikes 2021b). One Uyghur speaker, for instance, was able to explain or "admit" the feeling of *distance* they had begun to feel, over the past decade of increased state violence, between themselves and the bodies of any Han person before, during, and after a given interaction (even if the Han interlocutor was otherwise a "compassionate" and "good" person). The testimonies of Uyghur and Kazakh speakers here likewise moved at least some Han participants to reevaluate their "knowledge" about the so-called "educational camps" portrayed by state media as "benign 'vocational training centers' meant to rehabilitate alleged 'extremists'" (Gan 2018, as cited in S. Roberts 2020, 214).

The latter part of the conversation, in contrast, consisted of a two-sided dialogue in which Han and other participants responded to earlier commentaries, asked novel questions, and shared their affective experience within the immediate space-time of the Clubhouse room. As such, it afforded the co-creation of a space-time that, at least relatively speaking, moved beyond the kinds of Hantopic spaces represented by New Life and Li Wenliang's Weibo page. While dismissed as "one-sided" by Chinese state media outlets (Liu et al. 2021), others remarked upon the ways in which the interaction emerged as a disarming and unexpected dialogue between Uyghur, Kazakh, and Han Chinese citizens, among others (Byler 2021b; Kuo and Goldkorn

2021). It did, indeed, at least at times seem to become a uniquely *vulnerable* space that was generative in ways that cannot necessarily be assessed from a perspective that links value to "outcomes." Guldana Salimjan, a Kazakh Chinese citizen and gender studies scholar in Canada, for example—though first acknowledging how these kinds of encounters have often been critiqued "for letting states and settler societies off the hook"—went on to liken the conversation to a kind of spontaneous "Truth and Reconciliation" event within which the lived experience of marginalized and traumatized people was both *recognized* and *validated* (personal communication, as cited in Byler 2021a).

I do not presume to know the experience of all non-Han, nor even Han Chinese, citizens in the conversation. Upon reflection, however, one participant noted that there was very little "Hansplaining" in the space, a term they used to describe the normative communicative process mode in which Han citizens effectively silence Uyghur speakers "as if [their experience] was just their opinion and could be debated" (Byler 2021b). Despite this, there were times when I observed the encounter itself to be distinctly unsafe, not only in the sense of the fear that pervaded the contributions of Han speakers, many of whom recognized what was at stake and articulated their concerns about anonymity. Additionally, there were many moments when the conversation seemed not just clumsy, but painful and unsafe in a more concealed but nevertheless intimate sense. For instance, there were still many moments that arguably constituted the kind of *gaslighting* that anthropologist and somatic practitioner Kesha Fikes (2021a) observes often prevails in conversations that avoid acknowledgment of marginalized peoples' experience. There were numerous moments when Han speakers enacted what might be called a kind of "Han fragility," for example, by proposing simplified "solutions," defending their own previous ignorance, occupying the space of their allotted ten minutes with their own grief, or situating their fear under the current regime as the "same" as Uyghur and Kazakh participants. In the sense that the efforts Han speakers were making felt entirely unusual and "well-intentioned," perhaps even such moments felt like they inched toward justice. One might imagine, however, that these moments afforded neither safety nor a sense of belonging for non-Han interlocutors.

It is noteworthy, however, that the latter seven hours of the dialogue began with a specific chronotopic *request*, uttered by the anonymous Uyghur speaker cited in the epigraph above, inviting Han interlocutors to "stay with us." Underscoring how there is no "normal" to which one can possibly hope to return after this encounter, the conversation seemed to situate both Han and non-Han Chinese citizens in the same "space-time zone," so to speak, *without* collapsing difference into "sameness." Beyond the kinds of binary, scalar "state change" (Heritage 1984) in which Han participants expressed having moved from "not knowing" or "not believing" to both knowing and believing, the encounter thus afforded a nuanced form of emergent, collaborative, and intimate scalar inquiry on the part of Han participants. Pointing, again, to the ways in which ruptures in normative modes of operation "become times of questioning" (Zigon 2008, 59), the conversation on Clubhouse thus underscores the ways in which widespread disasters as well as ongoing atrocities and "absurdities" present people with a unique opportunity to *scrutinize* the present (B. Xu 2017; Hillenbrand 2020). Several speakers, specifically, highlighted the ways in which the conversation itself had motivated them to conduct a deeper inquiry into a range of intimate cultural chronotopes, including "governance," "family," "civilization," "quality," and "education," among others. Other speakers offered vulnerable portrayals of the ways in which they had come to recognize that they had "grown up in a lie," as one Han speaker put it, going on to describe the sense of loneliness and isolation this realization had created in relationships with family members and friends. Yet another mentioned the profound sense of relief and "warmth" they were experiencing in the space in terms of being able to connect with other Han citizens who were actively engaged in the process of questioning the state.

In this sense, many of the inquiries participants in the Clubhouse conversation articulated constituted emotionally saturated scaling projects through which they simultaneously situated themselves in relation to one another as well as the fakery of the past, the violence of the present, and the bleakness of the future when (re)examined through the lens of their new "comrades" and "friends" (as they were often addressed). In questioning both together and across difference, moreover, several Han participants also conducted novel interrogations of the embodied, relational ways in which they might contribute to unsettling—if not dismantling—the interconnected webs of violence and deceit held in place by a Han ethnic nationalism that orients to fear. One participant, for example, invoked the intimacy of the "grand narratives" offered by the state, positing that the "instincts" of many Han citizens to refuse to listen to the truth is based in an embodied fear that itself has been instilled by the state-generated narratives of "nationhood" and "harmony." Upon encountering the possibility that the stories propelled by state media are false, they said, "our first reaction is to return to the grand narrative, to return to the comforting embrace of authority." Being able to recognize that this instinct is itself an intimate, embodied form of deception that keeps people from listening to other people's stories, they then went on to propose that the instinct itself is also an obstacle that blocks an ability to *love*.

The conversation on Clubhouse, I have suggested, thus constituted a "break" of sorts in public secrecy, at least for (some of) the participants joining from mainland China (Pritzker 2021b). In comparison to the kinds of "conversations with ghosts" that I have discussed throughout this book, however, or the politically coded "photo-forms" examined by Hillenbrand (2020), *this* conversation was disarmingly explicit It also occurred, importantly, in a time-space that, at least relatively speaking, moved beyond the kinds of Hantopic spaces represented by New Life and Li Wenliang's Weibo page.

I have no idea whether any of the participants who attended the Clubhouse event had been to New Life. The first part of my conclusion nevertheless involves my own kind of anticipatory mode with regard to the possible ways in which learning to love as I have examined it throughout this book—in terms of scalar inquiry, embodied defrosting, and the interrogation of the ways in which entrenched forms of scalar intimacy have been shaped by political and patriarchal structures far beyond any individual or family—*might*, under some circumstances, constitute the groundwork for *becoming vulnerable* in the context of dialogues across difference: conversations that move, in other words, beyond the cis- and heteronormative Hantopia.

I want to state here—emphatically even—that I do not see the conversation on Clubhouse as constituting, in itself, "justice." Eleven hours of dialogue, in other words, did very little to generate any satisfying or immediate "solutions" to the ongoing violence being enacted by the state in Xinjiang Province, often with the explicit support and involvement of Han citizens (Byler 2018, 2021a-b, 2022; Grose 2019; S. Roberts 2020). Moments in the conversation, however, did offer a rare glimpse into the kind of "extimacy" that Fikes (2021a) suggests affords the possibility that dialogues across difference might themselves move in the direction of justice. Further developing the notion of extimacy as initiated by Jacques Lacan (1988) and David Pavón-Cuéllar (2014), Fikes explains that extimacy "is about allowing conceptual space for the outside to affect and move one's inner world in really intimate ways" (2021a, n.p.). Underscoring the spatiotemporal disjuncture that inevitably precedes encounters across difference (see also Knoblauch 2021), Fikes centers the complexity and "actual messiness" of the contemporary moment as it has been shaped by historically and culturally entrenched social hierarchies. She thus proposes that a practice of extimacy offers a foundation for the possibility that people might come together in an *interim* space-time of "mutual collapse" and "mutual reckoning with the unspoken" in a way that "creates space for something different, *something unknown*" (2021a, n.p.). Underscoring how even the best-intentioned efforts to "solve problems" can lead to the kind of *progressive dystopia* that Savannah Shange brilliantly casts as "the chicanery of the nonprofit industrial complex" in the United States (2019, 16 and 70), Fikes makes a plea here for a kind of embodied abolitionism that opens up the space for an extimate practice of despairing together. Casting extimacy and the embodied forms of communication it affords as a "sparring practice," however, Fikes also underscores how, without the cultivation of both *active awareness* and *somatic intelligence* over time, such encounters—even those enacted with the "best intentions"—can cause tremendous harm to people whose body-selves have been subject to racialization and gaslighting over the course of a lifetime.

In fleeting moments when the conversation seemed to situate both Han and non-Han Chinese citizens in the same "space-time zone"—without necessarily collapsing difference into "sameness"—it did in many ways feel like a "mutual collapse." In unsettling what Rosa (2020) might call *the indexical disorder* that holds injustice firmly in place as both scalar and intimate, such moments seemed to profoundly dismantle both "hope" and "harmony" in ways that afforded extimacy, vulnerability, and even transparency. Many of the inquiries enacted by Han participants, as well as the narratives of Uyghur and Kazakh participants, likewise constituted what Fikes frames as a "mutual reckoning with the unspoken." At several points, it also seemed like participants were engaging in the kind of somatic inquiries that Fikes situates as the basis for extimacy.

One participant who engaged with the ways in which Han embodied "instincts" to rest comfortably in the "embrace" of authority and "nationhood," for example, suggests how the kinds of embodied, relational scalar inquiry that I have examined in this book constitute at least a *partial* kind of embodied social justice, or at least an affordance for engaging in the kinds of collective action that do orient toward "real" justice. Indeed, while not seen as a *replacement* for collective social action that challenges legal, medical, or educational policies and practices, practitioners of embodied social justice attend to dismantling of racialized white (and I might add, Han) supremacy, patriarchy, and other oppressive regimes *within* bodies that are themselves differently positioned in terms of proximity to power (Menakem 2017; Hicks Peterson 2018; R. Johnson 2018; Haines 2019; Fikes 2021b; King 2021).

As I have discussed throughout this book, liberation psychology adopts a similar perspective on intimate and scalar inquiries conducted by those whose proximity to power requires more deconstructing in order to *hear* the voices of those who "[cry] out from the negative space of non-being for recognition, restitution, and justice" (Gaztambide 2019, 194–95). Gaztambide here turns toward Frantz Fanon, citing his assertion that "individual liberation is inert without the power of a collective affective experience" (1952, 112, as cited in Gaztambide 2019, 105). In his own words, cited in the epigraph to this chapter, Gaztambide thus describes how such an experience—or collective *practice* as Fikes's perspective emphasizes—allows people, which he frames as *we*, to "[struggle] through the web of lies to reach the other" and "begin to acknowledge . . . the calamity we are both caught up in. In this way, we restore a sense of our shared humanity, and 'connect the dots' to understand the world we must transform together" (2019, 174). It affords, in other words, the kind of love that bell hooks situates as "a choice to connect—to find ourselves in the other," even if only briefly (2000, 125).

The kind of embodied social justice that I describe here as *sometimes* and *possibly* occurring at New Life, in this sense, may serve as a tiny piece of an incomplete puzzle pointing the way toward the kind of love that moves, through collective action rather than simply political subjectivity, toward more equitable forms of justice. As noted in several chapters, then, the question becomes whether and how might these conversations incorporate a more nuanced engagement with the kinds of nonknowledge that are neither public nor secret, but which nonetheless impact the bodies of all Chinese citizens, regardless of their (perceived or real) proximity to power. Lest I seem too optimistic in my own, white-bodied enactment of progressive enthusiasm, however, my ultimate conclusion veers, more appropriately, in the direction of despair rather than dreaming.

CONCLUDING REFLECTIONS

I could, given the previous discussion, quite effortlessly center my ultimate conclusion around the absolute centrality, in both liberation psychology and embodied social justice, of explicit, scaffolded, and critical forms of "political education" (Haines 2019) or "mentalization" (Gaztambide 2019) in any practice that hopes to begin dismantling or even simply deconstructing the privilege-oppression matrix of global racial capitalism in the self or the world. It is important to keep in mind, however, that New Life was *not* a space for political organizing but, indeed, was a space for "comfort" and self-growth. Though I concur wholeheartedly with the implementation of more of these conversations within psychospiritual spaces, however, I want to return to the fundamental perspective in linguistic anthropology that orients to language in interaction (or encounters with text) as *always* both referential and pragmatic as well as indexical. But I also want to return to the observation that knowing how to *refer* without saying, or knowing how to "do indexicality," is often a critical skill in China. Indeed, public and outspoken dissidents in China are often subject to "disappearances," and their family members are equally at risk (I. Johnson 2017; B. Xu 2017; Chen 2019). While I am entirely on board with abdicating one's privilege by putting one's body on the line (Fikes 2021b), in China this kind of resistance—as one participant in the Clubhouse conversation noted—is often futile in the sense that it is crushed before it even begins. Or it is entirely performative. *Knowing how to refer without saying* is thus one of the key ways in which the kinds of "nonconfrontational activism" examined by Jing Wang (2019) are able to continue operating in China. For better or for worse.

To conclude, then, I want to condemn neither the interpersonal foci of New Life clientele nor even the implicitness that prevailed in conversations about governance and "justice" at New Life. I am further quite comfortable accepting that my "right role" in even engaging in this conversation, as a middle-class, white, cis-gendered woman who at least presents as heteronormative, is not to issue either condemnations or commands. I want to end, rather, by emphasizing my overall lack of optimism with regard to the possibility that the types of conversations that occurred on Clubhouse will become more widespread in China, whether they occur at New Life or elsewhere. Second, I want to acknowledge that even (or perhaps especially) when such conversations are institutionalized in official capacities, they often enact (at best) the kinds of nonperformative performativity identified by Sara Ahmed (2006). Perhaps more importantly, they often continue to enact harm upon the bodies of those whose emotional labor is recruited in order to soothe the racial guilt of participants whose privilege is systematically conferred upon them through the ongoing oppression of tokenized and marginalized participants (Anderson 2017; Menakem 2017; Di'angelo 2018). Third, I want to revisit my suggestion, above, that, in contrast to Han participants, Uyghur and Kazakh participants did not need to conduct the same kind of scalar inquiries into concepts and structures that have intimately excluded them from the start.[5]

Finally, I want to close by conducting one further inquiry into the ways in which, despite the sometimes-nuanced ways in which conversations at New Life interrogated "culture" as well as "fakery" in the present and violence in the past, their ultimate effectiveness was undermined by the ways in which they instantiated a uniform notion of able-bodied, heteronormative, Han "Chineseness." Likewise with the ways in which they oriented, ultimately, toward love and justice as "harmony." Pointing to the ways in which "harmonizing" discourses have historically been drawn upon throughout American history to manage potential conflict "by using tonality to model the 'spiritual mechanism' organizing utopian subjects: *solidarity*" (Fretwell 2020, 99; italics in original), the equation of love, justice, and *sameness* at New Life risks perpetuating an affective tonality that invokes the CCP's notion of the ethnic "pomegranate."[6] And so—while Karimzad and Catedral note that "(re)chronotopization is an ongoing and ever-present process, which allows for the possibility of positive change" (2021, 126) in much the same way as a kind of "emergent strategy" (brown 2017, Ritchie 2023),[7] it is important to acknowledge, here, that even deeply intimate rechronotopizations that are formulated within an anticipatory mode of trying to enact justice or even simply interrogating injustice in the present or future (or the past, as was often the case at New Life) also allows for the possibility of *negative* change. Or perhaps "positive change" that nevertheless instantiates the status quo in some other form.

Notes

INTRODUCTION

1. My roommate at one of the extended inner child retreats, for example, admitted that she had resisted participation in anything remotely like this because she was afraid that she would realize that, deep down, she *hated* her parents. For my roommate, this fear had turned out to be unfounded, but it underscores how intense is the hesitation and even terror of many participants, especially newcomers.

2. As I discuss in chapter 3, clinical therapist Wu Zhihong argues that most Chinese people are no more mature than six-month-old babies (Wu 2016). Wu's estimations of an epidemic of immaturity in China is often seen as outrageous, even heretical. His book, *Nation of Giant Infants*, was banned by the Chinese government in 2017, an action that, Yang notes, likely relates to his eviscerating critique of the ways in which the hierarchical family structure and harsh, exam-driven educational system in China as well as Confucianist ideologies more generally contribute to citizens' lack of maturity. Wu's assertions nevertheless resonate deeply with many individuals in China as well as abroad (see, e.g., Gao 2017). Many participants in the current study had furthermore either worked directly with Wu or used variations of his theories to understand themselves, their family, and the broader society in terms of both past and present structures of governance and dominant ideologies.

3. Following Jackson (1995), I refer, throughout this book, to "the world" in phenomenological rather than geographic terms. In speaking of participants "experience in the world," for example, I do not necessarily mean their experience beyond China, though in some cases that perspective does apply.

4. In this sense, this book is far from the only text in its genre that engages with the unspoken. Marsilli-Vargas (2022), for example, frames her book on psychoanalytic discourse in Argentina as focused on "a world traversed by listening to *that which is not* said but is still known" (24, italics in original).

5. According to quoteinvestigator.com, Gandhi never uttered this phrase precisely. Its broad uptake across multiple sectors, however, possibly traces back to a

1913 article in the *Gujarati Indian Opinion* focused on snakebites, in which Gandhi wrote that "We but mirror the world. All the tendencies present in the outer world are to be found in the world of our body. If we could change ourselves, the tendencies in the world would also change" (1964, 158; as cited in O'Toole 2017).

CHAPTER 2

1. 生命的不可思议, lit. "incredible life."
2. 转逆境为喜悦, lit. "turning adversity into joy."
3. 点亮自性之光 lit. "light up the light of the self."

CHAPTER 3

1. English original: http://www.robertaugustusmasters.com/my-grief-our-grief-the-grief/
2. Wu Zhihong 武志红, "Exercise Your Sixth Sense" 修炼你的第六感 *WeChat*, November 19, 2015.
3. The "hot spot" here points to the "hot seat" of Fritz Perls's encounter groups at Esalen (Wood 2008).
4. The Satir method is one of the most popular forms in the inner revolution in China (Zhang 2020) and was thus a form that many if not most New Life participants had engaged with. Originally developed in the United States by Virgina Satir, the method envisions the "I AM," or the integrated self, to lay, often dormant, beneath the multiple layers of one's "personal iceberg" (Akça-Koca 2017, Zhang 2020). As a fundamental wholeness and individuality that constitutes the spiritual basis of self-esteem (Akça-Koca 2017), the I AM at the core of the self also, however, constitutes a unique *individual* self who is simultaneously tied to what Satir discussed as a vastly more collective self or a "universal tree that connects [all] people at the roots" (Satir 1988, as cited in Akça-Koca 2017, 12). As Zhang notes, the Satir method is thus often framed as especially appropriate for *Chinese* people because of the ways in which it emphasizes the cultivation of an individual self at the same time as recognizing the fundamental relationality of the self (Zhang 2020, Yang and Lou 2013). In the United States and Europe, however, the Satir method is often invoked as an ideal modality for *westerners* because of the ways it addresses the kinds of loneliness and isolation that emerge from an orientation to "independence" and "individualism" (Earls 2007).
5. Unlike other forms of entirely free-form ecstatic dance, 5Rhythms involves a facilitator who leads groups of dancers, sometimes in specific exercises, through the "five rhythms." Moving from "flowing" to "staccato" to "chaos" to "lyrical," the fifth rhythm is understood as "stillness" (Roth 1997; Roth and Loudon 1998).

CHAPTER 5

1. As noted by Chao in chapter 3, men at New Life rarely expressed emotion as intensely as the women. Emotion was nonetheless present in the subtle physical reactions of men.

2. The extent to which Hellinger actually drew upon or appropriated specific Zulu practices has been debated (see, e.g., Mayer and Viviers 2016; Carnabucci 2015, 2018).

3. Menakem (2017) here also engages with the persistent embodied trauma of police officers, or "blue" Americans.

4. Ulsamer's 2009 text, presumably written in either German or English, is translated by prominent *jiapai* therapist Zheng Lifeng). Citations throughout this chapter, offered in English, are my own "back translations" from the Chinese.

CHAPTER 6

1. My clinical training is in Chinese medicine, including both acupuncture and Chinese herbal medicine. As part of my licensure requirements, however, I am also trained in emergency first aid.

2. As Diana Fu writes, the Chinese state's emphasis on "harmony" functions, at least in part, by "instilling in ordinary people a dread of chaos and disorder" (2020, n.p.).

3. The reasons for such separations differ across generation as well as geographical and socioeconomic divides in the past and present. Parents and children were apart during the 1970s, for example, because of political participation or persecution. In the countryside, the need for rural parents to travel to the cities for employment, beginning in the 1980s, has endured through the present. Among elite urban parents both in the past and present, on the other hand, demanding international jobs and the concomitant pressure to excel in one's career required parents to be away from their children for long stretches.

4. Though the couple had never done formal testing, it is commonly assumed that the woman, within a heterosexual marriage, is to blame for infertility. Sulin's guilt and shame had thus been amplified when, upon their divorce, her husband had gone on to sire a child with his new wife.

5. Enneagram courses focus on the study of the nine personality types, each one associated with one of the points in the nine-pointed "Enneagram."

CONCLUSION

1. https://www.weibo.com/u/1139098205?is_all=1
2. https://chinadigitaltimes.net/about/
3. https://chinadigitaltimes.net/chinese/638523.html
4. https://www.clubhouse.com

5. This is not to say, however, that they, perhaps more than anyone in China, deserve the kind of "comfort" afforded by spaces (and times) designated for healing wounds created and sustained by injustice (see Linklater 2014). The question of whether it is possible to conduct this kind of trauma work in mixed ethnoracial spaces, however, is debatable. As Resmaa Menakem suggests, the deep work of healing intergenerational trauma emerging from racialization and violence is best done in racially homogenous caucuses. This work then becomes, as Fikes (2021a) suggests, the basis for encounters where healing together emerges through the vulnerable process of establishing "extimacy."

6. "The pomegranate has become the defining image of minzu [ethnic] cohesion," writes Timothy Grose, describing how, in a 2014 speech in Xinjiang, Xi Jinping "encouraged China's minzu groups to nestle tightly as if they were pomegranate seeds" (2019, 2). Going on to interrogate "the pomegranate metaphor" (or chronotope, if you will), Grose observes that "[it] is only convincing if the fruit remains enclosed in its leathery outer skin . . . Once the seeds are exposed, they will loosen and fall to the ground with a delicate tap and gentle squeeze" (2019, 3). Here, Grose unveils the precarity underlying discourses of harmonious solidarity that undergird the oppressive structures of power that afford the very privilege and "comfort" that New Life offered to participants.

7. Emergent strategies "are ideas drawn from the natural worlds, as well as observations of human interactions and societies, about how to shape and shift complex systems through relatively simple, interconnected interactions" (Ritchie 2023, 63; see also brown 2017).

References

Agha, Asif. 2005. "Voice, Footing, Enregisterment." *Journal of Linguistic Anthropology* 15 (1): 38–59.
Agha, Asif. 2007. "Recombinant Selves in Mass Mediated Spacetime." *Language & Communication* 27 (3): 320–35.
Ahmed, Sara. 2006. "The Nonperformativity of Antiracism." *Meridians* 7 (1): 104–26.
Ahmed, Sara. 2007. "A Phenomenology of Whiteness." *Feminist Theory* 8 (2): 149–68.
Akça Koca, Dilek. 2017. "Spirituality-Based Analysis of Satir Family Therapy." *Spiritual Psychology and Counseling* 2: 121–42.
Akomolafe, Bayo. 2017. *These Wilds beyond Our Fences: Letters to My Daughter on Humanity's Search for Home*. Berkeley, Calif.: North Atlantic Books.
Albanese, Catherine L. 1999. "The Subtle Energies of Spirit: Explorations in Metaphysical and New Age Spirituality." *Journal of the American Academy of Religion* 67 (2): 305–25.
Althusser, Louis. 2008. *On Ideology*. London: Verso.
Anderson, Carol. 2017. *White Rage: The Unspoken Truth of Our Racial Divide*. New York: Bloomsbury.
Arendt, Hannah. 1958. *The Human Condition*. Chicago: University of Chicago Press.
Arendt, Hannah. 1971. "Thinking and Moral Considerations: A Lecture." *Social Research* 38 (3): 417–46.
Austin, J. L. (1962) 2003. *How to Do Things with Words*. Cambridge: Harvard University Press.
Bakhtin, Mikhail M. 1981. "Forms of Time and of the Chronotope in the Novel." In *The Dialogic Imagination*, edited by Michael Holquist, 84–258. Austin: University of Texas Press.
Bauman, Richard, and Charles Briggs. 2003. *Voices of Modernity: Language Ideologies and the Politics of Inequality*. Cambridge: Cambridge University Press.
Benjamin, Rich. 2009. *Searching for Whitopia: An Improbable Journey to the Heart of White America*. New York: Hyperion.

Besnier, Niko. 1990. "Language and Affect." *Annual Review of Anthropology* 19: 419–51.

Bloom, Mia, and Sophia Moskalenko. 2021. *Pastels and Pedophiles: Inside the Mind of Q-Anon*. Stanford, Calif.: Redwood Press.

Boal, Augusto. 1979. *Theatre of the Oppressed*. Translated by Charles A. McBride and Maria-Odilia Leal McBride. New York: Theatre Communications Group.

Bolinger, D. L. 1957. *Interrogative Structures of American English: The Direct Question*. Tuscaloosa: University of Alabama Press.

Bossler, Beverly. 2020. "Sexuality, Status, and the Female Dancer: Legacies of Imperial China." In *Corporeal Politics: Dancing East Asia*, edited by Katherine Mezur and Emily Wilcox, 24–43. Ann Arbor: University of Michigan Press.

Bradshaw, John. 1990. *Homecoming: Reclaiming and Championing Your Inner Child*. New York: Bantam Books.

Bregnbæk, Susanne. 2016. *Fragile Elite: The Dilemmas of China's Top University Students*. Stanford, Calif.: Stanford University Press.

brown, adrienne maree. 2017. *Emergent Strategy*. Chico, Calif.: AK Press.

Bruner, Jerome S. 2002. *Making Stories: Law, Literature, Life*. New York: Farrar, Straus and Giroux.

Bucholtz, Mary. 2007. "Variation in Transcription." *Discourse Studies* 9 (6): 784–808.

Butler, Judith. 2016. "Rethinking Vulnerability and Resistance." In *Vulnerability in Resistance*, edited by Judith Butler, Zeynep Gambetti, and Leticia Sabsay, 12–27. Durham: Duke University Press.

Butler, Judith, Zeynep Gambetti, and Leticia Sabsay. 2016a. *Vulnerability in Resistance*. Durham: Duke University Press.

Butler, Judith, Zeynep Gambetti, and Leticia Sabsay. 2016b. "Introduction." In *Vulnerability in Resistance*, edited by Judith Butler, Zeynep Gambetti, and Leticia Sabsay, 1–11. Durham: Duke University Press.

Butler, Octavia E. 1993. *Parable of the Sower*. New York: Four Walls Eight Windows.

Byler, Darren. 2018. "Violent Paternalism: On the Banality of Uyghur Unfreedom." *Asia-Pacific Journal* 24 (16): 1–15.

Byler, Darren. 2021a. *In the Camps: China's High-Tech Penal Colony*. New York: Columbia Global Reports.

Byler, Darren. 2021b. "'Truth and Reconciliation': Excerpts from the Xinjiang Clubhouse." *SupChina*. Accessed March 3, 2021.

Byler, Darren. 2022. *Terror Capitalism: Uyghur Dispossession and Masculinity in a Chinese City*. Durham: Duke University Press.

Capps, Lisa, and Elinor Ochs. 1995. *Constructing Panic: The Discourse of Agoraphobia*. Cambridge: Harvard University Press.

Carnabucci, Karen. 2015. "Cultural Appropriation: When to Borrow from the Indigenous, and When Might It Offend?" September 22. https://www.realtruekaren.com/blog/cultural-appropriation-when-to-borrow-from-the-indigenous-and-when-might-it-offend

Carnabucci, Karen. 2018. "The Challenge and Promise for Psychodrama and Family and Systemic Constellations." *Journal of Psychodrama, Sociometry, and Group Psychotherapy* 66 (1): 81–91.

Carr, E. Summerson. 2011. *Scripting Addiction: The Politics of Therapeutic Talk and American Sobriety*. Princeton: Princeton University Press.

Carr, E. Summerson, and Michael Lempert. 2016. "Introduction: Pragmatics of Scale." In *Scale: Discourse and Dimensions of Social Life*, edited by E. Summerson Carr and Michael Lempert, 1–22. Oakland: University of California Press.

Carrico, Kevin. 2017. *The Great Han: Race, Nationalism, and Tradition in China Today*. Oakland: University of California Press.

Chace, Charles, and Zhang Ting Liang, eds. 1997. *A Qin Bowei Anthology: Clinical Essays by Master Physician Qin Bowei*. Brookline, Mass.: Paradigm.

Cheek, Timothy. 2019. "Thought Reform." In *Afterlives of Chinese Communism: Political Concepts from Mao to Xi*, edited by Christian Sorace, Ivan Franceschini, and Nicholas Loubere, 287–92. Canberra: Australian National University Press.

Chen, Chih-Jou Jay. 2019. "Deriving Happiness from Making Society Better: Chinese Activists as Warring Gods." In *The Chinese Pursuit of Happiness: Anxieties, Hopes, and Moral Tensions in Everyday Life*, edited by Becky Yang Hsu and Richard Madsen. Oakland: University of California Press.

Cheng, Chen, and Bo Qin. 2011. "The Ancient Origins of Chinese Traditional Female Gender Role: A Historical Review from Pre-Qin Dynasty to Han Dynasty." 2011 International Symposium—Female Survival and Development, Jinan, China.

Cheng, Yinghong. 2019. *Discourses of Race and Rising China*. London: Palgrave Macmillan.

Chödrön, Pema (佩玛丘卓). 2013. *The Places That Scare You: A Guide to Fearlessness in Difficult Times* [转逆境为喜悦: 与恐惧共处的智慧]. Translated by Yinmeng Hu. Shen Zhen: 深圳报业集团出版社 [Shen Zhen Press Group Publishing House].

Clemente, Ignasi. 2013. "Conversation Analysis and Anthropology." In *The Handbook of Conversation Analysis*, edited by Jack Sidnell and Tanya Stivers, 688–700. West Sussex: Wiley Blackwell.

Coates, Ta-Nehisi. 2015. *Between the World and Me*. 1st ed. New York: Spiegel and Grau.

Cohen, Dan Booth. 2006. "'Family Constellations': An Innovative Systemic Phenomenological Group Process from Germany." *Family Journal: Counseling and Therapy for Couples and Families* 14 (3): 226–33.

Dai, Jinhua. 2018. *After the Post–Cold War: The Future of Chinese History*. Edited by Lisa Rofel. Sinotheory. Durham: Duke University Press.

Davis, Mark H. 2004. "Empathy: Negotiating the Border between Self and Other." In *The Social Life of Emotions*, edited by Larissa Z. Tiedens and Colin Wayne Leach, 19–42. Cambridge: Cambridge University Press.

del Pilar Blanco, María, and Esther Pereen. 2013. "Introduction: Conceptualizing Spectralities." In *The Spectralities Reader: Ghosts and Haunting in Contemporary Cultural Theory*, edited by María del Pilar Blanco and Esther Pereen, 1–28. London: Bloomsbury.

Delfino, Jennifer B. 2021. "White Allies and the Semiotics of Wokeness: Raciolinguistic Chronotopes of White Virtue on Facebook." *Journal of Linguistic Anthropology* 31 (2): 238–57.

Derrida, Jacques. 1994. *Specters of Marx*. New York: Routledge.

Desjarlais, Robert R. 2019. *The Blind Man: A Phantasmography*. Thinking from Elsewhere. New York: Fordham University Press.

Divita, David. 2019. "Recalling the Bidonvilles of Paris: Historicity and Authority among Transnational Migrants in Later Life." *Journal of Linguistic Anthropology* 29 (1): 50–68.

Duncan, Whitney. 2017. "'Dinámicas Ocultas': Culture and Psy-Sociality in Oaxacan 'Family Constellations' Therapy." *Ethos* 45 (4): 489–513.

Duncan, Whitney L. 2018. *Transforming Therapy: Mental Health Practice and Cultural Change in Mexico*. Nashville: Vanderbilt University Press.

Duranti, Alessandro. 2009. *Linguistic Anthropology: A Reader*. 2nd ed. Blackwell Anthologies in Social and Cultural Anthropology. Malden, Mass.: Wiley-Blackwell.

Duranti, Alessandro, and Charles Goodwin. 1992. *Rethinking Context: Language as an Interactive Phenomenon*. Vol. 11, *Studies in the Social and Cultural Foundations of Language*. Cambridge: Cambridge University Press.

Durkheim, Émile. (1912) 1995. *The Elementary Forms of Religious Life*. Translated by Karen Fields. New York: Free Press.

Earls, Charles Anthony. 2007. "The Detached Individual, the Dangerous Pair, and the Spirit of the Community: Josiah Royce on the Metaphysics of Mediation" *Pluralist* 2 (2): 119–43.

Evans, Harriet. 2008. *The Subject of Gender: Daughters and Mothers in Urban China*. Lanham, Md.: Rowman and Littlefield.

Evans, Harriet. 2012. "The Intimate Individual: Perspectives from the Mother-Daughter Relationship in Urban China." In *Chinese Modernity and the Individual Psyche*, edited by Andrew B. Kipnis, 119–48. New York: Palgrave Macmillan.

Evans, Harriet. 2020. *Beijing from Below: Stories of Marginal Lives in the Capital's Center*. Durham: Duke University Press.

Fang, Fang. 2020. *Wuhan Diary: Dispatches from a Quarantined City*. Translated by Michael Berry. New York: Harper Collins.

Farnell, Brenda. 1999. "Moving Bodies, Acting Selves." *Annual Review of Anthropology* 28: 341–73.

Farnell, Brenda, and Laura Graham. 2015. "Discourse-Centered Methods." In *Handbook of Methods in Cultural Anthropology*, edited by H. Russell Bernard and Clarence C. Gravlee, 391–438. London: Rowman and Littlefield.

Farquhar, Judith, and Qicheng Zhang. 2012. *Ten Thousand Things: Nurturing Life in Contemporary Beijing*. New York: Zone Books.

Farrelly, Paul J. 2017. "Finding It: Echoes of America in Taiwan's New Age." In *Eastspirit: Transnational Spirituality and Religious Circulation in East and West*, edited by Jørn Borup, 299–324. Leiden: Brill.

Farrelly, Paul J. 2019a. "Terry Hu: Writing Her Transition from Actor to New Age Authority in Taiwan." *Asian Ethnology* 78 (1): 53–73.

Farrelly, Paul J. 2019b. "Wisdom Light New Age Shop in Beijing." *Seeing Religion in China: Visual Essays of Religious Sites.*

Feng, Emily. 2022. "How a Deadly Fire in Xinjiang Prompted Protests Unseen in China in Three Decades." *National Public Radio.*

Feuchtwang, Stephan. 2013. "Political History, Past Suffering and Present Source of Moral Judgement in the People's Republic of China." In *Ordinary Ethics in China*, edited by Charles Stafford, 222–41. London: Bloomsbury.

Fikes, Kesha. 2021a. "'Extimacy' as Racial Transparency in the Embodied Relational Field." Embodied ZSocial Justice Summit, Online, January 30.

Fikes, Kesha. 2021b. "What Bodies Do in Social Movements." Module 3: Embodied Social Justice Certificate, April 19. Embody Lab. https://www.theembodylab.com/schedule/2022-embodied-social-justice-certificate

Fincher, Leta Hong. 2016. *Leftover Women: The Resurgence of Gender Inequality in China.* Asian Arguments. London: Zed Books.

Fincher, Leta Hong. 2019. "Property, Patriarchy, and the Chinese State." In *The Psychology of Women under Patriarchy*, edited by Holly F. Mathews and Adriana M. Monago, 195–210. Albuquerque: University of New Mexico Press.

Fincher, Leta Hong. 2021. *Betraying Big Brother: The Feminist Awakening in China.* London: Verso.

Fisher, Gareth. 2014. *From Comrades to Boddhisattvas: Moral Dimensions of Lay Buddhist Practice in Contemporary China.* Honolulu: University of Hawai'i Press.

Foucault, Michel. 1983. "The Subject and Power." In *Michel Foucault: Beyond Structuralism and Hermeneutics*, edited by Hubert L. Dreyfus and Paul Rabinow, 208–26. Chicago: University of Chicago Press.

Foucault, Michel. 1988. *Technologies of the Self: A Seminar with Michel Foucault.* Edited by Luther H. Martin, Huck Gutman, and Patrick H. Hutton. Amherst: University of Massachusetts Press.

French, Brigittine M. 2012. "The Semiotics of Collective Memories." *Annual Review of Anthropology* 41: 337–53.

Fretwell, Erica. 2020. *Sensory Experiments: Psychophysics, Race, and the Aesthetics of Feeling.* Durham: Duke University Press.

Freud, Sigmund. (1923) 1995. *The Ego and the Id: And Other Works (1923–1925).* London: Hogarth.

Friend, John M., and Bradley A. Thayer. 2017. "The Rise of Han-Centrism and What It Means for International Politics." *Studies in Ethnicity and Nationalism* 17 (1): 91–114.

Fu, Diana. 2020. "China Has a Playbook for Managing Coronavirus Chaos." *Foreign Policy*, May 5. Accessed June 21, 2020.

Gadamer, Hans-Georg. 1981. *Reason in the Age of Science.* Translated by Frederick G. Lawrence. Cambridge, Mass.: MIT Press.

Gal, Susan. 2002. "A Semiotics of the Public/Private Distinction." *differences: A Journal of Feminist Cultural Studies* 13 (1): 77–95.

Gal, Susan. 2016. "Scale-Making: Comparison and Perspective as Ideological Projects." In *Scale: Discourse and Dimensions of Social Life*, edited by E. Summerson Carr and Michael Lempert, 91–111. Oakland: University of California Press.

Gambetti, Zeynep. 2016. "Risking Oneself and One's Identity: Agonism Revisited." In *Vulnerability in Resistance*, edited by Judith Butler, Zeynep Gambetti, and Leticia Sabsay, 28–51. Durham: Duke University Press.

Gan, Nectar. 2018. "Xinjiang Camps: Top Chinese Official in First Detailed Admission of 'Training and Boarding' Centres." *South China Morning Post*, October 16.

Gandhi, Mahatma. 1964. *The Collected Works of Mahatma Gandhi, Volume XII, April 1913 to December 1914*. New Delhi: Publications Division, Ministry of Information and Broadcasting, Government of India.

Gao, Helen. 2017. "China's 'Giant Infants'." *New York Times*, August 8. Accessed July 10, 2020.

Gardner, Daniel K. 1996. "Zhu Xi on Spirit Beings." In *Religions of China in Practice*, edited by Donald S. Lopez. Princeton: Princeton University Press.

Gaztambide, Daniel José. 2019. *A People's History of Psychoanalysis: From Freud to Liberation Psychology*. Lanham, Md.: Lexington Books.

Gell, Alfred. 1998. *Art and Agency: An Anthropological Theory*. Oxford: Clarendon Press.

Gibson, James J. 1979. *The Ecological Approach to Visual Perception*. Boston: Houghton Mifflin.

Goffman, Erving. 1981. *Forms of Talk*. Philadelphia: University of Pennsylvania Press.

Good, Byron J., and Mary-Jo Delvecchio Good. 1994. "In the Subjunctive Mode: Epilepsy Narratives in Turkey." *Social Science & Medicine* 38 (6): 835–42.

Goodwin, Charles. 2018. *Co-Operative Action*. Cambridge: Cambridge University Press.

Goodwin, Marjorie Harness. 1990. *He Said, She Said: Talk as Social Organization among Black Children*. Bloomington: Indiana University Press.

Goodwin, Marjorie Harness, and Asta Cekaite. 2018. *Embodied Family Choreography: Practices of Control, Care, and Mundane Creativity*. New York: Routledge.

Goodwin, Marjorie Harness, and Charles Goodwin. 2000. "Emotion within Situated Activity." In *Linguistic Anthropology: A Reader*, edited by Alessandro Duranti, 239–57. Malden, Mass.: Blackwell.

Grose, Timothy. 2019. *Negotiating Inseparability in China: The Xinjiang Class and the Dynamics of Uyghur Identity*. Hong Kong: Hong Kong University Press.

Hall, Casey, Josh Horwitz, and Martin Quin Pollard. 2022. "Clashes in Shanghai as Covid Protests Flare across China." *Reuters*, November 27. Accessed December 14, 2022.

Haines, Staci K. 2019. *The Politics of Trauma: Somatics, Healing, and Social Justice*. Berkeley, Calif.: North Atlantic Books.

Haines, Staci. 2021. "Safety, Belonging, and Dignity: Connecting Personal and Social Change." Module 6: Embodied Social Justice Certificate Program, April 28.

Embody Lab. https://www.theembodylab.com/schedule/2022-embodied-social-justice-certificate

Hammer, Gili. 2018. "Dialogical Encounters with Disability in Integrated Dance Education." *Journal of Inclusive Practice in Further and Higher Education* 10 (1): 106–19.

Hammer, Gili. 2020. "Expanding Intersubjective Awareness: The Anthropology of Kinaesthetic Diversity." *Journal of the Royal Anthropological Institute* 16 (3): 554–74.

Hammer, Gili. 2021. "A Pirouette with the Twist of a Wheelchair: Embodied Translation and the Creation of Kinesthetic Commensurability." *American Anthropologist* 123: 292–304.

Haviland, John B. 2003. "Comments on 'The Meanings of Interjections in Q'eqchi Maya: From Emotive Reaction to Social and Discursive Action.'" *Current Anthropology* 44 (4): 480–81.

Heelas, Paul. 1996. *The New Age Movement: The Celebration of the Self and the Sacralization of Modernity*. Oxford: Blackwell.

Heelas, Paul. 2008. *Spiritualities of Life: New Age Romanticism and Consumptive Capitalism*. Malden, Mass.: Blackwell.

Hellinger, Bert. 1998. *Love's Hidden Symmetry*. Phoenix, Ariz.: Zeig, Tucker, & Theisen.

Hellinger, Bert. 2000. *Supporting Love: How Love Works in Couple Relationships*. Translated by Colleen Beaumont, edited by Johannes Neuhaser. Phoenix, Ariz.: Zeig, Tucker, & Theisen.

Hellinger, Bert. (2001) 2007. *Love's Own Truths: Bonding and Balancing in Close Relationships*. Translated by Maureen Oberli-Turner and Hunter Beaumont. Phoenix, Ariz.: Zeig, Tucker, & Theisen.

Hemphill, Prentis. 2020. "Embodied Activism (Panel Discussion)." Embodiment Conference, October 15. https://portal.theembodimentconference.org/sessions/embodied-activism-ff837d

Hendriks, Eric C. 2016. "China's Self-Help Industry: American(ized) Life Advice in China." In *Handbook of Cultural and Creative Industries in China*, edited by Michael Keane, 311–27. Cheltenham: Edward Elgar.

Heritage, John. 1984. "A Change-of-State Token and Aspects of Its Sequential Placement." In *Structures of Social Action: Studies in Conversation Analysis*, edited by J. Maxwell Atkinson and John Heritage, 299–345. Cambridge: Cambridge University Press.

Heritage, John. 2013. "Epistemics in Conversation." In *The Handbook of Conversation Analysis*, edited by Jack Sidnell and Tanya Stivers, 370–94. West Sussex: Wiley Blackwell.

Hershatter, Gail. 2004. "State of the Field: Women in China's Long Twentieth Century." *Journal of Asian Studies* 63 (4): 991–1065.

Herzfeld, Michael. 2016. *Cultural Intimacy: Social Poetics and the Real Life of States, Societies and Institutions*. 3rd ed. London: Routledge.

Hicks Peterson, Tessa. 2018. *Student Development and Social Justice: Critical Learning, Radical Healing, and Community Engagement*. London: Palgrave Macmillan.

Hillenbrand, Margaret. 2020. *Negative Exposures: Knowing What Not to Know in Contemporary China*. Sinotheory. Durham: Duke University Press.

Hird, Derek. 2018. "Smile Yourself Happy: *Zheng Nengliang* and the Discursive Construction of Happy Subjects." In *Chinese Discourses on Happiness*, edited by Gerda Wielander and Derek Hird, 106–28. Hong Kong: Hong Kong University Press.

Hirsch, Marianne. 2016. "Vulnerable Times." In *Vulnerability in Resistance*, edited by Judith Butler, Zeynep Gambetti, and Leticia Sabsay, 76–96. Durham: Duke University Press.

Hizi, Gil. 2018. "Gendered Self-Improvement: Autonomous Personhood and the Marriage Predicament of Young Women in Urban China." *Asia Pacific Journal of Anthropology* 19 (4): 298–315.

Hollan, Douglas. 1992. "Cross-Cultural Differences in the Self." *Journal of Anthropological Research* 48 (4): 283.

Hollan, Douglas. 2001. "Developments in Person-Centered Ethnography." In *The Psychology of Cultural Experience*, edited by C. Moore and H. F. Mathews, 48–67. Cambridge: Cambridge University Press.

Hollan, Douglas. 2005. "Mind and Experience in Tahiti, Nepal, and Beyond." *Ethos* 33 (4): 430–32.

hooks, bell. 1992. "Eating the Other: Desire and Resistance." In *Black Looks: Race and Representation*, edited by bell hooks, 21–29. Boston: South End Press.

hooks, bell. 2000. *All about Love: New Visions*. New York: William Morrow.

Hoskins, Andrew. 2011. "7/7 and Connective Memory: Interactional Trajectories of Remembering in Post-Scarcity Culture." *Memory Studies* 4 (3): 269–80.

Hu, Yinmeng (胡因梦). 2011. 生命的不可思议 [The journey of the soul]. Shen Zhen: 深圳报业集团出版社 [Shen Zhen Press Group Publishing House].

Huang, Claudia. 2016. "Dancing Grannies in the Modern City: Dance and Alternative Consumption in Urban China." *Asian Anthropology* 15 (3): 225–41.

Huang, Erin Y. 2020. *Urban Horror: Neoliberal Post-Socialism and the Limits of Visibility*. Durham: Duke University Press.

Huang, Hsuan-Ying. 2014. "The Emergence of the Psycho-Boom in Contemporary Urban China." In *Psychiatry and Chinese History*, edited by Howard Chiang, 183–204. London: Pickering and Chatto.

Illouz, Eva. 2008. *Saving the Modern Soul: Therapy, Emotions, and the Culture of Self-Help*. Berkeley: University of California Press.

Ingold, Tim, and Elizabeth Hallam. 2007. "Creativity and Cultural Improvisation: An Introduction." In *Creativity and Cultural Improvisation*, edited by Elizabeth Hallam and Tim Ingold, 1–24. Oxford: Berg.

Irvine, Judith T. 1990. "Registering Affect: Heteroglossia in the Linguistic Expression of Emotion." In *Language and the Politics of Emotion*, edited by Catherine A. Lutz and Lila Abu-Lughod, 126–61. Cambridge: Cambridge University Press.

Irvine, Judith T., and Susan Gal. 2000. "Language Ideology and Linguistic Differentiation." In *Regimes of Language*, edited by Paul V. Kroskrity, 35–83. Santa Fe, N.Mex.: School of American Research Press.

Ivy, Marilyn. 1993. "Have You Seen Me? Recovering the Inner Child in Late Twentieth-Century America." *Social Text* 37: 227–52.

Jacka, Tamara. 2009. "Cultivating Citizens: Suzhi (Quality) Discourse in the PRC." *positions* 17 (3): 523–35.

Jackson, Michael. 1995. *At Home in the World*. Durham: Duke University Press.

Jain, Andrea R. 2020. *Peace, Love, Yoga: The Politics of Global Spirituality*. New York: Oxford University Press.

Jankowiak, William, and Xuan Li. 2017. "Emergent Conjugal Love, Mutual Affection, and Female Marital Power." In *Transforming Patriarchy: Chinese Families in the Twenty-First Century*, edited by Gonçalo D. Santos and Stevan Harrell, 146–62. Seattle: University of Washington Press.

Jefferson, Gail. 2004. "Glossary of Transcript Symbols with an Introduction." In *Conversation Analysis: Studies from the First Generation*, edited by Gene H. Lerner, 13–31. Amsterdam: John Benjamins.

Jiang, Dong 江东. 2020. "The Dilemma of Chinese Classical Dance: Traditional or Contemporary?" In *Corporeal Politics: Dancing East Asia*, edited by Katherine Mezur and Emily Wilcox, 225–39. Ann Arbor: University of Michigan Press.

Johnson, Ian. 2017. *The Souls of China: The Return of Religion after Mao*. 1st ed. New York: Pantheon Books.

Johnson, Rae. 2018. *Embodied Social Justice*. New York: Routledge.

Johnson, Rae. 2023. *Embodied Activism: Engaging the Body to Cultivate Liberation, Justice, and Authentic Connection*. Berkeley: North Atlantic Books.

Johnston, James. 2013. "Filial Paths and the Ordinary Ethics of Movement." In *Ordinary Ethics in China*, edited by Charles Stafford, 45–65. London: Bloomsbury.

Joniak-Lüthi, Agnieszka. 2015. *The Han: China's Diverse Majority*. Seattle: University of Washington Press.

Karimzad, Farzad. 2020. "Metapragmatics of Normalcy: Mobility, Context, and Language Choice." *Language & Communication* 70: 107–18.

Karimzad, Farzad, and Lydia Catedral. 2018. "Mobile (Dis)Connection: New Technology and Rechronotopized Images of the Homeland." *Journal of Linguistic Anthropology* 28 (3): 293–312.

Karimzad, Farzad, and Lydia Catedral. 2021. *Chronotopes and Migration: Language, Social Imagination, and Behavior*. New York: Routledge.

Karl, Rebecca E. 2020. *China's Revolutions in the Modern World: A Brief Interpretive History*. London: Verso.

Kazan, Tina S. 2005. "Dancing Bodies in the Classroom: Moving toward Embodied Pedagogy." *Pedagogy* 5 (3): 379–408.

Keane, Webb. 2014. "Affordances and Reflexivity in Ethical Life: An Ethnographic Stance." *Anthropological Theory* 14 (1): 3–26.

Keane, Webb. 2016. *Ethical Life: Its Natural and Social Histories*. Princeton: Princeton University Press.

King, Sará. 2021. "The Science of Social Justice." Module 7: Embodied Social Justice

Certificate Program, May 3. Embody Lab. https://www.theembodylab.com/schedule/2022-embodied-social-justice-certificate

Kipnis, Andrew B. 2011. *Governing Educational Desire: Culture, Politics, and Schooling in China*. Chicago: University of Chicago Press.

Kitagawa, Chisato, and Adrienne Lehrer. 1990. "Impersonal Uses of Personal Pronouns." *Journal of Pragmatics* 14: 739–59.

Kleinman, Arthur. 1986. *Social Origins of Distress and Disease: Depression, Neurasthenia, and Pain in Modern China*. New Haven: Yale University Press.

Kleinman, Arthur, Yunxiang Yan, Jun Jing, and Lee Sing. 2011. *Deep China: What Anthropology and Psychiatry Tell Us about China Today*. Berkeley: University of California Press.

Knoblauch, Steven H. 2021. *Bodies and Social Rhythms: Navigating Unconscious Vulnerability and Emotional Fluidity*. London: Routledge.

Kockelman, Paul. 2006. "A Semiotic Ontology of the Commodity." *Journal of Linguistic Anthropology* 16 (1): 76–102.

Krauss, Chris. (1997) 2016. *I Love Dick*. London: Serpent's Tail.

Krishnamurti, Jiddu. (克里希那穆提). 2007. *This Light in Oneself (点亮自性之光)*. Translated by Yinmeng Hu. Shen Zhen: 深圳报业集团出版社 [Shen Zhen Press Group Publishing House].

Kuan, Teresa. 2015. *Love's Uncertainty: The Politics and Ethics of Child Rearing in Contemporary China*. Berkeley: University of California Press.

Kulick, Don, and Bambi B. Schieffelin. 2004. "Language Socialization." In *A Companion to Linguistic Anthropology*, edited by Alessandro Duranti, 349–68. Malden, Mass.: Blackwell.

Kuo, Kaiser, and Jeremy Goldkorn, 2021. "The Xinjiang Camps on Clubhouse." *Sinica* podcast, the China Project. https://thechinaproject.com/podcast/the-xinjiang-camps-on-clubhouse/

Kuo, Lily. 2020. "Wuhan Doctor Speaks Out against Authorities." *Guardian*, March 11. Accessed June 18, 2022.

Lacan, Jacques. 1988. *The Seminar of Jacques Lacan, Book I: Freud's Papers on Technique, 1953–1954*. Translated by John Forrester. edited by Jacques-Alain Miller. New York: W.W. Norton and Company.

Lam, Ling Hon. 2018. *The Spatiality of Emotion in Early Modern China: From Dreamscapes to Theatricality*. New York: Columbia University Press.

Larre, Claude, and Elisabeth Rochat de la Vallée. 1996. *The Seven Emotions: Psychology and Health in Ancient China*. Cambridge, U.K.: Monkey Press.

Leander, Kevin M. 2004. "'They Took Out the Wrong Context': Uses of Time-Space in the Practice of Positioning." *Ethos* 32 (2): 188–213.

Lee, Haiyan. 2023. *A Certain Justice: Toward an Ecology of the Chinese Legal Imagination*. Chicago: University of Chicago Press.

Lempert, Michael, and Sabina Perrino. 2007. "Entextualization and the Ends of Temporality." *Language & Communication* 27 (3): 205–11.

Levy, Robert, and Douglas Hollan. 1998. "Person-Centered Interviewing and Observation." In *Handbook of Methods in Anthropology*, edited by H. R. Bernard, 333–64. Walnut Creek, Calif.: Altamira Press.

Li, Jie. 2020. *Utopian Ruins: A Memorial Museum of the Mao Era*. Durham: Duke University Press.

Li, Yuan, and Rumsey Taylor. 2020. "How Thousands in China Gently Mourn a Coronavirus Whistle-Blower." *New York Times*, April 13. Accessed April 20, 2020.

Li, Zehou. 2010. *The Chinese Aesthetic Tradition*. Honolulu: University of Hawai'i Press.

Libby, Lisa K., and Richard P. Eibach. 2002. "Looking Back in Time: Self-Concept Change Affects Visual Perspective in Autobiographical Memory." *Journal of Personality and Social Psychology* 82 (2): 167–79.

Lin, Delia. 2012. "Working to Be Worthy: Shame and the Confucian Technology of Governing." In *Chinese Modernity and the Individual Psyche*, edited by Andrew B. Kipnis, 169–86. New York: Palgrave Macmillan.

Lin, Delia. 2017. *Civilising Citizens in Post-Mao China: Understanding the Rhetoric of Suzhi*. London: Routledge.

Lin, Delia, and Susan Trevaskes. 2019. "Creating a Virtuous Leviathan: The Party, Law, and Socialist Core Values." *Asian Journal of Law and Society* 6: 41–66.

Ling, Li. 2010. "Gentlemen and Petty Men." *Contemporary Chinese Thought* 41 (2): 54–65.

Link, E. Perry. 2013. *An Anatomy of Chinese: Rhythm, Metaphor, Politics*. Cambridge: Harvard University Press.

Linklater, Rennee. 2014. *Decolonizing Trauma Work: Indigenous Stories and Strategies*. Halifax, Nova Scotia: Fernwood Publishing.

Liu Xin, Cui Fandi, Li Qiao, and Chen Qingqing. 2021. "Clubhouse Is No 'Free Speech Heaven,' Say Chinese Mainland Users." *Global Times*, February 8. Accessed March 4, 2021.

Lo, Adrienne, and Heidi Fung. 2012. "Language Socialization and Shaming." In *The Handbook of Language Socialization*, edited by Alessandro Duranti, Elinor Ochs, and Bambi B. Schieffelin, 169–89. Malden, Mass.: Wiley-Blackwell.

Loizidou, Elena. 2016. "Dreams and the Political Subject." In *Vulnerability in Resistance*, edited by Judith Butler, Zeynep Gambetti, and Leticia Sabsay, 122–45. Durham: Duke University Press.

Low, Setha M. 2017. *Spatializing Culture: The Ethnography of Space and Place*. London: Routledge.

Lucia, Amanda J. 2020. *White Utopias: The Religious Exoticism of Transformational Festivals*. Oakland: University of California Press.

Lyons, Kate, and Farzad Karimzad. 2019. "Chronotopeography: Nostalgia and Modernity in South Delhi's Linguistic Landscape." *Sociolinguistic Studies* 13 (1): 83–105.

Ma, Zhiying. 2012. "Psychiatric Subjectivity and Cultural Resistance: Experience and Explanations of Schizophrenia in Contemporary China." In *Chinese Modernity and the Individual Psyche*, edited by Andrew B. Kipnis, 203–27. New York: Palgrave Macmillan.

Magee, Rhonda V. 2019. *The Inner Work of Racial Justice: Healing Ourselves and Transforming Our Communities through Mindfulness*. New York: Tarcher Perigee.

Manning, Paul. 2018. "Spiritualist Signal and Theosophical Noise." *Journal of Linguistic Anthropology* 28 (1): 67–92.

Marsilli-Vargas, Xochitl. 2014. "Listening Genres: The Emergence of Relevance Structures through the Reception of Sound." *Journal of Pragmatics* 69 (2014): 42–51.

Marsilli-Vargas, Xochitl. 2022. *Genres of Listening: An Ethnography of Psychoanalysis in Buenos Aires*. Durham: Duke University Press.

Martin, Fran. 2006. "Stigmatic Bodies: The Corporeal Qiu Miaojin." In *Embodied Modernities: Corporeality, Representation, and Chinese Cultures*, edited by Fran Martin and Larissa Heinrich, 177–94. Honolulu: University of Hawai'i Press.

Martín-Baró, Ignacio. 1976. "La Verdad de la Mentira." *Alternativa* 1: 1.

Mason, Katherine A. 2020. "When the Ghosts Live in the Nursery: Postpartum Depression and the Grandmother-Mother-Baby Triad in Luzhou, China." *Ethos* 48 (2): 149–70.

Mattingly, Cheryl. 2010. *The Paradox of Hope: Journeys through a Clinical Borderland*. Berkeley: University of California Press.

Mattingly, Cheryl. 2014. *Moral Laboratories: Family Peril and the Struggle for a Good Life*. Oakland: University of California Press.

Mattingly, Cheryl. 2019. "Defrosting Concepts, Destabilizing Doxa: Critical Phenomenology and the Perplexing Particular." *Anthropological Theory* 18 (4): 415–39.

Matza, Tomas Antero. 2018. *Shock Therapy: Psychology, Precarity, and Well-Being in Postsocialist Russia*. Durham: Duke University Press.

Mayer, Claude-Hélène, and Rian Viviers. 2016. "Constellation Work and Zulu Culture: Theoretical Reflections on Therapeutic and Cultural Concepts." *Journal of Sociology and Social Anthropology* 7 (2): 101–10.

McIntosh, Peggy. 1989. "White Privilege: Unpacking the Invisible Knapsack." *Peace and Freedom Magazine* (July/August), 10–12.

Menakem, Resmaa. 2017. *My Grandmother's Hands: Racialized Trauma and the Pathway to Mending Our Hearts and Bodies*. Las Vegas, Nev.: Central Recovery Press.

Menakem, Resmaa. 2022. *The Quaking of America: An Embodied Guide to Navigating Our Nation's Upheaval and Racial Reckoning*. Las Vegas: Central Recovery Press.

Mol, Annemarie, Ingunn Moser, and Jeannette Pols. 2010. "Care: Putting Practice into Theory." In *Care in Practice: On Tinkering in Clinics, Homes, and Farms*, edited by Annemarie Mol, Ingunn Moser, and Jeannette Pols. Bielefeld: transcript Verlag.

Murthy, Vivek Hallegere. 2020. *Together: The Healing Power of Human Connection in a Sometimes Lonely World*. New York: HarperCollins,.

Myers, Neely A. L. 2016. "Recovery Stories: An Anthropological Exploration of Moral Agency in Stories of Mental Health Recovery." *Transcultural Psychiatry* 53 (4): 427–44.

Nakassis, Constantine. 2016. "Anthropology in 2015: Not the Study of Language." *American Anthropologist* 118 (2): 330–45.

Ndefo, Nkem. 2021. "Embodied Approaches in Organizational Settings." Module 24: Embodied Social Justice Certificate Program, June 28. Embody Lab. https://www.theembodylab.com/schedule/2022-embodied-social-justice-certificate

Nelson, Eric S., and Yang Liu. 2016. "The Yijing, Gender, and the Ethics of Nature." In *The Bloomsbury Research Handbook of Chinese Philosophy and Gender*, edited by Ann Pang-White, 267–88. London: Bloomsbury.

Nussbaum, Martha Craven. 1994. *The Therapy of Desire: Theory and Practice in Hellenistic Ethics*. Princeton: Princeton University Press.

Ochs, Elinor. 1979. "Transcription as Theory." In *Developmental Pragmatics*, edited by Elinor Ochs and Bambi B. Schieffelin, 43–72. New York: Academic Press.

Ochs, Elinor. 2004. "Narrative Lessons." In *A Companion to Linguistic Anthropology*, edited by Alessandro Duranti, 269–89. Malden, Mass.: Blackwell.

Ochs, Elinor. 2012. "Experiencing Language." *Anthropological Theory* 12 (2): 142–60.

Ochs, Elinor, and Lisa Capps. 2001. *Living Narrative: Creating Lives in Everyday Storytelling*. Cambridge: Harvard University Press.

Ochs, Elinor, and Bambi Schieffelin. 1989. "Language Has a Heart." *Text* 1: 7–25.

Osburg, John. 2013. *Anxious Wealth: Money and Morality among China's New Rich*. Stanford: Stanford University Press.

O'Toole, Garson. 2017. "Be the Change You Wish to See in the World." QuoteInvestigator.com.

Papadopoulos, Renos K. 2018. "Home: Pardoxes, Complexities, and Vital Dynamism." In *Thinking Home: Interdisciplinary Dialogues*, edited by Sanja Bahun and Bojana Petrić, 53–70. London: Routledge.

Parish, Steven M. 2008. *Subjectivity and Suffering in American Culture: Possible Selves*. Culture, Mind, and Society. New York: Palgrave Macmillan.

Park, Joseph Sung-Yul. 2021. "Figures of Personhood: Time, Space, and Affect as Heuristics for Metapragmatic Analysis." *International Journal of the Sociology of Language*, no. 272, 47–73.

Parmentier, Richard J. 2007. "It's About Time: On the Semiotics of Temporality." *Language & Communication* 27 (3): 272–77.

Pavón-Cuéllar, David. 2014. "Extimacy." *Encyclopedia of Critical Psychology*, edited by Thomas Teo. New York: Springer. https://doi.org/10.1007/978-1-4614-5583-7_106

Peirce, Charles S.. 1992. *The Essential Peirce: Selected Philosophical Writings*. Edited by Nathan Houser and Christian J. W. Kloesel. 2 vols. Peirce Edition Project. Bloomington: Indiana University Press.

Perrino, Sabina. 2007. "Cross-Chronotope Alignment in Senegalese Oral Narrative." *Language & Communication* 27 (3): 227–44.

Perrino, Sabina, and Sonya E. Pritzker, eds. 2022. *Research Methods in Linguistic Anthropology*. London: Bloomsbury Academic.

Polsky, Andrew Joseph. 1991. *The Rise of the Therapeutic State*. The City in the Twenty-First Century. Princeton: Princeton University Press.

Pritzker, Sonya E. 2003. "The Role of Metaphor in Culture, Consciousness, and Medicine: A Preliminary Inquiry into Metaphors of Depression in Chinese and Western Medical and Common Languages." *Clinical Acupuncture and Oriental Medicine* 4 (1): 11–28.

Pritzker, Sonya E. 2007. "Thinking Hearts, Feeling Brains: Metaphor, Culture, and the Self in Chinese Narratives of Depression." *Metaphor and Symbol* 22 (3): 251–74.

Pritzker, Sonya E. 2011. "The Part of Me That Wants to Grab: Embodied Experience and Living Translation in U.S. Chinese Medical Education." *Ethos* 39: 395–413.

Pritzker, Sonya E. 2012. "Living Translation in US Chinese Medicine." *Language in Society* 41 (3): 343–63.

Pritzker, Sonya E. 2014. *Living Translation: Language and the Search for Resonance in U.S. Chinese Medicine*. New York: Berghahn Books.

Pritzker, Sonya E. 2016. "New Age with Chinese Characteristics? Translating Inner Child Emotion Pedagogies in Contemporary China." *Ethos* 44 (2): 150–70.

Pritzker, Sonya E. 2017. "Family Constellation Therapy and the Enregistering of Emotion in China." American Anthropological Association Annual Meeting, Washington, D.C., November 29–December 3.

Pritzker, Sonya E. 2018. "Desire with Chinese Characteristics: Scaling Intimacy in Narratives of Personal Psycho-Spiritual Development." Living Well in China conference, Irvine, CA, November.

Pritzker, Sonya E. 2019. "Ghosts in the Data: Family Constellation Therapy and the Anthropological Imaginary." American Anthropological Association, Vancouver, BC.

Pritzker, Sonya E. 2020. "Language, Emotion, and the Politics of Vulnerability." *Annual Review of Anthropology* 49: 241–56.

Pritzker, Sonya E. 2021a. "Intimacy, Political Subjectivity, and the Magical Power of Dr. Li Wenliang." MIT Department of Anthropology, Language and Technology Lab, Boston, September 17.

Pritzker, Sonya E. 2021b. "We Are Also Terrified: Han Political Subjectivity on Clubhouse." Speaking from the Heart: Translating Xinjiang's Diverse Voices, University of British Columbia Xinjiang Documentation Project, Vancouver, October 9.

Pritzker, Sonya E. 2023. "'What's Going On with My China?' Political Subjectivity, Scalar Inquiry, and the Magical Power of Li Wenliang." *American Anthropologist* 125 (1): 125–38.

Pritzker, Sonya E., and Yuan Bing. 2004. "The Apologetic Heart: Shame, Depression, and Bei Die in Chinese Culture and Medicine." *Journal of Chinese Medicine* 76: 9–14.

Pritzker, Sonya E., and Whitney L. Duncan. 2019. "Technologies of the Social: Family Constellation Therapy and the Remodeling of Relational Selfhood in China and Mexico." *Culture, Medicine, and Psychiatry* 43 (3): 468–95.

Pritzker, Sonya E., and Tony Hu. 2022. "'This Is China's Wailing Wall': Chronotopes and the Configuration of Li Wenliang on Weibo." *Language, Culture, and Society* 4 (2): 110–35.

Pritzker, Sonya E., and Kiki Q. Y. Liang. 2018. "Semiotic Collisions and the Metapragmatics of Culture Change in Dr. Song Yujin's 'Chinese Medical Psychology.'" *Journal of Linguistic Anthropology* 28 (1): 43–66.

Pritzker, Sonya E., and Sabina Perrino. 2020. "Culture Inside: Scale, Intimacy, and Chronotopic Stance in Personal Narratives." *Language in Society* 50: 365–87.

Pritzker, Sonya E., and Sabina Perrino. 2022. "Participant Observation and Fieldnotes in Linguistic Anthropology." In *Research Methods in Linguistic Anthropology*, edited by Sabina M. Perrino and Sonya E. Pritzker, 125–57. London: Bloomsbury Academic.

Puglionesi, Alicia. 2020. *Common Phantoms: An American History of Psychic Science*. Stanford: Stanford University Press.

Ramstead, Maxwell D., Samuel P. L. Veissiere, and Laurence J. Kirmayer. 2016. "Cultural Affordances: Scaffolding Local Worlds through Shared Intentionally and Regimes of Attention." *Frontiers in Psychology* 7.

Rapport, Nigel. 2018. "Anyone—Any Arthur, Sean or Stan: Home-Making as Human Capacity and Individual Practice." In *Thinking Home: Interdisciplinary Dialogues*, edited by Sanja Bahun and Bojana Petrić, 17–38. London: Routledge.

Ritchie, Andrea J. 2023. *Practicing New Worlds: Abolition and Emergent Strategies*. Chico, CA: AK Press.

Roberts, Daniel. 2013. "Same Dream, Different Beds: Family Strategies in Rural Zhejiang." In *Ordinary Ethics in China*, edited by Charles Stafford, 154–72. London: Bloomsbury.

Roberts, Margaret E. 2018. *Censored: Distraction and Diversion inside China's Great Firewall*. Princeton: Princeton University Press.

Roberts, Rosemarie A. 2013. "Dancing with Social Ghosts: Performing Embodiments, Analyzing Critically." *Transforming Anthropology* 21 (1): 4–14.

Roberts, Sean R. 2020. *The War on the Uyghurs: China's Internal Campaign against a Muslim Minority*. Princeton: Princeton University Press.

Rofel, Lisa. 2007. *Desiring China: Experiments in Neoliberalism, Sexuality, and Public Culture*. Durham: Duke University Press.

Rosa, Jonathan. 2019. *Looking Like a Language, Sounding Like a Race: Raciolinguistic Ideologies and the Learning of Latinidad*. Oxford: Oxford University Press.

Rosa, Jonathan. 2020. "(Dis)Possessing Race and LInguage: Rethinking Colonialism in the Learning of Latinidad." American Association of Applied Linguistics Annual Meeting, Online, March 28.

Rosa, Jonathan. 2021. "Indexical Disorder and the Diacritics of Raciolinguistic Life." Society for Linguistic Anthropology: Talking Politics Series, Online/Zoom.

Rose, Nikolas S. 1996. *Inventing Our Selves: Psychology, Power, and Personhood*. Cambridge: Cambridge University Press.

Roseneil, Sasha, Isabel Crowhurst, Tone Hellesund, and Mariya Stoilova. 2020. *The Tenacity of the Couple-Norm: Intimate Citizenship Regimes in a Changing Europe*. London: UCL Press.

Roth, Gabrielle. 1997. *Sweat Your Prayers: Movement as Spiritual Practice*. New York: J.P. Tarcher/Putnam.

Roth, Gabrielle, and John Loudon. 1998. *Maps to Ecstasy: A Healing Journey for the Untamed Spirit*. Novato, Calif.: Nataraj Pub.

Rudolph, Josh. 2020. "Coronavirus Martyr Li Wenliang's Digital 'Wailing Wall.'" *China Digital Times*. Accessed June 15, 2020.

Sabsay, Leticia. 2016. "Permeable Bodies: Vulnerability, Affective Powers, Hegemony." In *Vulnerability in Resistance*, edited by Judith Butler, Zeynep Gambetti, and Leticia Sabsay, 278–302. Durham: Duke University Press.

Samuels, Annemarie. 2018. "'This Path Is Full of Thorns': Narrative, Subjunctivity, and HIV in Indonesia." *Ethos* 46 (1).

Sang, Tze-lan D. 2006. "The Transgender Body in Wang Dulu's Crouching Tiger, Hidden Dragon." In *Embodied Modernities: Corporeality, Representation, and Chinese Cultures*, edited by Fran Martin and Larissa Heinrich, 98–114. Honolulu: University of Hawai'i Press.

Santos, Gonçalo D. 2016. "Multiple Mothering and Labor Migration in Rural South China." In *Transforming Patriarchy: Chinese Families in the Twenty-First Century*, edited by Gonçalo D. Santos and Stevan Harrell, 91–112. Seattle: University of Washington Press.

Santos, Gonçalo D., and Stevan Harrell. 2017. *Transforming Patriarchy: Chinese Families in the Twenty-First Century*. Seattle: University of Washington Press.

Satir, Virginia. 1988. *The New Peoplemaking*. Palo Alto, Calif.: Science and Behavior Books.

Schaedler, Luc. 2018. *A Long Way Home*. Go Between Films.

Seligman, Rebecca. 2014. *Possessing Spirits and Healing Selves: Embodiment and Transformation in an Afro-Brazilian Religion*. Culture, Mind, and Society. New York: Palgrave Macmillan.

Seligman, Rebecca. 2018. "Mind, Body, Brain, and the Conditions of Meaning." *Ethos* 46 (3): 397–417.

Seok, Bongrae. 2017. *Moral Psychology of Confucian Shame: Shame of Shamelessness*. Lanham, Md.: Rowman and Littlefield International.

Shange, Savannah. 2019. *Progressive Dystopia: Abolition, Antiblackness, + Schooling in San Francisco*. Durham: Duke University Press.

Shohet, Merav. 2017. "Troubling Love: Gender, Class, and Sideshadowing the 'Happy Family' in Vietnam." *Ethos* 45 (4): 555–76.

Shohet, Merav. 2018. "Two Deaths and a Funeral: Ritual Inscriptions' Affordances for Mourning and Moral Personhood in Vietnam." *American Ethnologist* 45 (1): 60–73.

Shohet, Merav, and Heather Loyd. 2022. "Transcription and Analysis in Linguistic Anthropology: Creating, Testing, and Presenting Theory on the Page." In *Research Methods in Linguistic Anthropology*, edited by Sabina M. Perrino and Sonya E. Pritzker, 261–95. London: Bloomsbury Academic.

Silverstein, Michael. 1979. "Language Structure and Linguistic Ideology." In *The Elements: A Parasession on Linguistic Units and Levels*, edited by Paul Clyne, William F. Hanks, and Carol L. Hofbauer. Chicago: Chicago Linguistic Society.

Simchai, Dalit, and Avihu Shoshana. 2018. "The Ethic of Spirituality and the Non-Angry Subject." *Ethos* 46 (1): 115–33.

Smith, Richard J. 2008. *Fathoming the Cosmos and Ordering the World: The Yijing (I-Ching, or Classic of Changes) and Its Evolution in China*. Charlottesville: University of Virginia Press.

Stafford, Charles. 2013. "Ordinary Ethics in China Today." In *Ordinary Ethics in China*, edited by Charles Stafford, 3–25. London: Bloomsbury.

Stivers, Tanya, Lorenza Mondada, and Jakob Steensig. 2011. *The Morality of Knowledge in Conversation*. Cambridge: Cambridge University Press.

Strozzi Heckler, Richard. 1993. *The Anatomy of Change: A Way to Move through Life's Transitions*. Berkeley: North Atlantic Books.

Sumartojo, Shanti, and Sarah Pink. 2019. *Atmospheres and the Experiential World: Theory and Methods*. London: Routledge.

Sutin, Angelina R., and Richard W. Robins. 2008. "When the 'I' Looks at the 'Me': Autobiographical Memory, Visual Perspective, and the Self." *Consciousness and Cognition* 17: 1386–97.

Szasz, Thomas. 1974. *The Myth of Mental Illness: Foundations of a Theory of Personal Conduct*. Rev. ed. New York: Harper & Row.

Szasz, Thomas. 2008. *Psychiatry: The Science of Lies*. Syracuse, N.Y.: Syracuse University Press.

Taussig, Michael. 1999. *Defacement, Public Secrecy, and the Labor of the Negative*. Stanford: Stanford University Press.

Taylor, Charles. 1989. *Sources of the Self: The Making of the Modern Identity*. Cambridge: Harvard University Press.

Teo, Thomas. 2018. "Homo Neoliberalus: From Personality to Forms of Subjectivity." *Theory & Psychology* 28 (5): 581–99.

Throop, C. Jason. 2014. "Moral Moods." *Ethos* 42 (1): 65–83.

Tolle, Eckhart. 2005. *A New Earth: Awakening to Your Life's Purpose*. New York: Dutton/Penguin Group.

Trouillot, Michel-Rolph. 1995. *Silencing the Past: Power and the Production of History*. Boston: Beacon Press.

Trouillot, Michel-Rolph. 2003. *Global Transformations: Anthropology and the Modern World*. New York: Palgrave Macmillan.

Tu, Wei-ming. 1985. *Confucian Thought: Selfhood as Creative Transformation*. Albany: State University of New York Press.

Tu, Wei-ming. 1994. "Embodying the Universe: A Note on Confucian Self-Realization." In *Self as Person in Asian Theory and Practice*, edited by Roger T. Ames, Wimal Dissanayake, and Thomas P. Kasulis, 177–86. Albany: State University of New York Press.

Turner, Edith L. B. 2012. *Communitas: The Anthropology of Collective Joy*. Contemporary Anthropology of Religion. New York: Palgrave Macmillan.

Turner, Victor W. 1969. *The Ritual Process: Structure and Anti-Structure*. London: Routledge and Kegan Paul.

Turner, Victor. 1985. *On the Edge of the Bush: Anthropology as Experience*. Tucson: University of Arizona Press.

Ulsamer, Bertold. 2005. *The Healing Power of the Past: The Systemic Therapy of Bert Hellinger*. Nevada City, Calif.: Underwood Books.

Ulsamer, Bertold. 2009. 家庭系统排列例如们 [The healing power of the past]. Translated by 郑立峰 [Zheng Li Feng]. Beijing: 化学工业出版社 Huaxue Gongye Chuban She [Chemical Industrial Press].

Wang, C. C. 1969a. ""Translator's Postscript [Yihouji]." *Literature Monthly* 34 (6): 4.

Wang, C. C. [as Ji Qing]. 1969b. "Your Child Really Isn't Yours" [Nide Haizi Bing Bushi Nide]. *The Woman* (May).

Wang, Jing. 2019. *The Other Digital China: Nonconfrontational Activism on the Social Web*. Cambridge: Harvard University Press.

Wei, John. 2020. *Queer Chinese Cultures and Mobilities: Kinship, Migration, and Middle Classes*. Hong Kong: Hong Kong University Press.

Wielander, Gerda. 2018a. "Introduction." In *Chinese Discourses on Happiness*, edited by Gerda Wielander and Derek Hird, 1–24. Hong Kong: Hong Kong University Press.

Wielander, Gerda. 2018b. "Happiness in Chinese Socialist Discourse: Ah Q and the 'Visible Hand.'" In *Chinese Discourses on Happiness*, edited by Gerda Wielander and Derek Hird, 25–43. Hong Kong: Hong Kong University Press.

Wielander, Gerda, and Derek Hird, eds. 2018. *Chinese Discourses on Happiness*. Hong Kong: Hong Kong University Press.

Wilce, James M. 2001. "Divining Troubles, or Divining Troubles? Emergent and Conflictual Dimensions of Bangladeshi Divination." *Anthropological Quarterly* 74 (4): 190–200.

Wilce, James M. 2009. *Language and Emotion*. Vol. 25, *Studies in the Social and Cultural Foundations of Language*. Cambridge: Cambridge University Press.

Wilce, James M. 2014. "Current Emotion Research in Linguistic Anthropology." *Emotion Review* 6 (1): 77–85.

Wilce, James M., and Janina Fenigsen. 2016. "Emotion Pedagogies: What Are They, and Why Do They Matter?" *Ethos* 44 (2): 81–95.

Williams, Raymond. 1977. *Marxism and Literature*. Marxist Introductions. Oxford: Oxford University Press.

williams, Rev. angel kyodo, Lama Rod Owens, and Jasmine Syedullah. 2016. *Radical Dharma: Talking Race, Love, and Liberation*. Berkeley, Calif.: North Atlantic Books.

Wirtz, Kristina. 2016. "The Living, the Dead, and the Immanent: Dialogue across Chronotopes." *Hau-Journal of Ethnographic Theory* 6 (1): 343–69.

Wolf, Margery. 1994. "Beyond the Patrilineal Self: Constructing Gender in China." In *Self as Person in Asian Theory and Practice*, edited by Roger T. Ames, Wimal Dissanayake. and Thomas P. Kasulis, 251–70. Albany: State University of New York Press.

Wolynn, Mark. 2016. *It Didn't Start with You: How Inherited Family Trauma Shapes Who We Are and How to End the Cycle*. New York: Penguin Books.

Wong, Jamie, Crystal Lee, Vesper Keyi Long, Di Wu, and Graham M. Jones. 2021. "'Let's Go, Baby Forklift!' Fandom Governance and the Political Power of Cuteness in China." *Social Media + Society* (April): 1–18.

Wong, Magdalena. 2020. *Everyday Masculinities in 21st-Century China: The Making of Able-Responsible Men*. Hong Kong: Hong Kong University Press.

Wood, Linda Sargent. 2008. "Contact, Encounter, and Exchange at Esalen: A Window onto Late Twentieth-Century American Spirituality." *Pacific Historical Review* 77 (3): 453–87.

Woodstock, Louise. 2005. "Vying Constructions of Reality: Religion, Science and 'Positive Thinking' in Self-Help Literature." *Journal of Media and Religion* 4 (3): 155–78.

Woolard, Kathryn A. 2013. "Is the Personal Political? Chronotopes and Changing Stances toward Catalan Language and Identity." *International Journal of Bilingual Education and Bilingualism* 16 (2): 210–24.

Wright, Kate. 2010. *The Rise of the Therapeutic Society: Psychological Knowledge and the Contradictions of Cultural Change*. Washington, D.C.: New Academia Publishing.

Wu, Cuncun, and Mark Stevenson. 2006. "Male Love Lost: The Fate of Male Same-Sex Prostitution in Beijing in the Late Nineteenth and Early Twentieth Centuries." In *Embodied Modernities: Corporeality, Representation, and Chinese Cultures*, edited by Fran Martin and Larissa Heinrich, 42–59. Honolulu: University of Hawai'i Pres.

Wu, David Y. H. 1994. "Self and Collectivity: Socialization in Chinese Preschools." In *Self as Person in Asian Theory and Practice*, edited by Roger T. Ames, Wimal Dissanayake, and Thomas P. Kasulis, 235–50. Albany: State University of New York Press.

Wu, Zhihong 武志红 2015. 修炼你的第六感 [Exercise your sixth sense]. Accessed November 19, 2015.

Wu, Zhihong 武志红. 2016. 巨婴国 [Nation of giant infants]. Hangzhou: Zhejiang People's Publishing House.

Xiang, Biao, and Qi Wu. 2022. *Self as Method: Thinking through China and the World*. Singapore: Springer Nature Singapore.

Xiao, Hui Faye. 2014. *Family Revolution: Marital Strife in Contemporary Chinese Literature and Visual Culture*. Seattle: University of Washington Press.

Xie, Kailing. 2021. *Embodying Middle Class Gender Aspirations: Perspectives from China's Privileged Young Women*. Singapore: Palgrave Macmillan.

Xu, Bin. 2017. *The Politics of Compassion: The Sichuan Earthquake and Civic Engagement in China*. Durham: Duke University Press.

Xu, Jing. 2017. *The Good Child: Moral Development in a Chinese Preschool*. Stanford: Stanford University Press.

Xu, Jing. 2020. "Tattling (*Gaozhuangi*) with Chinese Characteristics: Norm Sensitivity, Moral Anxiety, and 'the Genuine Child.'" *Ethos* 48: 29–49.

Yan, Yunxiang. 2009. *The Individualization of Chinese Society*. English ed. Oxford: Berg.
Yan, Yunxiang. 2013. "The Drive for Success and the Ethics of the Striving Individual." In *Ordinary Ethics in China*, edited by Charles Stafford, 263–91. London: Bloomsbury.
Yan, Yunxiang. 2016. "Intergenerational Intimacy and Descending Familism in Rural North China." *American Anthropologist* 118: 244–57.
Yan, Yunxiang. 2017. "Doing Personhood in Chinese Culture: The Desiring Individual, Moralist Self and Relational Person." *Cambridge Journal of Anthropology* 35 (2): 1–17.
Yan, Yunxiang. 2018. "Neo-Familism and the State in Contemporary China." *Urban Anthropology* 47 (3/4): 1–43.
Yang, Jie. 2015. *Unknotting the Heart: Unemployment and Therapeutic Governance in China*. Ithaca, NY: ILR Press.
Yang, Jie. 2018a. *Mental Health in China: Change, Tradition, and Therapeutic Governance*. China Today. Cambridge: Polity.
Yang, Jie. 2018b. "'Happy Housewives': Gender, Class, and Psychological Self-Help in China." In *Chinese Discourses on Happiness*, edited by Gerda Wielander and Derek Hird, 129–49. Hong Kong: Hong Kong University Press.
Yang, Jie. 2020. "Counselling and Confucianism in China: A New Twist on Tradition." In *The Routledge International Handbook of Global Therapeutic Cultures*, edited by Daniel Nehring, Ole Jacob Madsen, Edgar Cabanas, China Mills, and Dylan Kerrigan, 245–56. London: Routledge.
Yang, Li, and Vivian Lou. 2013. "Applying the Satir Model of Counseling in Mainland China: Illustrated with 20 Case Sessions." *Satir Journal of Counselling and Family Therapy* 1 (2013): 18–39.
Yang, Mayfair Mei-hui. 2020. *Re-Enchanting Modernity: Ritual Economy and Society in Wenzhou, China*. Durham: Duke University Press,.
Yang, Zi. 2017. "Xi Jinping and China's Traditionalist Restoration." *China Brief* 17 (9).
Yeh, Catherine. 2020. "Mei Lanfang and Modern Dance: Transcultural Innovation in Peking Opera, 1910s-1920s." In *Corporeal Politics: Dancing East Asia*, edited by Katherine Mezur and Emily Wilcox, 44–59. Ann Arbor: University of Michigan Press.
Zhang, Everett. 2015. *The Impotence Epidemic: Men's Medicine and Sexual Desire in Contemporary China*. Durham: Duke University Press.
Zhang, Li. 2008. "Private Homes, Distinct Lifestyles: Performing a New Middle Class." In *Privatizing China: Socialism from Afar*, edited by Li Zhang and Aihwa Ong, 23–40. Ithaca: Cornell University Press.
Zhang, Li. 2014. "Bentuhua: Culturing Psychotherapy in Postsocialist China." *Culture, Medicine, and Psychiatry* 38 (2): 283–305.
Zhang, Li. 2017. "The Rise of Therapeutic Governing in Postsocialist China." *Medical Anthropology* 36 (1): 6–18.
Zhang, Li. 2018. "Cultivating the Therapeutic Self in China." *Medical Anthropology* 37 (1): 45–58.

Zhang, Li. 2020. *Anxious China: Inner Revolution and Politics of Psychotherapy*. Oakland: University of California Press.

Zhang, Yanhua. 2007. *Transforming Emotions with Chinese Medicine: An Ethnographic Account from Contemporary China*. SUNY Series in Chinese Philosophy and Culture. Albany: State University of New York Press.

Zhang, Yanhua. 2014. "Crafting Confucian Remedies for Happiness in Contemporary China: Unraveling the Yu Dan Phenomenon." In *The Political Economy of Affect and Emotion in East Asia*, edited by Jie Yang, 31–44. London: Routledge.

Zhang, Yanhua. 2018. "Cultivating Capacity for Happiness as a Confucian Project in Contemporary China." In *Chinese Discourses on Happiness*, edited by Gerda Wielander and Derek Hird, 150–68. Hong Kong: Hong Kong University Press.

Zigon, Jarrett. 2008. *Morality: An Anthropological Perspective*. Oxford: Berg.

Zigon, Jarrett. 2009. "Morality and Personal Experience: The Moral Conception of a Muscovite Man." *Ethos* 37 (1): 78–101.

Index

able-responsible man, 21, 229–30
aesthetics, 10, 17, 26, 71, 77–79, 90–91, 94–95, 166, 255
affect. *See* emotion
affordances, 9–10; ethical affordances, 82, 183
agency, 5–6, 10, 13, 28, 43, 58, 78, 81, 90, 115–16, 118, 130, 141, 142, 147, 149, 150, 157–58, 160–66, 179, 208, 234, 241, 250–52; moral agency (*see* morality)
Agha, Asif, 12, 29, 36, 260
Ahmed, Sara, 3, 12, 36, 67, 100, 268
Akça-Koca, Dilek, 6, 272
Akomlafe, Bayo, 35, 69
Albanese, Catherine, 6
alchemy, 4, 29, 246–47, 251
Althusser, Louis, 201
ancestors: and embodiment, 190–93; see also suffering, intergenerational trauma; in family constellation therapy (*see* family constellation therapy); as ghosts, 7, 154–58; relationality with, 154, 236–39
Anderson, Carol, 217
anger: accessing anger, 15; in Chinese medicine, 35; expressing anger (*see* emotion, expressing emotion); in family constellations, 175; men's anger, 230; in New Age settings, 118; towards children, 130, 227, 237; towards parents, 2–3, 53, 225; unacknowledged anger, 102
anticipatory modes, 8, 27, 29, 53, 74, 75, 85, 123, 132, 147, 157, 166, 183, 205, 239, 241, 253, 265, 269
anxiety: anxious experience, 54, 63, 102, 143, 235; in Chinese society, 5; and shame, 198
Arendt, Hannah, 13, 37, 195, 204, 258
atmosphere, 26–28, 70–92, 95, 110, 112, 117–118, 162, 164, 183, 185, 191, 207, 231, 255
Austin, J.L., 12, 65
authority, 28, 117, 158, 179, 207, 251, 265–66

Bakhtin, Mikhail, 80, 82, 192, 225, 235, 242, 253
Bauman, Richard, 258
Benjamin, Rich, 21
Besnier, Niko, 103
Bloom, Mia, 195
Boal, Augusto, 186
Bolinger, D. L., 158
books, 58, 69, 72–73, 75, 82
Bossler, Beverly, 199

Bradshaw, John, 6, 106, 198
Bregnbæk, Susanne, 47, 132
Briggs, Charles, 258
brown, adrienne maree, 16, 19, 194, 269, 274
Bruner, Jerome, 37
Bucholtz, Mary, 24
Butler, Judith, 13, 38, 93, 95, 251
Butler, Octavia, ix
Byler, Darren, 22, 151, 187, 262–63, 265

Capps, Lisa, 37, 80
care, 47–50, 56, 125; care practices, 223; as control, 47–49, 128, 132, 197; and gender (*see* gender); as nourishment, 43; self-care, 86, 257–58
Carnabucci, Karen, 273
Carr, E. Summerson, 13, 35, 104
Carrico, Kevin, 12, 37–38, 40, 117, 121, 127, 137, 150, 175, 187, 195
Catedral, Lydia, 13, 36, 223, 269
Cekaite, Asta, 27, 95, 115
Chace, Charles, 135
chaos (*luan*), 40–41, 72, 131, 193, 207, 272
Cheek, Timothy, 138, 182
Chen, Chih-Jou Jay, 16, 268
Cheng, Chen, 21
Cheng, Yinghong, 21, 22, 150, 175, 187
China: contemporary Chinese society, 5
China Dream, 40
Chinese medicine, 23, 80, 135–36, 198
Chineseness, 18, 20–22, 28, 75, 79, 99, 127, 130, 133–50, 192–94, 207, 223, 269
Chödrön, Pema, 78
chronotopes, 11–12; chronotopal dilemmas, 34; contrasting chronotopes, 14, 133–51; *see* chronotopic contrasts; cultural chronotopes, 12–15, 35–37, 48, 52, 63–67, 86, 94, 99, 193, 256, 264; embodied chronotopes, 12, 36–37, 48, 99; and figures of personhood, 260; as flexible, 138; home chronotope, 26, 40–44, 73–75, 78–83, 84, 89–92, 232, 236, 255; horizon chronotopes, 26, 73–75, 78–83, 89–92; as intimate (*see* embodied chronotopes); as moral-relational, 224–25, 256; as orienting devices, 89–90; rechronotopization, 13, 241, 250–252, 269; and scalar inquiry (*see* scalar inquiry); and scalar intimacy (*see* scalar intimacy)
chronotopic contrasts: East/West, 89, 134, 138–42, 149–50, 197, 200, 210; inside/outside, 71–73, 78, 83, 89, 94; justiceo/injustice, 14; past/present, 132–134, 149–50, 239–240; public/private, 7, 9, 35, 89–90; tradition/modernity, 48, 115–16, 137, 141; urban/rural, 55–56, 143, 145–48, 149
Clemente, Ignasi, 24
Clubhouse, 30, 261–68
co-operative action. *See* interaction
Coates, Ta-Nahesi, 260
Cohen, Dan Booth, 171
collective development, 7, 26, 74, 87, 89, 119, 121
communitas, 161, other?
Confucianism, 63, 82, 97–98, 116, 149, 156, 198, 236, 247, 249, 271
consciousness, 118. 151, 230
context, 73
critical consciousness, 196, 218–19
criticism, 33–34, 207–8
critiquing the state. *See* scalar inquiry
Cultural Revolution, 17, 22, 32, 33–34, 131, 140, 144, 174, 177–78, 181, 207
culture: "Asian" culture, 197, 199; in anthropology, 11, 186; Chinese culture, 133–134, 136, 138, 140–143, 149, 221, 224, 240; cultural chronotopes (*see* chronotopes); as discursive resource, 138, 218, 256; interrogating culture, 27–28, 124–51, 269; *see also* scalar inquiry; and nationhood (*see*

nationhood); and scalar initmacy (*see* scalar intimacy); and suffering, 171–73; and translation, 79

Dai, Jinhua, 18, 152, 157, 199, 241
dance, 57, 110–21, 201–2
Daoism, 82, 247, 249
Davis, Mark H., 155
defrosting, 13, 28–29, 37, 86, 193–96, 200–36, 252, 256, 258, 265
del Pilar Blanco, Maria, 184
Delfino, Jennifer, 13
Derrida, Jaques, 1, 152, 161, 212
desire: as anticipatory mode (*see* anticipatory modes); as claustrophobia, 31, 35, 47, 51; and culture, 127, 210, 255; as expectation, 213–14; as experience in space-time, 33; for future, 28, 35, 53, 55–56, 108, 118, 128–33, 140, 145–50, 152, 154, 159–60, 187, 222, 241, 256; for home, 5, 39–44, 74; and intimacy, 129–30, 184; for justice, 8; for maturity (*see* maturity); and political subjectivity, 12; and power, 21; for resolution, 26, 37–39, 45, 62; for self-transformation, 216, 253; shared desires, 60; to understand the past, 181
Desjarlais, Robert, 161, 185
disentangling, 14, 26, 74, 92, 97, 117, 223, 250, 256
Divita, David, 12, 36
dreaming. *See* anticipatory mode; anticipatory modes
Duncan, Whitney, 4, 10, 34, 39, 74, 85, 95, 97, 107, 122, 154–56, 169–170, 174, 177, 186–87, 196, 257
Duranti, Alessandro, 10, 73
Durkheim, Émile, 119

Earts, Charles Anthony, 272
education, 37, 46–47, 52, 56, 132; and care, 48, 125; and emotions, 136; as form of governance, 48, 126–30, 132, 136, 144, 146, 159, 207, 224–25, 264; political education, 29, 122, 194, 196, 205, 218, 268; throughout the lifecourse, 47
Eiback, Richard, 107, 155
embodied social justice, 16, 19, 122, 194, 218, 266–69
embodiment: and agency (*see* agency); and chronotopes (*see* scalar intimacy); and collective experience, 182, 203; and culture, 171–74, 273; embodied awareness, 96, 26667; embodied capacity, 96; embodied defrosting (*see* defrosting); embodied encounters, 96–97, 100, 103, 106, 108, 119–22, 132, 157–58; embodied experience (tiyan), 14, 79, 144; embodied geography, 26–27, 89, 91–92, 95, 255; embodied inquiry (*see* scalar inquiry); embodied intimacy, 106, 212, 236; embodied memory, 114; embodied orienting devices, 5; embodied unconscious, 212; embodying the past, 110, 131, 175, 185, 193, 201, 209, 211; and emotion, 3, 105, 110, 115; *see also* emotion; in enactments at New Life, 7, 104–6, 109, 162, 188, 245; and family (*see* family); in family constellation therapy, 28, 156–58; feeling of disorientation, 5; and gender, 108, 174, 190, 229–32; and ghosts, 154–56; in interaction, 27, 95–97, 105, 131, 208; and intimacy (*see* intimacy); and justice (*see* embodied social justice); and memory (*see* memory); and metamorphosis (*see* metamorphosis); movement/dance, 116; and oppression/injustice, 122, 187, 211, 217; and political subjectivity, 192, 196, 200, 242, 257; and the self

embodiment (*continued*)
(*see* self); and self-development (*see* self-development); and shame (*see* shame); and space-time (*see* chronotopes); and suffering (*see* suffering)

emboiment: embodying the past, 108

emergent strategies, 269, 274

emotion: anger (*see* anger); in Chinese medicine, 135; and embodiment, 105, 110, 115; emotion realms, 95; emotion work, 237; emotional constraint, 135, 139; emotional excesses, 116; enacted emotion, 104; enregisterment of emotion, 95; expressing emotion, 2–3, 14–15, 41, 55, 62–66, 95, 111–18, 130–35, 139–40, 175, 221–22, 229–30; in family constellation therapy, 175; fear, 127 175, 198–99, 205, 230, 245, 263–64; and gender, 193, 228–30, 237, 273; guilt, 51–53, 102, 154, 172, 177, 214; and language, 41, 259; moral emotions, 197; and politics, 12, 259

Enneagram, 76, 210, 273

entangling differently, 8, 14–15, 27, 74, 82–83, 92, 97, 117, 190, 193–94, 215, 224, 228, 250, 257

equality, 129, 168, 186, 225, 232, 247

ethics. *See* morality

Evans, Harriet, 18, 98, 129, 187, 206

extimacy, 30, 265–66, 274

fakery, 8, 42, 56, 117, 145, 264, 269

family: as "home" (*see* home); the Chinese family, 134–38, 139–43, 235; cultural ideologies of, 4–5, 28, 37, 50, 131, 134–38, 233–34, 264, 271; familial self, 7; family harmony, 28, 160, 184; family karma, 161; family photographs (*see* photographs); family systems (*see* family constellation therapy); family values, 40–41; and gender (*see* gender); and governance, 147, 181, 182, 207, 224–25; and morality (*see* morality); and public secrecy, 208; *see also* public secrecy; and the self (*see* self)

family constellation therapy (*jiapai*), 7, 28, 34, 76, 85, 104, 152–87; as "time travel," 7; as "wrangling with ghosts," 7; representation of ancestors, 169

Fang, Fang, 259

Farnell, Brenda, 10, 24, 188, 191

Farquhar, Judith, 5, 18

Farrelly, Paul J., 16, 80, 81

fathers, 2, 8, 41, 46–48, 55, 162, 176, 205, 234–36

feminism, 16, 42, 246, 251–52

Feng, Emily, 260

Feuchtwang, Stephan, 18, 99, 144, 157, 176, 178, 199, 201, 207, 210

figures of personhood or person-types, 12, 224, 244, 260

Fikes, Kesha, 218, 261–63, 265–68, 274

filial piety, 3, 5, 46, 52, 100, 134, 255

Fincher, Leta Hong, 5, 18, 40, 41, 42, 237, 246, 251

Fisher, Gareth, 5, 39

Foucault, Michel, 10, 122, 201

fractacl recursivity, 89, 149

freedom, 19, 25, 119–21, 147–49, 173, 187, 216, 225

French, Brigittine, 131, 183

Fretwell, Erica, 269

Freud, Sigmund, 10, 19, 112, 218

Friend, John M., 21, 22, 150

Fu, Diana, 18, 193, 273

Fung, Heidi, 197, 200

Gadamer, Hans-Georg, 13

Gal, Susan, 73, 89–90, 139, 149

Gambetti, Zeynep, 38, 119

Gan, Nectar, 262

Gandhi, Mahatma, 15, 271–72

Gao, Helen, 271

Gardmer. Daniel K., 155
Gaztambide, Daniel José, 10, 19, 23, 122, 218, 255, 267–68
Gell, Alfred, 78, 162
gender: and citizenship, 5; cultural ideologies of gender, 5, 37, 63, 100, 159, 185, 199, 213, 229–32, 235, 240, 245; and embodiment (*see* embodiment); and emotion (*see* emotion); enacting different genders, 109–10; gender binary, 199, 228; gender differences, 108; gender hierarchies, 228–32; gender roles: in family constellation therapy, 174; men's gender roles, 41, 229–230, 240; men's work, 228–33; New Life clientele, 4, 25; and patriarchy (*see* patriarchy); gendered expression of emotion, 175; and the Great Self, 98–99, 236; heteronormativity (*see* heteronormativity); inversion of gender norms, 232; and marriage, 42, 235, 246, 252; same-sex relationships, 199; and shame (*see* shame); women's gender roles, 40–42, 63, 241, 246; in the Yijing, 248–51
ghosts: conversations with, 154–60, 265; hungry ghosts, 155; learning from, 152, 212; in the nursery, 130–31; in psychotherapy, 7; psychotherapy for, 155–56; and public secrecy, 166–71, 185, 186; resonance with (*ganying*), 156; wrangling with, 7, 18, 28, 152, 187, 252
Gibson, James J., 10
Goffman, Erving, 146, 222
Goldkorn, Jeremy, 262
Good, Byron, 34
Good, Mary Jo Delvecchio, 34
Goodwin, Charles, 11, 39, 60, 72, 87, 94, 115, 116, 122, 223, 250, 256
Goodwin, Marjorie, 27, 95, 103, 115
governance, 8, 10, 40, 48, 116–17, 132–33, 137, 143–44, 149, 151, 159. 182, 197, 199, 207–8, 224–25, 256, 264, 268, 271
Graham, Lauran, 10, 24
grandparents, 1, 75, 171, 172, 234, 236, 264
Great Leap Forward, 17, 131, 174
Grose, Timothy, 187, 265, 274
group therapeutic exercise: enactments, 103–5; mirroring exercises, 100–103; movement exercises, 110–21; *see also* dance; time travel, 7, 105–10, 155, 160
group therapeutic exercises, 1–3
growth (personal and/or spiritual growth), 16, 48, 76, 91, 145, 202, 209; *see also* self-development

Haines, Staci K., 16, 19, 23, 29, 96, 122, 172, 194, 204–5, 217, 218, 267–68
Hall, Casey, 260
Hallam, Elizabeth, 115
Hammer, Gili, 119
Han-centrism, 21
Hantopias, 20–22, 28, 87, 92, 122, 219, 261, 265
happiness, 18, 41, 55, 255
harmonization: in Chinese medicine, 135
harmony: "harmonious family," 28, 156–160, 184; "harmonious society," 18, 40–41, 117, 156, 193, 264–69; in ancient China, 136–38; *vs.* chaos, 18; as cultural ideology, 15, 39–41, 100; in family constellation therapy, 174; and gender, 193; as life goal, 246–51; social harmony, 92
Haviland, John B., 103
heart, 32–33, 43, 52, 78, 84, 201–2, 222, 238–40; in Chinese medicine, 135, 198; as embodied site for home, 43, 234–35; as seat of emotion, 56, 139
Heelas, Paul, 4, 6, 9, 15, 20, 38, 66, 69, 72, 91, 95, 115, 118, 181, 255

Hellinger, Bert, 7, 154–55, 157–58, 170–73, 176, 179, 273
Hemphill, Prentis, 218
Hendriks, Eric C., 10
Heritage, John, 158, 264
Hershatter, Gail, 199
Herzfeld, Michael, 17, 48, 127
heteronormativity, 41–42, 92, 119, 177, 219, 260, 265, 268, 269
Hicks Peterson, Tessa, 218, 267
hidden rules (*qian guize*), 215
Hillenbrand, Margaret-, 17, 18, 22, 28, 76–78, 131–32, 150, 157, 159, 166–68, 170–71, 183, 186–87, 201, 207–8, 210, 264–65
Hird, Derek, 10, 18, 86, 107, 147, 155, 156, 172, 175, 199, 215, 269
Hirsch, Marianne, 166
Hizi, Gil, 5, 9, 10, 246
Hollan, Douglas, 12, 99–100, 149, 198
home (*jia*), 5, 26, 32–35, 39–44, 46–54, 59, 62–63, 69–92, 165, 210, 232, 245, 255–56; being-at-home-in-the-world, 6, 42–44, 53–54, 72, 74, 78–79, 91–92, 216, 234; as cultural ideology, 5, 33, 39–44, 156; and gender, 245, 249; home chronotopes (*see* chronotopes); home-place, 5, 37, 40, 84; homecoming, 6, 74, 82, 106; as located inside the self, 43, 233–35
homosexuality, 226–27
hooks, bell, 1, 8, 21, 267
hope, 1, 9, 12, 15, 35, 52–53, 82, 90, 127, 164, 181, 184, 216, 239–41, 247, 250–51, 253, 266–68, *see also* anticipatory modes
horizons: circumscribed horizons, 9, 26, 38, 61, 66, 72, 246, 249, 255; horizon chronotope (*see* chronotopes); horizoned promises, 7
Horwitz, Josh, 260
Hoskins, Andrew, 159

Hu, Yinmeng [Terry Hu], 16, 78, 81
Huang, Claudia, 116, 119, 147, 150, 203
Huang, Erin, 41
Huang, Hsuan-Ying, 23, 82
Hui, Wen, 114

I AM, 113, 272
Illouz, Eva, 142, 216
imagination. *See* anticipatory modes
immaturity, 5, 32–33, 49, 271
indexicality, 11; in family constellation therapy, 166–76
Ingold, Tim, 115
injustice: in contemporary Chinese society, 54, 168, 186–87, 196, 215–16; and embodiment, 217; *see also* embodied social justice; as indexical disorder, 266; and inequality, 168; interrogating injustice, 22, 269; *see also* scalar inquiry; in the past, 8, 15, 54, 177, 196, 216; and racial/ethnic homogeneity, 21
inner child therapy, 1–2, 6–7, 12, 76, 96, 105–10, 122, 229–30, 245, 271
inner revolution, 14, 20, 26, 79, 127, 222, 272
interaction: as "container," 39; across difference, 119, 262–63; and atmosphere (*see* atmosphere); and chronotopes (*see* chronotopes); as co-operative action, 11, 29, 39, 60, 71–72, 87, 92, 94, 109, 115–16, 122, 223, 250–51, 256; as constraint, 38; and embodiment, 27, 95–97, 105, 131, 208; in family constellation therapy (*see* family constellation therapy); implicit interaction, 9, 11, 17, 205, 251; and indexicality (*see* indexicality); informal interaction at New Life, 222, 229, 252; and interrogation (*see* scalar inquiry); in linguistic anthropoogy (*see* language); as peopled opportuni-

ties (*see* peopled opportunities); and power, 99, 122, 178, 208; reconfiguring of relationships in interaction, 15; and ritual, 94; and scalar inquiry (*see* scalar inquiry); and scalar intimacy (*see* scalar intimacy); and scaling projects, 12–13; and shame, 200; as wrangling with ghosts, 7, 18, 152–87
intercorporeality, 7, 95–96, 100, 105–6, 120–22, 155, 168, 170, 176, 256
intersubjectivity, 27, 71, 95, 103, 119, 122, 155–56, 170, 256
intimacy: cultural ideologies of, 97–100, 129–33, 134–43, 147–50, 159–60; cultural intimacy, 17, 48, 127; embodied intimacy (*see* embodiment); enregisterment of intimacy, 95–97, 103, 106, 155; in ethnographic interviews, 39; and extimacy (*see* extimacy); with ghosts, 154–60; in group exercises, 94–97 (*see* psysociality); and home chronotopes, 40–44, 75–92; and injustice, 128; in interaction, 67, 252–54; intergenerational intimacy, 129, 223, 236; intimacy with the past, 108, 183, 213, 238–39; intimate geography, 72–75, 78, 85–92, 208–9; intimate relationships, 32, 52, 162–66, 170–82, 202–3, 225–29, 234; and politics, 207–8; and scalar inquiry (*see* scalar inquiry); scalar intimacy (*see* scalar intimacy)
Irvine, Judith, 89, 95, 139, 149
Ivy, Marlyn, 4, 105

Jacka, Tamara, 130
Jackson, Michael, 6, 34, 42, 43, 72, 74, 91, 216, 234, 271
Jain, Andrea R., 15, 217
Jankowiak, William, 5
Jefferson, Gail, 24
Jiang, Dong, 116

Johnson, Ian, 9, 16, 268
Johnson, Rae, 16, 18, 19, 122, 172, 194, 218, 258, 267
Johnston, James, 206
Joniak-Lüthi, Agnieszka, 5, 40
justice: enacting justice, 8, 187, 218, 261, 267–269; and equality, 129, 225; and ethnocentrism in China, 20–22; and freedom, 225; in the future (*see* anticipatory modes); high *vs.* low justice, 8, 20, 186–87, 224; implicit justice, 15–21; social justice, 20, 25, 258; and somatics, 23

Karimzad, Farzad, 13, 36, 39, 75, 79, 223, 269
Karl, Rebecca, 18, 124, 126, 148, 149, 177, 181
Kazan, Tina, 119
Keane, Webb, 10, 82
King, Sará, 16, 19, 194, 218, 267
Kipnis, Andrew B., 48, 127, 225
Kirmayer, Laurence, 10
Kitagawa, Chisato, 105
Kleinman, Arthur, 23, 135
Knoblauch, Steven H., 95, 266
Kockelman, Paul, 75
Krauss, Chris, 31, 35
Krishna Das, 69–70
Krishnamurti, Jiddu, 78, 81
Kuan, Teresa, 10, 18, 22, 37, 48, 51, 53, 130–31, 143, 150, 193, 237
Kulick, Don, 147
Kuo, Kaiser, 262
Kuo, Lily, 259

Lacan, Jacques, 11, 30, 35, 265
Lam, Ling Hon, 95
language, 10–11, 17, 35–36, 65–66, 117, 256; and emotion (*see* emotion); language ideologies, 65–66; language-as-interaction, 11; language-

language (continued)
　in-interaction (see interaction); in linguistic anthropology, 10–11, 24, 35–36, 268; in psychoanalysis, 117; and secrecy, 17, 166
Larre, Claude, 135
Leander, Kevin, 36
learning to live, 7–8, 152, 157, 161
learning to love, 3–9, 15, 18, 20, 22–23, 26, 65, 74, 91, 129, 150, 157, 194, 203, 210, 212–14, 222, 228, 231, 250, 255, 257, 265
Lee, Haiyan, 8, 186, 224
Lehrer, Adirenne, 105
Lempert, Michael, 12, 13, 35, 36
Levy, Robert, 12
Li, Jie, 19, 131, 159, 176
Li, Wenliang, 30, 259
Li, Xuan, 5
Li, Yuan, 259
Li, Zehou, 63, 77, 78
Libby, Lisa K., 107, 155
liberation psychology, 19, 218, 267
Lin, Delia, 3, 8, 10, 40, 48, 132, 137, 186, 199, 224
linguistic anthropology, 10–11
Link, Perry E., 84
Linklater, Renee, 274
listening, 65–66, 71, 100, 103, 115, 128, 159, 194, 271; genres of listening, 103, 115, 159, 194
Liu, Xin, 262
Liu, Yang, 249
Lo, Adrienne, 197, 200
Loizidou, Elena, 8, 10, 27, 132, 147, 150
Lou, Vivian, 118, 272
love, 32, 42, 78, 96, 100, 120, 209–10, 261; as affective current across bodies, 7; capacity to, 94, 96, 265; as care, 50–52; in Chinese history, 238–239; as connection, 267; during Cultural Revolution, 207–8; and culture, 111, 139–140, 206–7; as ethic, 151; expression of love, 111, 139–40, 163; in family constellation therapy, 157, 164, 169; in family systems, 111, 139–140, 157; learning to love, 3–9, 15, 18, 20, 22–23, 26, 65, 74, 91, 129, 150, 157, 194, 203, 210, 212–14, 222, 228, 231, 250, 255, 257, 265; love's promise, 1; mother love, 234–36; in New Age, 118; and politics, 22, 28–30, 267–69; as relationality, 118; self-love, 69, 214, 240, 244
Low, Setha, 78, 79
Lucia, Amanda, 15, 20–21, 172
Lyons, Kate, 69, 75

Ma, Zhiying, 10
Magee, Rhonda, 16, 19, 194
Manning, Paul, 158
marriage, 32, 37, 42, 45, 162, 164, 177, 211, 214, 235, 240, 242, 246, 273
Marsilli-Vargas, Xochitl, 47, 65, 71, 103, 112, 115, 159, 194, 271
Martin-Baró, Ignacio, 19, 23
Martin, Fran, 199
Marxism, 230
Mason, Katherine, 48–49, 128, 130, 178
Mattingly, Cheryl, 10, 13, 37, 39, 97, 185–86, 196, 219, 257–58
maturity: becoming mature, 44, 53–54, 206, 220, 231, 249, 250; as cultural discourse, 46, 117, 133; and personal growth (see self-development)
Matza, Tomas, 4, 10, 39, 74, 95
Mayer, Claude-Hélene, 273
McIntosh, Peggy, 151
memory, 27, 54, 83, 114, 152, 159, 188, 191, 197, 256
Menakem, Resmaa, 173, 175, 198, 209, 218, 267, 269, 273, 274
metamorphosis, 192, 196, 210, 217, 225–26, 235, 242, 253
minor publics, 168, 186

Mol, Annemarie, 220, 223
morality: and aesthetics (*see* aesthetics); Chinese values, 40; and chronotopes (*see* chronotopes); Confucian ethics (*see* Confucianism); as consciousness, 118, 151; distance between moral discourse and everyday experience, 9; and embodiment, 34, 37, 118, 195; ethical affordances, 82, 183; ethical imagination, 130, 181; ethical objects, 82; ethical subjectivity, 10, 130, 237; and gender, 116; and governance (*see* governance); as mode of being-in-world, 39; moral agency, 10, 58, 130, 150, 237, 241; moral chronotopes (*see* chronotopes); moral compass, 56; moral dilemmas, 63; moral discourses and norms, 3, 22, 33, 36–37, 40–41, 56, 89, 97, 100, 116, 244; moral emotions, 197; moral experimentation, 39; moral geography, 26–27, 36, 51–52, 72–75, 84–85, 90–92, 95, 149, 249; moral ideologies, 258; moral injury, 197; moral person-types, 12, 224, 260; moral personhood, 36–37, 42, 60–63; moral stance, 65–66, 129, 147, 243; peopled opportunities (*see* peopled opportunities); and politics, 18; in relation to immorality, 56; and scalar inquiry (*see* scalar inquiry); and shame (*see* shame); social morality (daode), 140–42, 150; as value entanglement, 132
Moser, Ingunn, 220, 223
Moskalenko, Sophia, 195
mother-daughter relationships. *See* mothers
motherhood, mothering, 37, 128–33, 233–41, 243–49
mothers, 1–3, 8, 24, 33, 34, 45–52, 109–10, 124–30, 153, 162–64, 169–71, 176–77, 204–6, 213, 219222, 224–27, 233

mothers-in-law, 46–47, 81, 128, 162
Murthy, Vivek, 147, 150
music, 69–70, 76, 83, 90, 110–18, 201–3
Myers, Neely, 5, 39, 46, 51, 67

Nakassis, Constantine, 11
narrative, 31–68; and chronotopes (*see* chronotopes); coherent narratives, 48; cultural narratives, 4–5, 22, 28, 38, 49–50, 100, 116, 131, 133, 138, 141–43, 145, 149, 177, 181–82, 184, 207–8, 264–66; and desire, 26, 31–68, 226; in interaction, 38–39, 59–66, 122; narrative potential, 67–68; narratives of transformation (*see* metamorphosis); open-ended narratives, 48–49, 58, *see also* subjunctivity; and scalar inquiry (*see* scalar inquiry); and scalar intimacy (*see* scalar intimacy); search for resolution, 45–48, 125, 127; as telling suffering, 34, 35–38, 67–68; tentativeness, subjunctivity, 25–26, 34–36, 39
nationhood. *See* political subjectivity
Ndefo, Nkem, 16, 19, 194
Nelson, Eric, 249
New Age, 4, 16, 79, 118, 230
New Life Center: clientele, 4–5; physical, moral, relational geography, 26–27, 51–52, 73, 84–85, 91–92, 94–95, 166, 208
Nussbaum, Martha, 186

O'Toole, Garson, 272
Ochs, Elinor, 11, 24, 37, 48, 59, 80, 83, 103
Osburg, John, 63

Papadopoulos, Renos, 42, 43
parent-child separations, 206–7, 273
Parish, Steven, 35
Park, Joseph, 260
Parmentier, Richard, 211

patriarchy, 29, 42, 116, 129, 174, 213, 220–54
Pavón-Cuéllar, David, 30, 265
Peirce, Charles S., 11
peopled opportunities, 39, 51, 67
Pereen, Esther, 184
permeability, 97, 103–5, 155, 158, 220, 222, 224, 228, 242, 253
perplexing particulars, 10, 97, 185, 257
Perrino, Sabina, 10, 12, 24, 35–36, 38, 99, 133, 192, 224, 238–40, 242, 254
phenomenological posture, 158, 170
photographs: family photographs, 28, 52, 160; at New Life, 76; photo-forms, 17–18, 166–71, 184–87, 265; and temporality, 161
Pink, Sarah, 8, 26, 27, 71–72, 74, 75, 90, 92, 132, 147, 183, 185, 255
play, 6, 115
political mentalization, 19, 122
political subjectivity, 10, 22, 28, 29–30, 36, 123, 143, 147, 150–51, 184, 192, 196, 200, 242, 254, 256–57, 267
politics, 15, 41, 132, 138, 152, 161, 166, 178, 205, 219, 258–59, 262
Pollard, Martin Quin, 260
Pols, Jeannette, 220, 223
Polsky, Andrew, 10
positive energy (*zheng nengliang*), 18, 235
possibility. *See* anticipatory modes
Pritzker, Sonya, 10, 12, 13, 23–24, 34, 35, 36, 47, 71, 79, 80, 95, 99, 103–7, 122, 132–33, 135, 155–56, 160, 169, 174, 177, 187, 198, 224, 240, 242, 245, 254, 257, 259–60, 261–62, 265
progress, 116, 139–42, 181
psychological anthropology, 12
psychology: in China, 10, 14 79–91; Chinese medical psychology, 23–24
psychotherapy, 4; family constellation therapy (*see* family constellation therapy); and gender, 232; for ghosts (*see* ghosts); group practice in, 10, 156; history of psychoanalysis, 10, 19; image therapy, 143–44; and individualism, 104–6, 122, 142; inner child therapy (*see* inner child therapy); music therapy, 203; pendulum therapy, 210–11; and politics, 10, 19, 65–67, 114–15; psysociality (*see* psysociality); and remaking of self, 33–35, 66–68; somatic psychotherapy, 173; taking inventory, 104; tapping therapy, 214–15; therapeutic governance, 10; therapeutic language (*see* language)
psysociality, 85, 97, 103, 196, 222
public secrecy, 17–22, 28, 114, 132, 138, 143, 150, 157, 166–71, 175–78, 184–87, 208, 212, 265
Puglionesi, Alicia, 158

quality (*suzhi*), 129–30, 187, 237, 264

racism in China. *See* Han-centrism
Ramstead, Maxwell J., 10
Rapport, Nigel, 43, 84
relationships: with authority figures, 7; *see also* "governance"; with children, 7–8, 42, 48, 94, 118, 125–29, 131–32, 137–38, 144–47, 170, 174, 225–27, 229, 235–38; guanxi, 54, 56, 215; with mothers-in-law (*see* mothers-in-law); with parents, 1–3, 5, 7–8, 14, 32, 42, 45–53, 55, 102, 126–31, 134–35, 139, 163, 171, 175, 177–78, 202–6, 214, 220–26, 236, 238–39, 243, 256, 271; with partners/spouses, 5, 8, 42, 45–46, 52, 59, 81, 86, 94, 125, 128, 162, 164–65, 211, 213–14, 231, 235, 240–52
religion, 215. *See* spirituality
reported speech, 47
revelation, 17, 52, 144, 159, 167
Ritchie, Andrea J., 269, 274

ritual boundary-making, 83–90
ritual theater, 186
Roberts, Daniel, 224
Roberts, Rosemarie, 114, 119, 166
Roberts, Sean, 22, 262, 265
Robins, Richard, 107, 155
Rochat del Vallée, Elisabeth, 135
Rofel, Lisa, 22, 28, 131, 150, 176–78, 181, 183, 207, 208
Rosa, Jonathan, 27, 90, 127, 133, 139, 149, 218, 231, 266
Roseneil, Sasha, 12
Roth, Gabrielle, 116, 118, 120, 234, 272
Rudolph, Josh, 259

Sabsay, Leticia, 38, 105, 220, 224, 228, 242, 254
Samuels, Annemarie, 26, 34, 38, 39, 67
Sang, Tze-lan, 199
Santos, Gonçalo, 18, 29, 129–130, 181, 222–23, 225, 228
Satir method, 144, 210, 212, 272
Satir, Virginia, 6, 113
scalar inquiry, 12–15, 29–30, 37; as "defrosting," 195–96; as "ethics of trying," 53; in dialogue, 18–20; as entangling differently (*see* entangling differently); as interrogation of cultural chronotopes, 74, 150; online, 259–65; as rechronotopization, 13; and theory-building (*see* theory-building)
scalar intimacy, 12–15, 29–30, 33, 134, 149, 210; and agency, 12–13, 242, 254; and chronotopes, 36; in dialogue, 18–20, 239; and gender, 41; as intimate, embodied, 35–36; in narrative, 38, 46; *see* narrative; online, 25965; and political subjectivity, 12, 36; as scaling project, 35, 52, 192
Schaedler, Luc, 114
Schieffelin, Bambi, 103, 147

self: developing the self (*see* self-development); expressing inner self, 57; the extended self, 97, 108, 121–22; in family constellation therapy, 154–155; Great Self (dawo), 27, 92, 96–100, 191, 203, 236; and permeability (*see* permeability); True Self, 6, 104, 120
self-development: as "becoming mature" (*see* maturity); as collective development (*see* collective development); psychospiritual self-development (*xinling chengzhang*), 1, 5, 20, 42, 76, 87, 172, 181–92, 201, 206, 216, 222
Seligman, Rebecca, 36
Seok, Bongrae, 98, 197–98
shame, 55–57, 104, 144, 172, 197–201, 204–218, 236, 273; in Chinese medicine, 198–99; in Confucianism, 198–200; conversations about, 206, 208; and gender, 199; healing shame, 205; political shame, 199–200, 207; and relationships, 204; shaming practices, 200, 205; transmission of shame, 201; in western culture, 198–200
Shange, Savannah, 258, 266
Shohet, Merav, 24, 26, 34, 37, 59, 71
Shoshana, Avihu, 118
Silverstein, Michael, 66
Simchai, Dalit, 118
situation (qing), 130, 237–38, 241
Smith, Richard, 247, 249
social action, 10, 25, 30, 186, 257–58, 260, 266
somatics, 19, 23, 194
space. *See* atmosphere
spirituality, 4, 6, 14; commodification, 21, 75; in contemporary China, 215, 230; and harmony, 269; Indian spirituality, 76–77, 82, 200; New Age spirituality, 4, 79; and politics, 15–16; and self-help, 217; spiritual freedom,

spirituality (*continued*)
120, 147, 187; spiritual growth (*see* self-development); spiritual horizons, 91; spiritual travel, 76; spiritualism, 158; subjective life spirituality, 9
Stafford, Charles, 10, 127, 181
stance, 65–66, 129, 140, 141, 179, 181, 190, 198, 201
Stevenson, Mark, 199
Stivers, Tanya, 65
Strozzi Heckler, Richard, 194
subconscious, 43, 190, 212, 215, 234
subjunctivity, 26, 53, 159
success, 33, 139, 215
suffering: childhood suffering, 53–58, 105–6; and circumscribed horizons (*see* horizons); as collective, 29, 209, 210–17; in contemporary Chinese society, 5, 34; and culture (*see* culture); and desire (*see* desire); exploitation of, 91; as feeling of disorientation or being "off-time," 46; and gender/patriarchy, 233, 241–42; as injustice, 149–50, 262; and inquiry, 53, 65; as intergenerational trauma, 172–178, 190–94, 209, 238; making sense of, 26; as normal, 60–61; in relationships, 44–53, 129–31; telling suffering (*see* narrative); transforming suffering, 182
Sumartojo, Shanti, 8, 26, 27, 71–72, 74, 75, 90, 92, 132, 147, 183, 185, 255
Sutin, Angelina, 107, 155
Szasz, Thomas, 10

Taiwan, 4, 16, 79, 80–81, 98
Taussig, Michael, 17
Taylor, Charles, 26, 37, 71, 79, 81
Taylor, Rumsey, 259
technologies of the self, 10
technologies of the social, 122, 156
temporality: and atmosphere (*see* atmosphere); biographical time, 211; *see also* "chronotopes"; considering the future/possible futures, 29, 34–35, 38, 52–53, 58, 90, 108, 131–132, 149–50, 181, 183, 237, 246–49, 253, 269; cultural time, 160, 172–76, 211; experience of time, 112, 153, 161–62, 179–80; in family constellation therapy (*see* family constellation therapy); and feeling at-home-in-the-world, 42; and healing, 7–8; and meaning, 11; and personal transformation, 217; relating to the past, 50, 53–56, 105–10, 115, 131, 136–38, 143–44, 154–57, 184–85, 191, 203–4, 208, 234–35, 238; relating to the present, 8–9, 28, 46, 50, 65, 74, 106, 108, 131–33, 137–38, 168, 171–73, 183, 185–87, 208, 213, 216, 225, 269; and relationality (*see* relationships); in scalar intimacy (*see* scalar intimacy); and spatiality (*see* chronotopes); suffering as feeling "off-time," 26, 33–35, 37, 66–67; time talk, 133; time travel, 105–10, 160; *see also* "group therapeutic exercise"; time-space online, 260–62
Teo, Thomas, 114
texts. *See* books
Thayer, Bradley A., 21, 22, 150
theory-building, 8, 27, 90, 127, 145, 148–49, 183, 200, 231, 241, 250
therapy. *See* psychotherapy
Throop, Jason, 39
Tiananmen Square massacre, 17, 167, 175
tinkering, 29, 220–54
Tolle, Eckhart, 79, 201
touch, 27, 95, 106, 202, 256
translation: bentuhua, 79, 135; living translation, 79–80, 135; New Life texts, 79; translation of Chinese medicine, 23
trauma. *See* suffering

Trevaskes, Susan, 3, 28
Trouillot, Michel-Rolph, 21, 124, 148
Tu, Wei-ming, 97
Turner, Edith, 118
Turner, Victor, 186

Ulsamer, Bertold, 172–6, 273
uncertainty, 13, 26, 38–9, 53, 64, 67, 93, 129, 146, 214, 215

Vessier, Samuel, 10
virtual private networks, 179
vulnerability, 67, 115, 119, 120, 166, 168, 185, 195, 242, 259, 266

Wang, C.C., 16, 80, 81
Wang, Jing, 20, 268
Wei, John, 42, 199
Weilander, Gerda, 10, 18, 40, 42, 55, 99, 117, 137, 145, 156
Western culture
Whitopias, 21
Wilce, James, 71, 103, 239
Williams, Raymond, 3
williams, Reverend angel Kyodo, 16, 19, 172, 194, 218
Wirtz, Kristina, 12, 36, 137
witnessing, 120, 131, 154, 155–156, 162, 164, 167, 174, 184, 186, 191, 243; and labor, 170; third-person self-witnessing, 155
Wolf, Margery, 98, 233, 236
Wolynn, Mark, 7, 154, 158, 174
Wong, Jamie, 13
Wong, Magdalena, 5, 18, 118, 229–30, 240

Wood, Linda Sargent, 15, 272
Woodstock, Louise, 80, 217
Woolard, Kathryn, 192, 211
Wright, Kate, 4, 10, 19, 196
Wu, Cuncun, 199
Wu, David, 128, 132
Wu, Zhihong, 96, 271, 272

Xiang, Biao, 37
Xiao, Hui Faye, 40
Xie, Kailing, 5, 18, 40–42, 63, 118, 130, 241
Xinjiang, 22, 151, 260–61, 265, 274
Xu, Bin, 16, 260, 264, 268
Xu, Jing, 47, 118, 132, 215

Yan, Yunxiang, 15, 18, 46 129, 132, 181
Yang, Jie, 4, 9, 10 16, 18, 40, 41, 55, 82, 97, 156, 215, 216, 246
Yang, Li, 118, 272
Yang, Mayfair, 127, 155, 156
Yang, Zi, 18
Yeh, Catherine, 116
Yijing (Book of Changes), 248–51; Kun, 247–52; Qian, 247–52

Zhang, Defen (Tiffany Chang), 16
Zhang, Everett, 41, 199, 229, 230
Zhang, Li-1, 4–5, 9, 14, 18, 20, 22, 26, 66, 74, 79, 82, 91, 92, 95, 97–8 99, 135, 138, 156, 182
Zhang, Li-2, 216, 222–23, 232, 257
Zhang, Qicheng, 5, 18
Zhang, Ting Liang, 135
Zhang, Yanhua, 9
Zigon, Jarrett, 10, 39, 264